# A Short Course in MEDICAL TERMINOLOGY

FOURTH EDITION

Judi L. Nath, PhD
Professor
Lourdes University

Kelsey P. Lindsley, RPh, PharmD
Pharmacist, Preceptor
Clinical Practitioner

Wolters Kluwer

Philadelphia • Baltimore • New York • London
Buenos Aires • Hong Kong • Sydney • Tokyo

*Acquisitions Editor:* Jonathan Joyce
*Development Editor:* Amy Millholen
*Editorial Coordinator:* John Larkin
*Editorial Assistant:* Tish Rogers
*Marketing Manager:* Leah Thomson
*Production Project Manager:* David Saltzberg
*Design Coordinator:* Holly Reid McLaughlin
*Manufacturing Coordinator:* Margie Orzech
*Prepress Vendor:* S4Carlisle Publishing Services

Fourth edition


9 8 7 6 5 4 3 2

Printed in China

**Library of Congress Cataloging-in-Publication Data**

Names: Nath, Judi Lindsley, author.
Title: A short course in medical terminology / Judi L. Nath, Ph.D., Lourdes University, Kelsey P. Lindsley, R.Ph., Pharm.D.
Description: Fourth edition. | Philadelphia: Wolters Kluwer Health, [2019] | Revision of: Short course in medical terminology / C. Edward Collins, Text and Academic Authors Association, St. Petersburg, Florida. | Includes index.
Identifiers: LCCN 2017044655 | ISBN 9781496351470 (paperback)
Subjects: LCSH: Medicine—Terminology. | Medical sciences—Terminology. | BISAC: MEDICAL / Dictionaries & Terminology.
Classification: LCC R123 .C594 2019 | DDC 610.1/4—dc23 LC record available at https://lccn.loc.gov/2017044655



LWW.com

RRS1903

*This book is dedicated*
*to my students and colleagues*
*at Lourdes University,*
*who continue to provide inspiration*
*and support. Thank you!*

-JUDI L. NATH

*This book is dedicated to my parents,*
*who have always loved and supported me*
*and who accepted dishwashing*
*in exchange for rent*
*while I was working on this book.*

-KELSEY P. LINDSLEY

# New to This Edition

This new edition builds on the foundation established in the previous three editions. The reader will find the writing style of this edition easy to follow, with special focus given to ensuring that each page is user friendly and accessible to all levels of learning. As educators, we wanted to be sure that students found the content manageable, interesting, and understandable.

## APPROACH AND CONTENT ORGANIZATION

This section outlines the global changes that were made throughout the entire textbook as well as the chapter-by-chapter changes. We begin with those changes across the chapters.

### Global Changes

- The narrative has been modernized to make the text more user-friendly and approachable for students.
- The chapter headings have been standardized to appear in a consistent order so material is presented utilizing a consistent style.
- The topics in the study table were also standardized so that the order follows a predictable sequence.
- Study Tables may contain terms that are not in the narrative; however, all bold-faced terms in the narrative are found in the Study Tables. The book would become unwieldy with text if the terms in the tables were also in the narrative. We have selected the most relevant terms for inclusion in the tables.
- The end-of-chapter exercises have been standardized, so that from chapter-to-chapter exercises are presented in the same order.
- Chapter 15 The Special Senses of Sight and Hearing has been moved to appear directly after Chapter 7 The Nervous System. This order makes sense from a functional perspective and matches other current anatomy and physiology books. Rearranging the topics in this manner also allows the book to be used in tandem with an anatomy and physiology course.
- All terminology has been updated per current medical usage. *Stedman's Medical Dictionary*, *Terminologia Anatomica*, *Terminologia Histologica*, *Terminologia Embryologica*, and leading medical journals were used to standardize the medical terms, so that they are current and match terms used in common practice.
- Pronunciations match *Stedman's Medical Dictionary*. Although *Stedman's Medical Dictionary* uses a diacritic format whereby signs and symbols are used with letters to indicate pronunciations, the pronunciations given in this book are those used for oral communication so we used phonetic pronunciations.
- Appendixes A through E have been updated so the information is the most current, nationally recognized.
- The artwork has been updated and revised extensively to be accurate and contemporary. We also improved the text–art integration to enhance the student learning experience.

- Citations from image captions have been removed, so that the reader is not distracted from the image and its learning opportunity.
- Unnecessarily long table titles were shortened to make table titles easier for students to read and understand.
- More photos were added for realism and interest.
- The phrase "word elements" was changed to "word parts" to avoid ambiguities when some word parts served double functions, as in sometimes a word part was a root and a prefix. This change also enabled consistency.
- Quick Checks were updated to provide benchmarks within the chapter for students to assess retention of information.
- Sidebar Information was updated with interesting facts. It is also designed so that it is a "point-able feature" and there is at least one per chapter.
- Material from Crossword Puzzles and Chapter Quizzes has been folded into the End-of-Chapter Exercises.

## Revised Table of Contents

Chapter 1 Analyzing Medical Terms
Chapter 2 Common Prefixes and Suffixes
Chapter 3 Organization of the Body
Chapter 4 The Integumentary System
Chapter 5 The Skeletal System
Chapter 6 The Muscular System
Chapter 7 The Nervous System
Chapter 8 The Special Sense of Sight and Hearing
Chapter 9 The Endocrine System
Chapter 10 The Cardiovascular System
Chapter 11 The Lymphatic System and Immunity
Chapter 12 The Respiratory System
Chapter 13 The Digestive System
Chapter 14 The Urinary System
Chapter 15 The Reproductive System

## Basic Chapter Outline Template

1. Learning Outcomes (changed from learning objectives)
2. Introduction
3. Word Parts Related to the XXX System
4. Structure and Function
5. Quick Check (at lease one per chapter)
6. Disorders Related to the XXX System
7. Diagnostic Tests, Treatments, and Surgical Procedures
8. Practice and Practitioners
9. The XXX System Abbreviation Table
10. Sidebar (at least one per chapter)
11. The XXX System Study Table (alphabetized within subheadings)
    - Structure and Function
    - Disorders
    - Diagnostic Tests, Treatments, and Surgical Procedures
    - Practice and Practitioners
12. End-of-Chapter Exercises—not all exercises may be present, but the order of exercises is maintained
    - Exercise X-X Labeling
    - Exercise X-X Word Parts

- Exercise X-X Word Building
- Exercise X-X Matching
- Exercise X-X Multiple Choice
- Exercise X-X Fill in the Blank
- Exercise X-X Abbreviations
- Exercise X-X Spelling
- Exercise X-X Case Study

## Chapter-by-Chapter Changes

### *Chapter 1 Analyzing Medical Terms*

- New Art: Figure 1-1
- New Word Parts: non-
- New Terms: etymology and language sense
- Deleted Word Part: cleric
- Added new Quick Check

### *Chapter 2 Common Prefixes and Suffixes*

- Changed chapter title from Common Suffixes and Prefixes to Common Prefixes and Suffixes and changed the order of presentation in the chapter so that prefixes are introduced before suffixes and to match the new chapter title
- New Word Parts: a-, an-, anti-, -cele, -cyte, de-, dis-, -eal, -edema, -emesis, -emia, -ism, -lith, -lysis, -oid, -opsy, -pathy, -phobia, -plasia, -poesis, -rrhea, -sclerosis, -stasis, -stenosis, -stomy, tic, and –tome
- Added new Quick Check

### *Chapter 3 Organization of the Body*

- Changed chapter title from The Body's Organization to Organization of the Body
- New Art: Figures 3-1, 3-2, 3-3, 3-4, 3-5, 3-6, and 3-7
- New Word Parts: gastr/o and thorac/o
- New Terms: abdominal cavity, anatomy, caudal, cephalad, cervix, coccyx, coronal plane, cranial, lumbus, pelvic cavity, physiology, sacrum, thorax, and ventral
- Deleted Terms: anatomical terms of location, dorsal cavity, and midsagittal
- Added new Quick Check

### *Chapter 4 The Integumentary System*

- New Art: Figures 4-1, 4-6, and 4-10
- New Word Parts: adipo- and -oma
- New Terms: arrector pili muscles, benign, bulla, carcinoma, decubitus ulcers, edema, erythematous, fissure, hypodermis, integumentary system, malignant, plaque, pruritic, prurigo, and wheal

### *Chapter 5 The Skeletal System*

- New Art: Figures 5-1, 5-2, 5-8, 5-9, 5-10, 5-11, 5-12, 5-13, 5-14, and new images for Table 5-3
- New Terms: appendicular skeleton, axial skeleton, carpal bones, closed fracture, compound fracture, compact bone, cranial suture, cranium, epiphyseal plate, hip bone, joint, kinesiologists, lateral malleolus, ligaments, tendons, medial malleolus, neoplasms, occupational therapists, open fracture, osseous tissue, physical therapists, simple fracture, spongy bone, sternum, synovial fluid, synovial joint, tarsal bones, thoracic cage, and vertebral column
- New Abbreviations: MRI and NSAID
- Deleted Abbreviations: CTS and LE
- Deleted Terms: chondrodynia and dactylomegaly
- Deleted Word Parts: cheir/o and -desis

### *Chapter 6 The Muscular System*

- Deleted Table 6-2 because it is in Chapter 5
- Reorganized comparative art in Figure 6-1
- Added new Sidebar on dysphagia and dysphasia
- New Art: Figures 6-2 and 6-5
- New Abbreviations: ALS, FX, MD, NSAID, and PT
- Deleted Abbreviations: CTD, DMD, and DTR
- New Terms: agonist, Duchenne dystrophy, dysphagia, fascicle, muscle fibers, paresis, skeletal muscle, and striated muscle
- Deleted Terms: myoparesis, tenalgia, tenontoplasty, tendoplasty, and tenoplasty

### *Chapter 7 The Nervous System*

- New Art: Figures 7-1, 7-3, 7-5, 7-6, 7-8, and Labeling Exercise 7-1
- New Abbreviations: AD, CSF, CT, DM, MRI, and PD
- Deleted Abbreviations: IQ, OBS, PERRLA, SAD, and TENS
- New Terms: demyelination, lesion, seizure, sympathetic nervous system, and parasympathetic nervous system
- Term Changes: changed brain stem to brainstem per *Terminologia Anatomica*, changed petit mal seizure to absence seizure
- Added a new sidebar on the difference between psychiatrist and psychologist
- Deleted Terms: subsystems

### *Chapter 8 The Special Senses of Sight and Hearing*

- New Art: Figures 8-2, 8-3, 8-4, 8-8, 8-9, and Labeling Exercise 8-1
- New Abbreviations: EOM, LASIK, and O.D.
- Deleted Abbreviations: ASL, dB, ECCE, ERG, ICCE, and PVD
- New Terms: auditory tube, cones, external acoustic meatus, deaf, extra-ocular muscles, eyebrows, eyelashes, eyelids, lacrimal ducts, lacrimal fluid, lacrimal glands, lacrimal sac, laser-assisted in situ keratomileusis (LASIK), lateral angle of eye, medial angle of eye, orbit, refraction, rods, and scleral buckle
- Term Changes: inner canthus changed to medial angle of the eye, outer canthus changed to lateral angle of the eye, outer ear changed to external ear, inner ear changed to internal ear, external auditory canal changed to external acoustic meatus, and eustachian tube changed to auditory tube per *Terminologia Anatomica*
- Deleted Word Parts: dacryocyst/o, irit/o, and phak/o

### *Chapter 9 The Endocrine System*

- New Art: Figure 9-1, 9-3, 9-4, 9-5, 9-6, 9-7, and Labeling Exercise 9-1
- New Abbreviations: $T_3$, $T_4$, CT, PTH, and GTT
- Deleted Abbreviations: BS, IDDM, and NIDDM
- New Terms: corticosteroids, fasting blood sugar (FBS), goiter, exophthalmos, hypothalamus, pineal gland, glands, polydipsia, polyuria, and thyroid-stimulating hormone (TSH)

### *Chapter 10 The Cardiovascular System*

- New Art: Figures 10-5, 10-6, and 10-7
- Deleted Abbreviations: CP, ICU, $Rh^+$, and $Rh^-$
- New Terms: apex, atrioventricular valves, coronary artery disease, embolus, heartbeat, pulmonary circuit, and systemic circuit
- Deleted Terms: arteritis, cardiodynia, cardiomalacia, pericardial sac, and phagocyte

### Chapter 11 The Lymphatic System and Immunity

- New Art: Figures 11-1, 11-2, 11-3, 11-4, and Labeling Exercise 11-1
- New Abbreviations: EBV
- Deleted Abbreviations: CBC, HLA, and RIA
- Deleted Figure: former Figure 10-1
- New Terms: allergy, autoimmune disease, elephantiasis, immunization, lymph node, lymphography, pathogen, systemic lupus erythematosus, vaccination, and vaccine

### Chapter 12 The Respiratory System

- Changed The Nose heading to The Nose, Nasal Cavity, and Paranasal Sinuses; changed The Pharynx heading to The Pharynx and Tonsils; added new section on The Diaphragm
- Added new Sidebar on the common cold viruses
- New Word Part: adeno-
- New Art: Figures 12-1, 12-3, 12-4, 12-6, 12-7, 12-8, 12-9, and Labeling Exercise 12-1
- New Abbreviations: BP, c/o, F, ICU, P, T and A, URI, VC, and WBC
- Deleted Abbreviations: T&A changed to T and A
- Deleted Figure: former Figure 11-4
- New Table 12-2 Pulmonary Volumes and Capacities
- New Terms: cyanosis, lungs, nasal cavity, nasal septum, nose, paranasal sinuses, tonsils, and ventilation

### Chapter 13 The Digestive System

- New Art: Figures 13-1, 13-2, 13-3, 13-5, and Labeling Exercise 13-1
- Changed common bile duct to bile duct per *Terminologia Anatomica*
- New Abbreviations: NG and UGIS
- Deleted Abbreviations: GB, GBS NGT, and UGI
- New Terms: absorption, bile duct, digestion, elimination, esophagogastroduodenoscopy, irritable bowel syndrome, and lower esophageal sphincter
- Deleted Terms: common bile duct and fundus

### Chapter 14 The Urinary System

- New Art: Figures 14-1, 14-3, and Labeling Exercise 14-1
- Changed perirenal fat to perinephric fat or pararenal fat body per *Terminologia Anatomica*
- Added information on the nephron, glomerulus, and glomerular filtration rate
- New Abbreviations: ARF and CRF
- Deleted Abbreviations: BPH and PSA
- New Terms: antibiotic, calyx, kidney transplant, micturition, nephropexy, renal corpuscle, renal cortex, renal medulla, renal pelvis, and renal tubule

### Chapter 15 The Reproductive System

- New Art: Figures 15-1, 15-4, 15-6, 15-7, and Labeling Exercise 15-1
- New Sidebar on meiosis and mitosis
- Changed amniotic sac to amnion per *Terminologia Anatomica*
- Changed spermatozoon and spermatozoa to sperm per *Terminologia Histologica*
- New Abbreviations: A, C-section, EDC, EDD, G, HIV, P, Pap smear, STD, and STI
- Deleted Abbreviations: DUF, HRT, HSG, IUD, PMS, TAH, and VD
- New Terms: abortus, amnion, amniotic fluid, amniotic sac, clitoris, glans, foreskin, fundus, labium majus, labium minus, umbilical cord, urologist, and vulva

## OTHER RESOURCES

Online ancillary materials complement the text and provide additional support for student learning.

### *Student Resources:*

- Question Bank, with a variety of exercise types to reinforce chapter material
- Educational Games, such as crossword puzzles, hangman, and word-building challenges
- Audio Glossary
- Flash Cards, including Flash Card Generator
- Chapter Quizzes
- Final Exam

### *Instructor Resources:*

- PowerPoint slides and Lesson Plans include useful information to facilitate presentation of material by instructors.
- Test Generator, with more than 500 questions to test students' knowledge of terms, their meanings, and abbreviations.
- Handouts include additional puzzles and games for additional student practice.

# Author's Preface

Welcome to the field of medical terminology. This workbook-textbook is written to teach the language of medicine in an engaging and meaningful way. It is written to represent the real world so that you can move seamlessly from the classroom to actual practice. The approach is based on research that demonstrates how students learn best. To that end, we used a three-pronged approach: (1) immersion—the terms are presented in context; (2) chunking—the material is given in manageable units; and (3) practice—exercises that allow you to check your knowledge. Learning word parts is also an essential component of learning the terms. If you learn the tables of word parts, you will be well on your way to knowing medical terms you have never encountered, because you can figure out the terms by breaking them into their component word parts. This will be quite useful, because not every word you will encounter in your careers is found in this book, but you will be equipped with the knowledge to understand their meaning. We also encourage you to pay special attention to the analysis sections in the Study Tables, as these provide interesting, foundational information for forming medical terms.

While learning medical terminology, you will also learn some basic anatomy (body structures), physiology (body functions), and pathology (body diseases). Because medical terms describe the human body in health and in disease, attaining an elementary understanding of these topics will help you retain a working memory of medical language.

Learning medical terms can be easy if you approach the subject from a proper perspective. Begin by telling yourself that medical terms do not make up a separate language. Medical terms are simply words that you can add to your vocabulary. As with all words, medical words are meant to convey information.

As you enter a medical profession, you will be communicating with other medical professionals and with patients. Therefore, your job will include choosing words and sentence structures that convey accurate information and reflect a professional attitude. That is to say, both your communication skills and your attitude toward patients are very important. As you are about to discover, learning medical terminology can be easy at times and challenging at others. However, if you use the textbook and its ancillaries to their fullest, you will be well on your way to mastering medical terminology.

***Judi L. Nath, Ph.D.***
Professor
Lourdes University
Sylvania, Ohio

***Kelsey P. Lindsley, R.Ph., Pharm.D.***
Pharmacist, Preceptor
Clinical Practitioner
Port Clinton, Ohio

# User's Guide

*A Short Course in Medical Terminology*, Fourth Edition, was developed to provide an easy, efficient, and effective way to learn medical terminology. This User's Guide introduces the features of the book that help the learning experience.

A **logical organization** guides students through the basics of medical terminology, word parts, and word analysis.

**Chapters 1 and 2** introduce the basics of word building and set the foundation for learning terms.

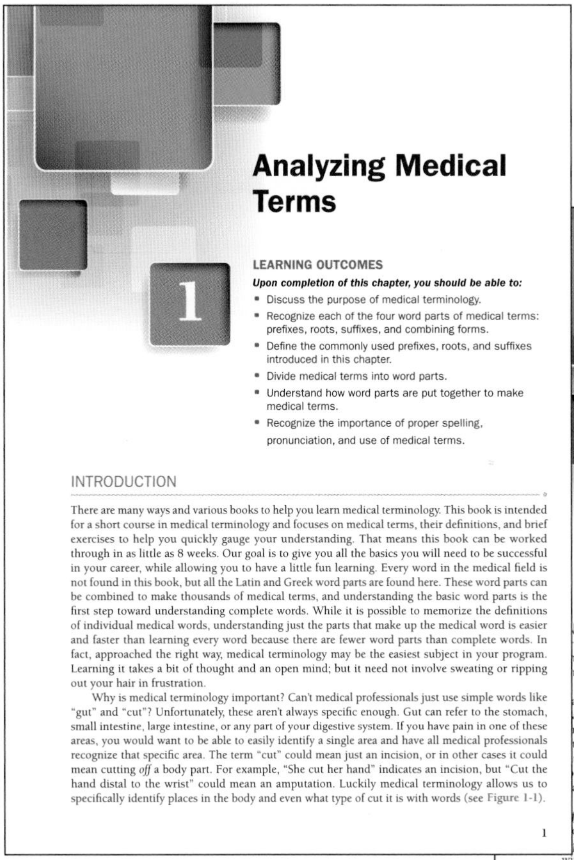

1

Analyzing Medical Terms

LEARNING OUTCOMES

***Upon completion of this chapter, you should be able to:***

- Discuss the purpose of medical terminology.
- Recognize each of the four word parts of medical terms: prefixes, roots, suffixes, and combining forms.
- Define the commonly used prefixes, roots, and suffixes introduced in this chapter.
- Divide medical terms into word parts.
- Understand how word parts are put together to make medical terms.
- Recognize the importance of proper spelling, pronunciation, and use of medical terms.

INTRODUCTION

There are many ways and various books to help you learn medical terminology. This book is intended for a short course in medical terminology and focuses on medical terms, their definitions, and brief exercises to help you quickly gauge your understanding. That means this book can be worked through in as little as 8 weeks. Our goal is to give you all the basics you will need to be successful in your career, while allowing you to have a little fun learning. Every word in the medical field is not found in this book, but all the Latin and Greek word parts are found here. These word parts can be combined to make thousands of medical terms, and understanding the basic word parts is the first step toward understanding complete words. While it is possible to memorize the definitions of individual medical words, understanding just the parts that make up the medical word is easier and faster than learning every word because there are fewer word parts than complete words. In fact, approached the right way, medical terminology may be the easiest subject in your program. Learning it takes a bit of thought and an open mind; but it need not involve sweating or ripping out your hair in frustration.

Why is medical terminology important? Can't medical professionals just use simple words like "gut" and "cut"? Unfortunately, these aren't always specific enough. Gut can refer to the stomach, small intestine, large intestine, or any part of your digestive system. If you have pain in one of these areas, you would want to be able to easily identify a single area and have all medical professionals recognize that specific area. The term "cut" could mean just an incision, or in other cases it could mean cutting *off* a body part. For example, "She cut her hand" indicates an incision, but "Cut the hand distal to the wrist" could mean an amputation. Luckily medical terminology allows us to specifically identify places in the body and even what type of cut it is with words (see Figure 1-1).

1

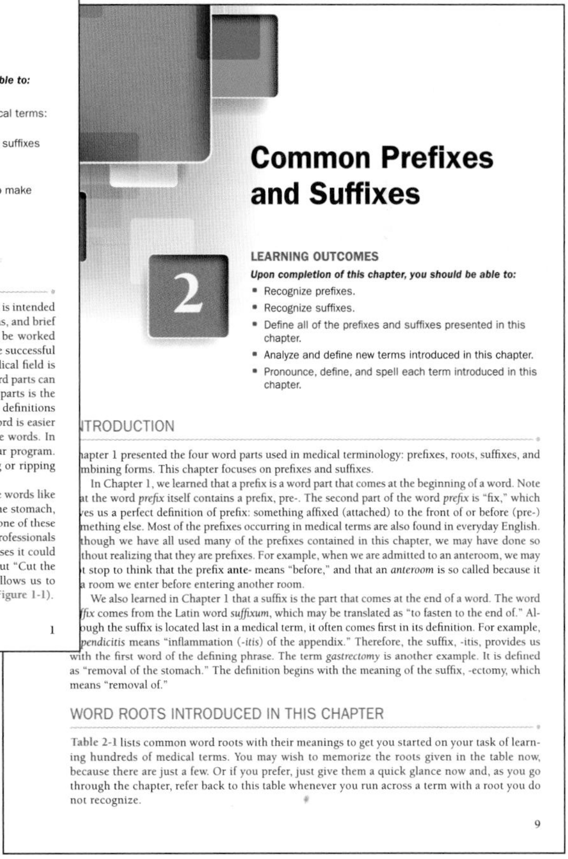

2

Common Prefixes and Suffixes

LEARNING OUTCOMES

***Upon completion of this chapter, you should be able to:***

- Recognize prefixes.
- Recognize suffixes.
- Define all of the prefixes and suffixes presented in this chapter.
- Analyze and define new terms introduced in this chapter.
- Pronounce, define, and spell each term introduced in this chapter.

ITRODUCTION

hapter 1 presented the four word parts used in medical terminology: prefixes, roots, suffixes, and mbining forms. This chapter focuses on prefixes and suffixes.

In Chapter 1, we learned that a prefix is a word part that comes at the beginning of a word. Note at the word *prefix* itself contains a prefix, pre-. The second part of the word *prefix* is "fix," which ves us a perfect definition of prefix: something affixed (attached) to the front of or before (pre-) mething else. Most of the prefixes occurring in medical terms are also found in everyday English. though we have all used many of the prefixes contained in this chapter, we may have done so thout realizing that they are prefixes. For example, when we are admitted to an anteroom, we may t stop to think that the prefix **ante-** means "before," and that an *anteroom* is so called because it a room we enter before entering another room.

We also learned in Chapter 1 that a suffix is the part that comes at the end of a word. The word *ffix* comes from the Latin word *suffixum*, which may be translated as "to fasten to the end of." Al- ough the suffix is located last in a medical term, it often comes first in its definition. For example, *pendicitis* means "inflammation (-*itis*) of the appendix." Therefore, the suffix, -itis, provides us with the first word of the defining phrase. The term *gastrectomy* is another example. It is defined as "removal of the stomach." The definition begins with the meaning of the suffix, -ectomy, which means "removal of."

WORD ROOTS INTRODUCED IN THIS CHAPTER

Table 2-1 lists common word roots with their meanings to get you started on your task of learning hundreds of medical terms. You may wish to memorize the roots given in the table now, because there are just a few. Or if you prefer, just give them a quick glance now and, as you go through the chapter, refer back to this table whenever you run across a term with a root you do not recognize.

9

**Chapters 3–15** offer an overview of each body system and introduce terms that identify the structure and function of that system along with terms that name system disorders, diagnostic tests, treatments, surgical procedures, practice, and practitioners.

## LEARNING OUTCOMES

***Upon completion of this chapter, you should be able to:***

- Recognize prefixes.
- Recognize suffixes.
- Define all of the prefixes and suffixes presented in this chapter.
- Analyze and define new terms introduced in this chapter.
- Pronounce, define, and spell each term introduced in this chapter.

Each chapter opens with a statement of **learning outcomes**. These are measurable educational aims and objectives that indicate what you should be able to do after completing the chapter.

An introduction and a tabular presentation of **Word Parts** related to a specific body system are presented next.

TABLE 3-1 WORD PARTS RELATED TO BODY ORGANIZATION

| Word Part | Meaning |
|---|---|
| anter/o | front, anterior |
| cerv/o | neck |
| chondr/o | cartilage |
| cyt/o, -cyte | cell |
| dors/o | back |
| gastr/o | stomach, abdomen |
| inguin/o | groin |
| my/o | muscle |
| myel/o | spinal cord |
| neur/o | nerve, neuron |
| poster/o | posterior, back |
| proxim/o | near |
| super/o | superior |
| thorac/o | chest (thorax) |
| trans- | across |

**Word Parts Exercises** offer you an opportunity to quickly review the word parts before moving on to new material.

**Word Parts Exercise**

After studying Table 3-1, write the meaning of each of the word parts.

| WORD PART | MEANING |
|---|---|
| 1. trans- | 1. ______ |
| 2. dors/o | 2. ______ |
| 3. proxim/o | 3. ______ |
| 4. chondr/o | 4. ______ |
| 5. anter/o | 5. ______ |
| 6. my/o | 6. ______ |
| 7. super/o | 7. ______ |
| 8. cerv/o | 8. ______ |
| 9. inguin/o | 9. ______ |
| 10. myel/o | 10. ______ |

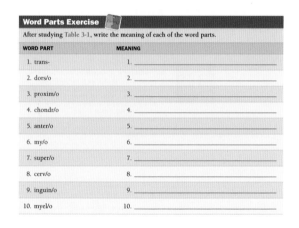

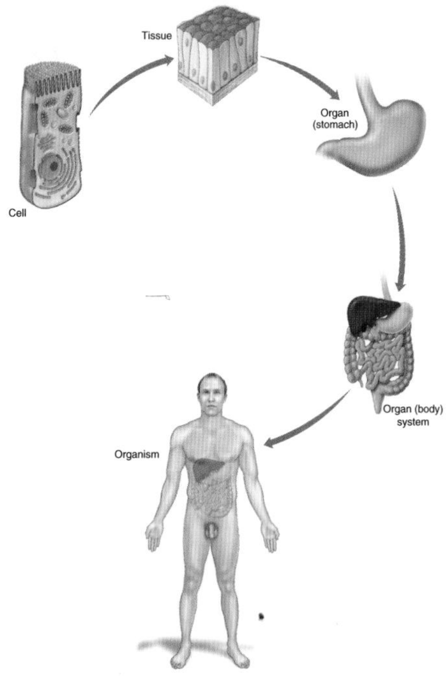


**Structure and Function** sections with **full-color illustrations** help you learn basic anatomy and physiology using tight text–art integration.

**Quick Check**

Fill in the **Suffix**, and write the resulting word in the **Term** column. The word that appears in boldface type in the **Meaning** column is a clue.

| PREFIX | ROOT | SUFFIX | TERM | MEANING |
|---|---|---|---|---|
| sub- | cutane/o | ________ | ________ | **adjective** meaning "below the skin" |
| no prefix | melan/o | ________ | ________ | a pigment-producing **cell** |
| no prefix | seb/o | ________ | ________ | **adjective** referring to sebum, which may be described as an **oil or fat** |

**Quick Checks** exercises help reinforce your knowledge of term parts before studying disorders related to the body systems.

All body system chapters include an **Abbreviations Table**, which lists common abbreviations and their meanings used in the chapter.

**Abbreviation Table** THE INTEGUMENTARY SYSTEM

| ABBREVIATION | MEANING |
|---|---|
| BSA | body surface area |
| I&D | incision and drainage |
| SLE | systemic lupus erythematosus |
| UV | ultraviolet |

Doesn't topical mean "relating to a particular topic," such as a topic in the news? Occasionally, the meaning of an English word changes when a segment of the population begins using it to mean something other than its traditional meaning. The word *topical* is such a word. However, its "medical" meaning most likely came first, given that its medical use dates back to the 17th century. Still, dictionaries include the notation *medical* alongside it, probably because English speakers may do a mental double take when encountering its medical use for the first time. Medical terms that fall into this category are identified throughout this book so that, as a medical professional, you will be aware of the possible confusion their use may cause, especially among patients.

**Sidebars** appear throughout to highlight interesting facts about medical terms and words in general.

**Study Table** THE INTEGUMENTARY SYSTEM

| TERM AND PRONUNCIATION | ANALYSIS | MEANING |
|---|---|---|
| **Structure and Function** | | |
| adipose tissue (AD-ih-pohs TISH-yoo) | from the Latin word *adeps* (fat) | fatty tissue |
| arrector pili muscles (uh-REK-tor PYE-lye MUS-elz) | from the Latin meaning "that which raises" + *pilus* (hair) + *musculus* (muscle) | bundles of smooth muscle fibers attached to hair follicles that cause the hairs to stand on end causing characteristic "goose bumps" |
| avascular (ay-VAS-kyuh-lahr) | *a-* (without); from the Latin word *vasculum* (small vessel) | without blood vessels |
| corium (KO-ree-uhm) | Latin for skin | synonym for dermis |
| cutaneous (cue-TAYN-ee-uhs) | from the Latin word *cutis* (skin) | adjective referring to the skin |
| cuticle (CUE-tih-kuhl) | from the Latin word *cutis* (skin) | the thin band of tissue that seals the nail to the skin |
| dermis (DUR-mis) | from the Greek word *derma* (skin) | inner layer of skin |
| epidermis (ep-ih-DUR-mis) | *epi-* (upon); *dermis* (skin) | outer layer of the skin |
| free edge (FREE EJ) | from German *frei* (free) | distal region at which the nail ends |
| hair follicles (HAIR FAWL-ik-uhlz) | from the Latin word *folliculus* (a small sac) | small sacs in the skin from which hair grows |
| hypodermis (high-poh-DER-mis) | from the Greek word *hypo* (under); *dermis* (skin) | layer immediately beneath the epidermis; also called the subcutaneous layer |
| integumentary system (in-teg-yoo-MEN-tuh-ree SIS-tem) | from the Latin word *integumentum* (a covering) | the membrane covering the body, including the epidermis, dermis, hair, nails, and glands |
| keratin (KERR-uh-tin) | from the Greek word *keras* (horn) | protein that forms hair, nails, and the tough outer layer of skin |

All body system chapters include a **Study Table** summarizing terms for reinforcement of the material in an easy-to-reference format. Some terms in the table are not found in the running narrative, but are important to include, or the terms are used in the end-of-chapter case study.

**End-of- Chapter Exercises** and a **Case Study** close out each chapter to maximize learning. Exercises include figure labeling, word building, matching, multiple choice, fill-in-the-blank, short answer, true/false, and spelling. The Case Study provides real world application of medical terms and gives you an opportunity to interact with the chapter material as you would in a clinical setting.

## END-OF-CHAPTER EXERCISES

### EXERCISE 1-1 DEFINING TERMS

**Combine the suffix *-logy* with the proper root to indicate the following medical specialties:**

1. Specialty dealing with heart disease ____________________
2. Specialty that deals with the problems of aging and diseases in the elderly ____________________
3. Specialty dealing with blood diseases ____________________
4. Specialty dealing with skin ailments ____________________
5. Specialty dealing with nervous system disorders ____________________
6. Specialty dealing with mental disorders ____________________

### EXERCISE 1-2 ANALYZING TERMS

**Analyze the following terms by putting the roots and suffixes in the appropriate columns. Then, write a definition for each term.**

| TERM | ROOT | SUFFIX | DEFINITION |
|---|---|---|---|
| 1. neuropathy | ________ | ________ | ____________________ |
| 2. psychology | ________ | ________ | ____________________ |
| 3. pathogenic | ________ | ________ | ____________________ |
| 4. neuralgia | ________ | ________ | ____________________ |
| 5. systemic | ________ | ________ | ____________________ |
| 6. psychiatrist | ________ | ________ | ____________________ |
| 7. pediatrician | ________ | ________ | ____________________ |
| 8. iatrogenic | ________ | ________ | ____________________ |
| 9. cardialgia | ________ | ________ | ____________________ |
| 10. neuritis | ________ | ________ | ____________________ |

### EXERCISE 10-9 CASE STUDY

**Read the case and answer the questions that follow.**

**BRIEF HISTORY:** The patient is a 56-year-old male who had been complaining of recurrent chest pain when performing mild activities at home. The chest pain subsides when he lies down. He also has experienced shortness of breath (SOB) when carrying in the groceries and climbing up one set of stairs. He has a history of high BP.

**EMERGENCY ROOM VISIT:** The patient arrives at the emergency room with angina pectoris that is relieved by rest, a BP of 180/110 mm Hg, and SOB. An EKG is performed, which indicates that the patient is having atrial arrhythmias and an MI. He is given aspirin and started on antiarrhythmics, diuretics, vasodilators, and oxygen. He is admitted to the CCU for observation and treatment.

**DIAGNOSIS:** Hypertension, an MI, and atrial fibrillation.

1. Define angina pectoris. ____________________
2. What does the acronym SOB stand for? ____________________
3. What is hypertension? ____________________
4. What is an EKG? ____________________
5. What type of pharmacologic intervention is used with this patient? Define each drug classification. ________ ____________________
6. What is an MI? What are the two roots in myocardial, and what do they mean? ____________________
7. Define atrial fibrillation. ____________________

# Reviewers

The authors and publisher would like to thank the following individuals who helped to review this textbook:


**Rhonda Anderson**
Instructor
Phlebotomy
Greenville Technical College
Greenville, South Carolina

**Marianne Demsky**
Instructor
Human Resources
Johns Hopkins Hospital
Baltimore, Maryland

**Patricia Ketcham**
Director of Nursing Laboratories
School of Nursing
Oakland University
Rochester, Michigan

**Amie Mayhall**
Instructor
Medical Office Careers
Olney Central College
Olney, Illinois

**Ashita Patel**
Instructor
Medical Assisting
Wake Technical Community College
Raleigh, North Carolina

**Lona Sandon**
Assistant Professor
Clinical Nutrition
UT Southwestern Medical Center
Dallas, Texas

**Karen K. Smith**
Assistant Professor
Health Information Management Program
University of Arkansas for Medical Sciences, College of Health Professions
Little Rock, Arkansas

**Jonette Talbott RN, MSN, NP-C**
Professor and Program Director
Practical Nursing
Southside VA Community College
Alberta, Virgina

**Margaret Tiemann**
Instructor—Retired
Health Information Technology
St. Charles Community College
Cottleville, Missouri

**Rafael Tolentino**
Chief Academic Officer
Nursing & Health Allied
Homestead Schools, Inc.
Torrance, California

# Acknowledgments

With sincere gratitude, I wish to acknowledge all the hard work done by the members of the editorial staff of Wolters Kluwer. Writing and publishing a textbook requires more than putting fingers to the keyboard. The printed book represents the work of many dedicated individuals, without whom this project could not be completed. To begin, thanks to exceptional editor, Jonathan Joyce, for bringing this book to my attention and encouraging me to work on it. To editorial coordinator, John Larkin, thank you for being my point person; you were always quick to respond and helpful with your responses. Special appreciation is extended to developmental editor, Amy Millholen, who has been at my side for several titles, providing expert advice and direction. A round of applause goes to the Wolters Kluwer sales and marketing team led by marketing manager, Leah Thomson.

We also offer posthumous heartfelt indebtedness to C. Edward Collins, the original author of this book. Through three editions you were the pen behind the pages; may this work be a testament to your legacy.

# Contents

# 1

# Analyzing Medical Terms

## LEARNING OUTCOMES

***Upon completion of this chapter, you should be able to:***

- Discuss the purpose of medical terminology.
- Recognize each of the four word parts of medical terms: prefixes, roots, suffixes, and combining forms.
- Define the commonly used prefixes, roots, and suffixes introduced in this chapter.
- Divide medical terms into word parts.
- Understand how word parts are put together to make medical terms.
- Recognize the importance of proper spelling, pronunciation, and use of medical terms.

## INTRODUCTION

There are many ways and various books to help you learn medical terminology. This book is intended for a short course in medical terminology and focuses on medical terms, their definitions, and brief exercises to help you quickly gauge your understanding. That means this book can be worked through in as little as 8 weeks. Our goal is to give you all the basics you will need to be successful in your career, while allowing you to have a little fun learning. Every word in the medical field is not found in this book, but all the Latin and Greek word parts are found here. These word parts can be combined to make thousands of medical terms, and understanding the basic word parts is the first step toward understanding complete words. While it is possible to memorize the definitions of individual medical words, understanding just the parts that make up the medical word is easier and faster than learning every word because there are fewer word parts than complete words. In fact, approached the right way, medical terminology may be the easiest subject in your program. Learning it takes a bit of thought and an open mind; but it need not involve sweating or ripping out your hair in frustration.

Why is medical terminology important? Can't medical professionals just use simple words like "gut" and "cut"? Unfortunately, these aren't always specific enough. Gut can refer to the stomach, small intestine, large intestine, or any part of your digestive system. If you have pain in one of these areas, you would want to be able to easily identify a single area and have all medical professionals recognize that specific area. The term "cut" could mean just an incision, or in other cases it could mean cutting *off* a body part. For example, "She cut her hand" indicates an incision, but "Cut the hand distal to the wrist" could mean an amputation. Luckily medical terminology allows us to specifically identify places in the body and even what type of cut it is with words (see Figure 1-1).

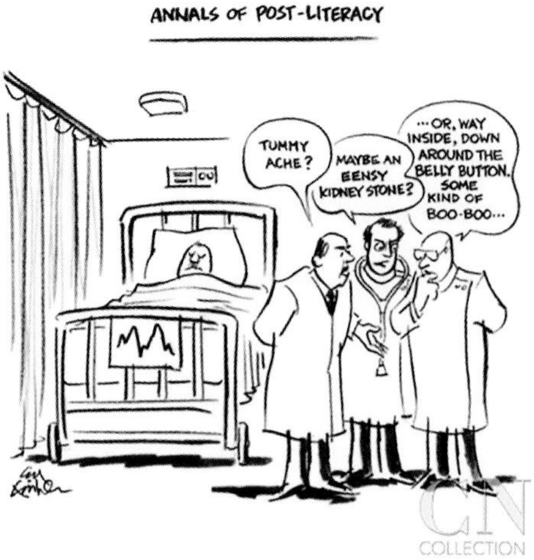


**FIGURE 1-1** This cartoon demonstrates the value of standardized medical terms.

The foundation of medical terminology is rooted in learning the four basic word parts: **prefixes, roots**, **suffixes**, and **combining forms**. You'll learn how to distinguish among these word parts in order to combine them into meaningful medical terms.

First, let's examine some medical term characteristics. Most medical terms are derived from Latin and Greek languages. While this may make them seem "foreign," 75% of *all English words* are derived from Latin and Greek. When you look up a term in the dictionary, its **etymology**, or word origin, is usually given along with its definition. For example, *dementia* is an impairment of cognitive function marked by memory loss. It comes from the Latin word, *demens*, which means "out of one's mind."

## ACQUIRING AND USING LANGUAGE SENSE

Accurate communication in any specialty field depends on *language sense*. **Language sense** is knowing what words mean and forecasting the effects their combinations will produce. This is a two-part definition. First, we have to understand what the word we're using means. Second, we have to trust that the person listening to what we're saying also understands the meaning of the words that we're using. While this is important in everyday language, it is especially important with medical terminology where misunderstanding can have drastic effects on patients.

> Who decides what the "correct" anatomic term is? A system of anatomic naming known as *Terminologia Anatomica* is considered the international standard for terminology that deals with human anatomy. It was created by the Federative Committee on Anatomical Terminology and first published in 1998. It is essentially an anatomy dictionary that gives the Latin base of the word along with the accepted English term. It has standardized anatomy-related terminology and is a great resource.

What does language sense have to do with learning medical terms? First, words have parts, and examining those parts forces the learner to see and hear words in a new way. That is, the person becomes conscious of words as words. You'll have to think about each part of the word and then put it all together to understand how the parts make up the whole. Second, the ability to use words well involves learning the phonetic and grammatical codes that make complex communication possible. This means using proper pronunciation and using medical terminology correctly in a sentence. Medical terminology is probably one of your first exposures to clinical culture. So congratulations! This is your first step toward success in the medical field!



## MEDICAL TERM PARTS

Nearly every medical term contains one or more *roots*. It may also contain one or more *prefixes* and one or more *suffixes*. When you start combining parts into words, you will also use a *combining form* of a root. This means a single medical term may consist of one part or several parts, but every part of a term behaves in one of three ways: root, prefix, or suffix. The good—and maybe surprising—news is that these three parts also make up all other English words. The even better news is that as an English speaker, you already know a lot of these parts, especially prefixes and suffixes.

Here is the order of word parts used in forming words: prefixes first, roots second, and suffixes last, assuming a word contains all three parts. If a **prefix** is present, it appears at the beginning of the term. A root is next. The **root** is found in the middle of the word, and they form words by adding prefixes or suffixes to them. **Suffixes** are always the endings of words. A **combining form** is used in combination with another word part that is distinct from a prefix or suffix that adjusts the sense or function of the word.

Some words, such as *nontraditional*, contain all three word parts. The prefix is **non-** (not), the root is **tradition** (established customs or norms), and the suffix **-al** (makes the word an adjective meaning "relating to"). This word is thus an adjective meaning "not relating to customs or norms."

> **EXAMPLE:** There are movements that encourage women to seek *nontraditional* occupations such as firefighting.

Some words contain only two parts, such as *traditionist.* Tradition is the root and –ist is the suffix that refers to "adhering to a system of beliefs or customs." So, a traditionist is a person with established beliefs or customs.

> **EXAMPLE:** Mr. Brown, who asked that boys in his classroom removed their hats, was considered a traditionist.

Other words contain other combinations, such as *nontradionalist* (the prefix **non-** = not; the root **tradition** = established customs or norm; the suffix **-al** = adjective form meaning relating to; and another suffix **–ist** = refers to adhering to a system of beliefs or customs). So, a *nontraditionalist* is a person without established beliefs or customs.

> **EXAMPLE:** Mrs. Brown, who didn't mind boys wearing hats in her classroom, was considered a nontradionalist.

Here is a medical term that has two roots: psychopath (**psycho** and **path**). *Psychopath* is a medical term that has become a common English word. It refers to a person who has a severe psychological disorder. One might contend that *path* is a suffix because in the term psychopath, it comes last. If we consider that the word part *path* comes to us from the English word **pathos**, which means sorrow, suffering, or tragedy, then maybe we ought to identify it as a root. However, as it comes at the end of some terms, is it not also a suffix? The best answer to that question is, "Who cares?" You may call it a root or a suffix, and it doesn't really matter as long as you know what it means and where it goes in a particular term. The bottom line is that prefix, root, and suffix identification is a convenient way to look at and decipher terms; and most of the time, assigning the labels of prefix, root, and suffix to a word's parts leads to an acceptable definition. If the parts vary a little now and then, don't despair; the universe will go on.

## ANALYZING TERMS

Learning to pick out prefixes, roots, and suffixes, as is done for you in Table 1-1, will permit you to define many, or even most, medical terms. Before going any further, we must deal with what has been traditionally referred to as a fourth word part: the **combining form**. A combining form is simply a root that includes one or more vowels tacked onto the end of it to make a root–suffix combination pronounceable, as in the word *psychology*. The main root is *psych* (mind), and the suffix is *-logy* (study of). But "psychlogy" doesn't flow as well as psychology, thus we insert the "o" to create a more English-sounding word. So, as the example shows, the combining form concept is all about vowels, consonants, and pronunciation. A problem thus arises. That problem is that we remember a word (or a word part, for that matter) in two ways: by recalling the sound it makes when we hear it spoken and by the sound a visual combination of its letters makes when we see it written.

When I asked a colleague how she pronounced the prefix **iatro-**, which means physician, she said, "eye-a-tro." Another colleague pronounced it, "eye-at-ur," and a French friend of mine insisted on, "eye-att-re" with a clipped final vowel sound, as in *Louvre*.

This book will introduce roots with their potential combining vowels added with forward slashes (/) separating them from the rest of the root.

**EXAMPLE:** card/i/o

By the way, it would make equal sense to introduce them as follows:

**EXAMPLE:** card; cardi; cardio (all three are, phonetically speaking, roots.)

You can learn a great deal from Table 1-1. To begin with, the terms **cardialgia**, **cardiology**, and **carditis** not only show the three forms of the root for heart (**card**, **cardi**, and **cardio**) but also introduce you to three important suffixes: -**algia**, -**logy**, and -**itis**.

- -algia = pain
- -logy = study of
- -itis = inflammation

**TABLE 1-1** ANALYSIS OF EXAMPLE WORDS

| Term | Prefix | Root | Suffix | Term Meaning |
| --- | --- | --- | --- | --- |
| cardialgia | | cardi (heart) | -algia (pain) | pain in the heart; also, heartburn (a digestive disorder) |
| cardiology | | cardio (heart) | -logy (study of) | study of the heart and its disorders |
| carditis | | card (heart) | -itis (inflammation) | inflammation of the heart |
| diagnosis | dia- (across; through) | *gnosis* (Greek word meaning "knowledge") | | discovery of the cause of signs and symptoms |
| iatrogenic disease | | iatro (physician); gen (origin, cause) | -ic (adjective suffix) | disease caused by health care (whether an individual worker, particular institution, or the system as a whole) |
| psychopath | | psycho (mind); path (disease) | | person with a (serious) mental disease |

These three suffixes occur in many medical terms. For example, when you learn a new root, such as **neur/o**, which means nerve, you will know the meanings of **neuralgia**, **neurology**, and **neuritis**:

- neuralgia = pain in a nerve
- neurology = the study of the nervous system; also the specialty dealing with diagnosis and treatment of nervous system disorders
- neuritis = inflammation of a nerve



## Quick Check

**Using your knowledge of prefixes, roots, and suffixes, see if you know which word parts make up a medical word you may not yet know. Intracranial means pertaining to the area within the skull.**

Intracranial: prefix = ________ root = ________ suffix = ________

Discerning readers may have noted that the suffix -logy is in the same category as the suffix -path. Although they both may be regarded as suffixes, we might also note that -logy is a root that comes to us from the Greek word *logos*, meaning "word"—not as in "a" word so much as in "the" word, that is, an explanation of things. That final meaning is why we define it as "study of" in Table 1-1. You may also recognize this root in common English words such as logic and logical.

In summary, you now know the first part of the definition of every term ending with any of the three suffixes introduced in the table. For *-algia*, the definition will begin with "pain in... ." It is important to note here that a second suffix, *-dynia*, also denotes pain. These two suffixes are sometimes interchangeable and sometimes not. Eventually, you will become familiar with instances in which one or the other is appropriate or at least most common.

For *-logy*, the definition will usually begin with "study of..."

For -itis, the definition will begin with "inflammation of..."

The term **diagnosis** introduces the prefix **dia-**, which means through, across, or between. You may have noticed that *dia-* appears in words you already know and use frequently, such as <u>dia</u>meter, a straight line running *through* the center point of a circle; <u>dia</u>gonal, a straight line running between opposite corners of a rectangle; and <u>dia</u>logue, people speaking words to each other across a space.

The word dialogue provides an example of how words change meaning when speakers or writers misunderstand their origins. This word has also come to refer to a conversation between two people because someone mistakenly interpreted the prefix to be *di*, meaning two, and other writers and speakers followed suit.

The medical term **diagnosis** refers to the determination of the presence of a disease or other disorder *through* consideration of signs, symptoms, and medical test results. That definition might seem to stretch the point of the word "through" until you learn that *gnosis* is the Greek word for knowledge. In other words, diagnosis is a procedure leading to a judgment "through knowledge." The verb **diagnose** represents a departure in one respect from the etymology of the term diagnosis. As with all back-formed verbs, clarity is easily lost. In this case, fuzziness comes about because "knowledge" (a noun) identifies something we know, whereas declaring (a verb) that we know it is something else entirely.

**Iatr/o** is a root that means physician, and **gen/o** (from a Greek word *gennao*, meaning the production of something) refers to origin or cause. The addition of **-ic** to gen forms **genic**, an adjective suffix meaning "originating from" or "caused by." Thus, an *iatrogenic disorder* is, literally speaking, "a disorder caused by a physician." In general use, the term *iatrogenic* refers to a disorder, disease, or ailment caused by any medical treatment or practitioner, such as a side effect from a drug or complications following surgery.

Another form of the root iatr/o is **iatr**, which may be coupled with other roots and several suffixes: **y**, **ic**, **ics**, **ist**, and **ician**. Here are examples of words formed from iatr, y, ic, ist, and ician:

| Term | Part | Meaning |
|---|---|---|
| psychiatry | psych + iatr + y | specialty dealing with disorders of the mind (in this case the *y* **does not** act as an adjective suffix) |
| psychiatric | psych + iatr + ic | adjective form of psychiatry |
| psychiatrist | psych + iatr + ist | specialist in psychiatry |
| geriatrics | ger + iatr + ics | specialty in disorders of the elderly |
| pediatrician | ped +iatr +ician | specialist in children's disorders |

The root psycho comes from the Greek word *psyche*, which means soul or mind. The suffixes **-ist** and **-ician** mean practitioner, and the suffixes **-y** and **-ics** mean practice. The final two items in the list introduce two new roots: **ger/o** and **ped/o**, the meanings of which you may deduce from the meanings of the terms **geriatrics** and **pediatrician**. The root *ger/o* (also sometimes **ger/onto**) comes from the Greek word *geron*, which means old man. The root *ped/o* is derived from the Greek word *pais*, which means child.

See Tables 1-2, 1-3, and 1-4, which list a sampling of roots, suffixes, and prefixes. Study these so you can start building and defining terms.

**TABLE 1-2 WORD ROOTS TO BEGIN BUILDING TERMS**

| Word Root | Meaning |
|---|---|
| arthr/o | joint |
| card/i/o | heart |
| derm/o/ato | skin |
| gen/o | origin, cause, formation |
| ger/o/onto | old age |
| hem/a/ato | blood |
| iatr/o | physician |
| muscul/o | muscle |
| natal | birth; born |
| neur/o | nerve |
| os/teo | bone |
| path/o | disease |
| ped/ia | child |
| phren/o | diaphragm, mind |
| psych/o | mind |
| skelet/o | skeleton |
| tend/o, ten/o | tendon |

**TABLE 1-3 PREFIXES TO BEGIN BUILDING TERMS**

| Prefix | Meaning |
|---|---|
| epi- | upon, following, or subsequent to |
| micro- | small |
| peri- | around |
| post- | after |
| pre- | before |

**TABLE 1-4 SUFFIXES TO BEGIN BUILDING TERMS**

| Suffix | Meaning |
|---|---|
| -al | adjective suffix |
| -algia | pain |
| -dynia | pain |
| -gen, -genesisa | origin, cause, formation |
| -ic | adjective suffix denoting of |
| -itis | inflammation |
| -logy | study of |
| -pathy | disease |
| -scope | viewing, an instrument used for viewing |

# END-OF-CHAPTER EXERCISES

## EXERCISE 1-1 DEFINING TERMS

**Combine the suffix *-logy* with the proper root to indicate the following medical specialties.**

1. Specialty dealing with heart disease ____________
2. Specialty that deals with the problems of aging and diseases in the elderly ____________
3. Specialty dealing with blood diseases ____________
4. Specialty dealing with skin ailments ____________
5. Specialty dealing with nervous system disorders ____________
6. Specialty dealing with mental disorders ____________

## EXERCISE 1-2 ANALYZING TERMS

**Analyze the following terms by putting the roots and suffixes in the appropriate columns. Then, write a definition for each term.**

| TERM | ROOT | SUFFIX | DEFINITION |
|---|---|---|---|
| 1. neuropathy | | | |
| 2. psychology | | | |
| 3. pathogenic | | | |
| 4. neuralgia | | | |
| 5. systemic | | | |
| 6. psychiatrist | | | |
| 7. pediatrician | | | |
| 8. iatrogenic | | | |
| 9. cardialgia | | | |
| 10. neuritis | | | |

## EXERCISE 1-3 FILL IN THE BLANK

**Fill in the blank with the correct answers.**

1. The prefix *peri-* denotes _______________.
2. The suffix *-logy* means _______________.
3. The word root derm/o refers to _______________.
4. The medical term *osteoarthritis* contains two _______________ and one _______________.
5. The suffix *-logy* is derived from the Greek word _______________, which means _______________.
6. Tendonitis refers to the _______________ of a _______________.
7. A prenatal examination is one that occurs _______________ the birth of a child.
8. _______________ is indicated by the suffixes -algia and _______________.
9. Inflammation is indicated by the suffix _______________.
10. The study of mental and emotional disorders is called _______________.

# 2

# Common Prefixes and Suffixes

## LEARNING OUTCOMES

***Upon completion of this chapter, you should be able to:***

- Recognize prefixes.
- Recognize suffixes.
- Define all of the prefixes and suffixes presented in this chapter.
- Analyze and define new terms introduced in this chapter.
- Pronounce, define, and spell each term introduced in this chapter.

## INTRODUCTION

Chapter 1 presented the four word parts used in medical terminology: prefixes, roots, suffixes, and combining forms. This chapter focuses on prefixes and suffixes.

In Chapter 1, we learned that a prefix is a word part that comes at the beginning of a word. Note that the word *prefix* itself contains a prefix, pre-. The second part of the word *prefix* is "fix," which gives us a perfect definition of prefix: something affixed (attached) to the front of or before (pre-) something else. Most of the prefixes occurring in medical terms are also found in everyday English. Although we have all used many of the prefixes contained in this chapter, we may have done so without realizing that they are prefixes. For example, when we are admitted to an anteroom, we may not stop to think that the prefix **ante-** means "before," and that an *anteroom* is so called because it is a room we enter before entering another room.

We also learned in Chapter 1 that a suffix is the part that comes at the end of a word. The word *suffix* comes from the Latin word *suffixum*, which may be translated as "to fasten to the end of." Although the suffix is located last in a medical term, it often comes first in its definition. For example, *appendicitis* means "inflammation (*-itis*) of the appendix." Therefore, the suffix, -itis, provides us with the first word of the defining phrase. The term *gastrectomy* is another example. It is defined as "removal of the stomach." The definition begins with the meaning of the suffix, -ectomy, which means "removal of."

## WORD ROOTS INTRODUCED IN THIS CHAPTER

Table 2-1 lists common word roots with their meanings to get you started on your task of learning hundreds of medical terms. You may wish to memorize the roots given in the table now, because there are just a few. Or if you prefer, just give them a quick glance now and, as you go through the chapter, refer back to this table whenever you run across a term with a root you do not recognize.

**TABLE 2-1** COMMON WORD ROOTS AND MEANINGS

| Word Root | Meaning |
|---|---|
| arter/i/o | artery |
| arthr/o | joint |
| card/i/o | heart |
| derm/at/o | skin |
| gen/i/o | origin, cause, formation |
| ger/o/onto | old age |
| hem/a/t/o | blood |
| iatr/o | physician |
| muscul/o | muscle |
| neur/o | nerve, nerve tissue |
| oste/o | bone |
| path/o | disease |
| ped/i/o | child |
| phren/o | diaphragm, mind |
| psych/o | mind |
| skelet/o | skeleton |
| spin/o | spine |
| tend/i/n/o | tendon |



## CATEGORIES OF PREFIXES

Not all medical terms include a prefix, but when one is present, it is critical to the term's meaning. For example, **hyper**glycemia (high blood sugar) and **hypo**glycemia (low blood sugar) are conditions that are exact opposites. Confusing those two prefixes creates errors. Two other similar-sounding prefix pairs prone to creating errors are ante- and anti-. The prefix *ante-* means "before," and the prefix *anti-* means "against."

| Term | Part | Meaning |
|---|---|---|
| hypoglycemia | prefix: hypo- = low<br>root: glyc/o- = sugar<br>suffix: -emia = condition | low blood sugar |
| antecubital | prefix: ante- = before<br>root: cubitum = elbow | anterior to the elbow |
| anticoagulant | prefix: anti- = against<br>root: coagulant = substance that causes blood to clot | preventing coagulation (clotting) |

Dividing prefixes into functional categories makes them easier to learn. There are five logical divisions:

- Prefixes of time or speed
- Prefixes of direction
- Prefixes of position
- Prefixes of size or number
- Prefixes of negation

**TABLE 2-2 PREFIXES OF TIME OR SPEED**

| Prefix | Refers to | Example | Meaning |
|---|---|---|---|
| ante-, pre- | before | antepartum, premature | before birth, before full development |
| brady- | abnormally slow rate of speed | bradycardia | abnormally slow heartbeat |
| neo- | new | neonatal | newborn (adjective) |
| post- | after | postscript | a written thought added after the main message |
| tachy- | rapid, abnormally high rate of speed | tachycardia | abnormally fast heartbeat |



Seeing prefixes in words we already know helps us learn their meanings quickly and enables us to understand medical terms we encounter later on. For that reason, common English words are included as examples in some of the following paragraphs and tables.

## Prefixes of Time or Speed

Prefixes denoting time or speed are used in everyday English. **Pre**historic and **post**graduate are common words with a prefix relating to time. Prefixes denoting speed, such as tachy- (fast) and brady- (slow), are often used to describe heart rate. Table 2-2 lists prefixes related to time or speed.

## Prefixes of Direction

The word **ab**normal is an example of a word containing a prefix that signifies direction. We use such prefixes in everyday life without bothering to analyze them. For example, we normally would not take the time to think about the prefix **contra-** (against) in the word contradiction, yet we understand its meaning. Prefixes related to direction are listed in Table 2-3.

## Prefixes of Position

**Infra**structure (*infra-* means inside or below), **inter**state (*inter-* means between), and **para**legal (*para-* means alongside) are all words we frequently use that include prefixes of position. Having these prefix meanings already in our working vocabularies makes it easier to learn their medical uses. Prefixes of position are commonly used during diagnostic and treatment procedures. Table 2-4 lists prefixes relating to position.

**TABLE 2-3 PREFIXES OF DIRECTION**

| Prefix | Refers to | Example | Meaning |
|---|---|---|---|
| ab- | away from, outside of, beyond | abnormal | not normal |
| ad- | toward, near to | adjective | toward a noun |
| con-, sym-, syn- | with, within | congenital, sympathetic, synthetic | with (or at) birth, with feeling toward, with the same idea or purpose |
| contra- | against | contraband | substance against the law |
| dia- | across, through | diameter | a line through the middle |

**TABLE 2-4 PREFIXES OF POSITION**

| Prefix | Refers to | Example | Meaning |
|---|---|---|---|
| ec-, ecto-, ex-, exo- | outside | extraction | removal to the outside |
| en- | inside | encephalopathy | disease inside the head, brain disease |
| endo- | within | endoscopy | visual examination of the inside of some part of the body |
| epi- | upon, subsequent to | epigastric | adjective referring to something above the stomach |
| extra- | beyond | extracellular | adjective referring to something outside a cell or cells |
| hyper- | above, beyond normal | hyperglycemia | high blood sugar |
| hypo- | low, below, below normal | hypogastric | region beneath the stomach |
| infra- | inside or below | infrarenal | adjective referring to something below the kidneys |
| inter- | between | interosseous | between bones |
| intra- | inside, within | intracerebral | inside the cerebrum |
| meso- | middle | mesothelioma | tumor arising from the mesothelium |
| meta- | beyond | metacarpal | the bone beyond the carpus; one of five bones in either hand |
| pan- | all or everywhere | pancarditis | general inflammation of the heart |
| para- | alongside, near | paraplegia | paralysis of the lower half of the body |
| peri- | around | perivascular | in the tissues surrounding a vessel |
| retro- | backward, behind | retrosternal | adjective referring to something behind the sternum |



## Prefixes of Size and Number

A **semi**annual (semi- means "half," annual means "yearly") sale is one that occurs every 6 months. The **uni**corn (uni- means "one") is a fictitious creature that has one horn. Prefixes of size and number are very common. Table 2-5 lists prefixes related to size and number.

**TABLE 2-5 PREFIXES OF SIZE AND NUMBER**

| Prefix | Refers to | Example | Meaning |
|---|---|---|---|
| bi- | two | biannual | twice per year |
| di-, dipl- | two, twice | diplopia | double vision |
| hemi- | half | hemiplegia | paralysis of one body side |
| macro- | big | macrocyte | big cell |
| micro- | small | microscope | instrument to view small objects |
| mono- | one | monocyte | cell with one nucleus |
| olig-, oligo- | a few, a little | oliguria | scant urine production |
| pan- | all or everywhere | pancarditis | whole heart inflammation |
| poly- | many | polydactyly | more than five hand or foot digits |

**TABLE 2-5 PREFIXES OF SIZE AND NUMBER** *(continued)*

| Prefix | Refers to | Example | Meaning |
|---|---|---|---|
| quadri- | four | quadriplegia | paralysis of all four limbs |
| semi- | half, partial | semiannual | occurring every half year |
| tetra- | four | tetradactyl | having only four hand or foot digits |
| tri- | three | triceps | three-headed muscle |
| uni- | one | unicellular | one-celled |

### Prefixes of Negation

Negation means absence or opposite of something. These include words like antidepressant (anti- means "against") and decriminalize (de- means "without"). Table 2-6 lists prefixes related to negation.



#### Quick Check

**Define each prefix and state whether it refers to time, speed, position, direction, number, or negation.**

1. anti- ____________________
2. hyper- ____________________
3. tachy- ____________________

## CATEGORIES OF SUFFIXES

Dividing suffixes into functional categories makes them easier to learn than they would be otherwise. A suffix adds to or changes a root in one of four different ways. Suffixes:

- Signify a medical condition.
- Signify a diagnostic term, test information, or surgical procedure.
- Name a medical practice or practitioner.
- Convert a noun to an adjective.

The suffix -stenosis, for example, indicates a narrowing or blockage in a body part, which is a condition. Consider the term arteriostenosis. Because the root arter/i/o means artery, we may conclude that arteriostenosis is a narrowing of an artery. Note how this term is divided into word parts:

| Term | Part | Meaning |
|---|---|---|
| arteriostenosis | root: arter/i/o = artery<br>suffix: -stenosis = narrowing | narrowing of an artery |

**TABLE 2-6 PREFIXES OF NEGATION**

| Prefix | Refers to | Example | Meaning |
|---|---|---|---|
| a-, an- | not | anuria | not able to urinate |
| anti- | against, opposed | antibiotic | drug that inhibits microbes |
| de- | without | dehumidifier | device that removes water |
| dis- | remove | disable | put out of action |

## Suffixes Signifying Medical Conditions

The suffix **-porosis**, which means porous, is added to the root **oste/o**, to form the term **osteoporosis**, which means "a porous condition of bone." See Table 2-7 for more examples.

**TABLE 2-7 SUFFIXES THAT SIGNIFY MEDICAL CONDITIONS**

| Suffix | Meaning of the Suffix | Example | Meaning of the Example |
|---|---|---|---|
| -algia, -dynia | pain | arthralgia, arthrodynia | pain in a joint |
| -cele | protrusion, hernia | rectocele | hernia of the rectum |
| -cyte | cell | leukocyte | white blood cell |
| -ectasis, -ectasia | expansion or dilation | angiectasis | dilation of a vessel |
| -edema (also a standalone word) | excessive fluid | angioedema | fluid buildup that causes swelling under the skin |
| -emesis | vomiting | hematemesis | vomiting of blood |
| -emia | blood | uremia | urea in the blood |
| -iasis | condition or state | cholelithiasis, sometimes also spelled "chololithiasis" | stones in the gallbladder or bile ducts |
| -ism | a condition of, a process, or a state of | hypothyroidism | condition characterized by thyroid hormone deficiency |
| -itis | Inflammation | appendicitis | inflammation of the appendix |
| -lith | stone, calculus, calcification | pneumolith | a stone in the lung |
| -lysis | disintegration, breaking down | hemolysis | rupture of red blood cells |
| -malacia | softening | osteomalacia | softening of the bones |
| -megaly | enlargement | gastromegaly | enlargement of the stomach |
| -oid | resembling or like | opioid | substance that resembles opium |
| -oma | tumor | gastroma | tumor of the stomach |
| -osis | abnormal condition | osteoporosis | condition of porous bones |
| -pathy | disease | myopathy | disease of the muscle |
| -penia | reduction of size or quantity | leukopenia | low number of white blood cells |
| -phobia | fear | carcinophobia | fear of cancer |
| -plasia | abnormal formation | neoplasia | abnormal growth of cells |
| -plegia | paralysis | hemiplegia | paralysis on one side of the body |
| -pnea | breathing | tachypnea | rapid breathing |
| -poiesis | producing | erythropoiesis | production of red blood cells |
| -porosis | porous condition | osteoporosis | porous |
| -ptosis | downward displacement | nephroptosis | downward displacement of a kidney |
| -rrhage | flowing forth | hemorrhage | significant discharge of blood from blood vessels |
| -rrhea | discharge | rhinorrhea | discharge from the nose (runny nose) |

**TABLE 2-7 SUFFIXES THAT SIGNIFY MEDICAL CONDITIONS** *(continued)*

| Suffix | Meaning of the Suffix | Example | Meaning of the Example |
|---|---|---|---|
| -rrhexis | rupture | hysterorrhexis | rupture of the uterus |
| -sclerosis | hardness | atherosclerosis | hardening of the arteries |
| -spasm | muscular contraction | angiospasm | muscular contraction of a vessel |
| -stasis | level, unchanging | thermostasis | a constant, consistent internal body temperature |
| -stenosis | a narrowing | arteriostenosis | narrowed arteries |

## Suffixes Signifying Diagnostic Terms, Test Information, or Surgical Procedures

Suffixes that form terms related to test information, diagnoses, and procedures are often attached to a root that signifies a body part. The term **appendectomy** is an example. The suffix **-ectomy** means "removal of," and **append** is the root for appendix. Thus, the term means "removal of the appendix." Table 2-8 lists common suffixes that signify diagnostic terms, test information, or surgical procedures.

## Suffixes That Name a Medical Practice or Practitioner

Some suffixes relating to a medical practice or practitioner are derived from the Greek word *iatros*, which means "physician" or "medical treatment." This Greek word is the source of the

**TABLE 2-8 SUFFIXES THAT SIGNIFY DIAGNOSTIC TERMS, TEST INFORMATION, OR SURGICAL PROCEDURES**

| Suffix | Refers to | Example |
|---|---|---|
| -centesis | surgical puncture | thoracentesis |
| -desis | surgical binding | arthrodesis |
| -ectomy | surgical removal | appendectomy |
| -gen, -genic, -genesis | origin, producing | osteogenic |
| -gram | a recording, usually by an instrument | electrocardiogram |
| -graph | instrument for making a recording | electrocardiograph |
| -graphy | act of graphic or pictorial recording | electrocardiography |
| -meter | instrument for measuring | audiometer |
| -metry | act of measuring | audiometry |
| -opsy | examination | autopsy |
| -pexy | surgical fixation | hysteropexy |
| -plasty | surgical repair | rhinoplasty |
| -rrhaphy | suture | herniorrhaphy |
| -scope | instrument for viewing | arthroscope |
| -scopy | act of viewing | arthroscopy |
| -stomy | artificial or surgical opening | tracheostomy |
| -tome | instrument for cutting | dermatome |
| -tomy | incision | colotomy |
| -tripsy | crushing | lithotripsy |

**TABLE 2-9 SUFFIXES THAT SIGNIFY MEDICAL PRACTICE AND PRACTITIONERS**

| Suffix | Refers to | Example |
|---|---|---|
| -ian | specialist | pediatrician |
| -iatrics | medical specialty | pediatrics |
| -iatry | medical specialty | psychiatry |
| -ics | medical specialty | orthopedics |
| -ist | specialist in a field of study | orthopedist |
| -logy | study of | gynecology |

root iatr/o. For practical purposes, you may consider the root *iatr* as an integral part of the suffixes **-iatric** and **-iatr**, as in the terms *geriatrics*, *psychiatric*, *psychiatry*, *psychiatrist*, *pediatrics*, and *pediatrician*. Although both *-ician* and *-ist* are used in referring to a specialist, the suffix *-ist* is perhaps the more common one. An example is **gerontologist**, a physician who diagnoses and treats disorders of aging.

Terms denoting a field or medical specialty may also end with the suffix **-logy**. Table 2-9 lists the suffixes for medical practice and practitioners.



> Root, prefix, or suffix? The word part **gen** can act as a suffix or a root, but, as is the case with **iatro-**, it combines nicely with several suffixes and may be considered as a part of them. Terms formed with **-genic** are adjectives, because of the **-ic** ending. As we will see later, **-ic** can act as a suffix by itself, too.

## Suffixes That Denote Adjectives

As with suffixes that signify medical practice and practitioners, suffixes used to create adjective forms are not governed by a clear set of rules. Nevertheless, there are some rules that come into play, such as the rules of English pronunciation. For example, we replace the final letter, *x*, in the word appendix with a *c* to form the adjective *appendicitis* because "appendixitis" does not sound much like an English word.

In creating adjectives, we also sometimes change noun terms that name specialties. For example, *psychiatry* and *pediatrics* are the names of specialties. Dropping the *y* from psychiatry and adding the adjective suffix -ic converts the specialty name to an adjective:

psychiatri**c** medicine
psychiatri**c** hospital

With *pediatrics*, on the other hand, all we need to do to form the adjective is drop the *s*:

pediatri**c** medicine
pediatri**c** hospital

Examples of adjective suffixes are listed in Table 2-10.

Prefixes and suffixes presented in this chapter will become familiar as you progress through the next chapters on body systems. Review the following study tables and do the self-testing exercises.

**TABLE 2-10 SUFFIXES THAT DENOTE ADJECTIVES**

| Suffix | Refers to | Example |
|---|---|---|
| -ac, -al, -an, -aneous, -ar, -ary, -eal, -eous, -iac, -iatric, -ic, -ical, -oid, -otic, -ous, -tic, -ular | converts a root or noun to an adjective | geriatric, orthopedic, ocular |

**Study Table** COMMON PREFIXES

| PREFIX | MEANING | EXAMPLE |
|---|---|---|
| a-, an- | not | anemic |
| ab- | away from, outside of, beyond | abnormal |
| ad- | toward, near to | addiction |
| ante-, pre- | before | antepartum, premature |
| anti- | against, opposed | antibiotic |
| bi- | two | bipolar |
| brady- | abnormally slow rate of speed | bradycardia |
| con-, sym-, syn- | with | congenital, sympathetic, synarthrosis |
| contra- | against | contralateral |
| de- | not | deodorant |
| di-, diplo- | two, twice | dipole |
| dia- | across, through | diagnosis |
| dis- | remove | disinfect |
| dys- | painful, bad, difficult | dyspnea |
| ec-, ecto- | outside, away from | ectopy |
| en- | inside | endosteum |
| endo- | within | endoderm |
| epi- | upon, subsequent to | epigastric |
| ex-, exo- | outside | exoskeleton |
| extra- | beyond | extrasystole |
| hemi- | half | hemiplegia |
| hyper- | above, beyond normal | hypergastric |
| hypo- | below, below normal | hypogastric |
| infra- | inside or below | infrastructure |
| inter- | between | intercostal |
| intra- | inside | intracerebral |
| macro- | big | macrophage |
| meso- | middle | mesothelium |
| meta- | beyond | metacarpal |
| micro- | small | microscope |
| mono-, uni- | one | monocyte |
| neo- | new | neoplasm |
| olig-, oligo- | a few, a little | oliguria |
| pan- | everywhere | pandemic |
| para- | alongside, near | paraplegia |

*(continued)*

**Study Table** COMMON PREFIXES (*continued*)

| PREFIX | MEANING | EXAMPLE |
|---|---|---|
| peri- | around | perimeter |
| post- | after | postsynaptic |
| quadri- | four | quadriceps |
| retro- | backward, behind | retroperitoneal |
| semi- | half, partial | semiconscious |
| tachy- | rapid | tachycardia |
| tetra- | four | tetradactyl |
| tri- | three | triceps |
| uni- | one | unilateral |

**Study Table** COMMON SUFFIXES

| SUFFIX | MEANING | EXAMPLE |
|---|---|---|
| -ac, -al, -an, -aneous, -ar, -ary, -eal, -eous, -iac, -iatric, -ic, -ical, -oid, -otic, -ous, -tic, -ular | converts a root or a noun term to an adjective | geriatric, orthopedic, ocular, dental, cutaneous, cyanotic, atrial, cardiac, ureteral |
| -algia, -dynia | pain | urodynia |
| -cele | protrusion, hernia | rectocele |
| -centesis | surgical puncture | thoracentesis |
| -cyte | cell | leukocyte |
| -desis | surgical binding | arthrodesis |
| -ectasis, -ectasia | expansion or dilation | angiectasis |
| -ectomy | surgical removal | appendectomy |
| -edema | excessive fluid in intracellular tissues | angioedema |
| -emesis | vomiting | hematemesis |
| -emia | blood | uremia |
| -genic | origin, producing | osteogenic |
| -gram | a recording, usually by an instrument | electrocardiogram |
| -graph | instrument for making a recording | electrocardiograph |
| -graphy | act of graphic or pictorial recording | electrocardiography |
| -ian, -iatrist, -ist, -logist, -logy, -ics, -iatry, -iatrics | specialty of, study of, practice of | geriatrist, pediatrician, gynecology |
| -iasis | condition or state | cholelithiasis |
| -ism | a condition of, a process, or a state of | gigantism, hyperthyroidism |

**Study Table** COMMON SUFFIXES (*continued*)

| SUFFIX | MEANING | EXAMPLE |
|---|---|---|
| -itis | inflammation | appendicitis |
| -lith | stone, calculus, calcification | pneumolith |
| -lysis | disintegration | hemolysis |
| -malacia | softening | osteomalacia |
| -megaly | enlargement | gastromegaly |
| -meter | device for measuring | audiometer |
| -metry | act of measuring | audiometry |
| -oid | resembling or like | android, mucoid |
| -oma | tumor | gastroma |
| -opsy | visual examination | biopsy |
| -osis | abnormal condition | osteoporosis, arthrosis |
| -pathy | disease | cardiopathy |
| -penia | reduction of size or quantity | leukopenia |
| -pexy | surgical fixation | hysteropexy |
| -phobia | fear | claustrophobia |
| -plasia | abnormal formation | chondroplasia |
| -plasty | surgical repair | rhinoplasty |
| -plegia | paralysis | hemiplegia |
| -pnea | breath, respiration | tachypnea |
| -poiesis | producing | erythropoiesis |
| -porosis | porous condition | osteoporosis |
| -ptosis | downward displacement | nephroptosis |
| -rrhage | flowing forth | hemorrhage |
| -rrhaphy | suture | herniorrhaphy |
| -rrhea | discharge | diarrhea |
| -rrhexis | rupture | hysterorrhexis |
| -sclerosis | hardness | arteriosclerosis |
| -scope | instrument for viewing | arthroscope |
| -scopy | act of viewing | arthroscopy |
| -spasm | muscular contraction | arteriospasm |
| -stasis | level, unchanging | hemostasis |
| -stenosis | a narrowing | arteriostenosis |
| -stomy | permanent opening | colostomy |
| -tome | instrument for cutting | osteotome |
| -tomy | incision | osteotomy |
| -tripsy | crushing | lithotripsy |

## END-OF-CHAPTER EXERCISES

### EXERCISE 2-1 ADDING PREFIXES OF TIME OR SPEED

Form a new word by adding each prefix in the list to the word appearing next to it. Then write the meaning of the new word in the space to the right. Refer to a dictionary as needed.

| PREFIX | WORD | NEW WORD | MEANING |
|---|---|---|---|
| 1. ante- | room | | |
| 2. neo- | classic | | |
| 3. post- | glacial | | |
| 4. pre- | dominant | | |
| 5. tacho- | meter | | |

### EXERCISE 2-2 ADDING PREFIXES OF DIRECTION

Form a new word by adding each prefix in the list to the word appearing next to it. Then write the meaning of the new word in the space to the right. Refer to a dictionary as needed.

| PREFIX | WORD | NEW WORD | MEANING |
|---|---|---|---|
| 1. ab- | normal | | |
| 2. ad- | joining | | |
| 3. con- | centric | | |
| 4. contra- | lateral | | |
| 5. dia- | gram | | |
| 6. sym- | pathetic | | |
| 7. syn- | thesis | | |

### EXERCISE 2-3 ADDING PREFIXES OF POSITION

Form a new word by adding each prefix in the list to the word or word part appearing next to it. Then write the meaning of the new word in the space to the right. Refer to a dictionary as needed.

| PREFIX | WORD/WORD PART | NEW WORD | MEANING |
|---|---|---|---|
| 1. ec- | centric | | |
| 2. ecto- | morph | | |

| | | | |
|---|---|---|---|
| 3. en- | slave | ____________ | ____________ |
| 4. endo- | cardial | ____________ | ____________ |
| 5. epi- | demic | ____________ | ____________ |
| 6. ex- | change | ____________ | ____________ |
| 7. exo- | sphere | ____________ | ____________ |
| 8. extra- | terrestrial | ____________ | ____________ |
| 9. hyper- | sensitive | ____________ | ____________ |
| 10. hypo- | thesis | ____________ | ____________ |
| 11. infra- | structure | ____________ | ____________ |
| 12. inter- | collegiate | ____________ | ____________ |
| 13. intra- | mural | ____________ | ____________ |
| 14. meso- | sphere | ____________ | ____________ |
| 15. meta- | physics | ____________ | ____________ |
| 16. pan- | orama | ____________ | ____________ |
| 17. para- | legal | ____________ | ____________ |

## EXERCISE 2-4 ADDING PREFIXES OF SIZE OR NUMBER

**Form a new word by adding each prefix in the list to the word or word part appearing next to it. Then write the meaning of the new word in the space to the right. Refer to a dictionary as needed.**

| PREFIX | WORD/WORD PART | NEW WORD | MEANING |
|---|---|---|---|
| 1. bi- | annual | ____________ | ____________ |
| 2. hemi- | sphere | ____________ | ____________ |
| 3. macro- | cosm | ____________ | ____________ |
| 4. micro- | scope | ____________ | ____________ |
| 5. mono- | rail | ____________ | ____________ |
| 6. olig- | archy | ____________ | ____________ |
| 7. quadri- | lateral | ____________ | ____________ |
| 8. semi- | annual | ____________ | ____________ |

| | | | |
|---|---|---|---|
| 9. tri- | angle | | |
| 10. uni- | cycle | | |

## EXERCISE 2-5 COMBINING ROOTS AND SUFFIXES THAT DENOTE MEDICAL CONDITIONS

**Build new words by combining the correct form of each of the roots with the suffixes appearing next to it. Suffixes and their definitions may be found in the Common Suffixes Study Table in this chapter. Then write the meaning of the new word in the space to the right. Refer to a medical dictionary as needed.**

| ROOT | SUFFIX | NEW WORD | MEANING |
|---|---|---|---|
| 1. card/i/o | -cele | | |
| | -dynia | | |
| | -ectasia | | |
| | -itis | | |
| | -malacia | | |
| | -megaly | | |
| | -ptosis | | |
| | -plegia | | |
| | -rrhexis | | |
| | -spasm | | |
| 2. dermat/o | -itis | | |
| | -oma | | |
| | -megaly | | |
| | -osis | | |
| 3. hem/o, hemat/o | -lysis | | |
| | -genesis | | |
| | -oma | | |
| | -osis | | |
| 4. neur/o | -algia | | |
| | -ectasis | | |
| | -itis | | |
| | -oma | | |

| | | | |
|---|---|---|---|
| 5. oste/o | -dynia | ______ | ______ |
| | -oma | ______ | ______ |
| | -malacia | ______ | ______ |
| | -penia | ______ | ______ |
| | -porosis | ______ | ______ |
| | -itis | ______ | ______ |
| 6. psych/o | -osis | ______ | ______ |

## EXERCISE 2-6 COMBINING ROOTS AND SUFFIXES THAT DENOTE DIAGNOSTIC TERMS, TEST INFORMATION, OR SURGICAL PROCEDURES

**Build new words by combining the correct form of each of the roots with the suffixes appearing next to it. Suffixes and their definitions may be found in the Common Suffixes Study Table in this chapter. Then write the meaning of the new word in the space to the right. Refer to a medical dictionary as needed.**

| ROOT | SUFFIX | NEW WORD | MEANING |
|---|---|---|---|
| 1. card/i/o | -genic | ______ | ______ |
| | -gram | ______ | ______ |
| | -graph | ______ | ______ |
| | -graphy | ______ | ______ |
| | -pathy | ______ | ______ |
| | -rrhaphy | ______ | ______ |
| 2. dermat/o | -plasty | ______ | ______ |
| 3. hemat/o | -genesis | ______ | ______ |
| | -metry | ______ | ______ |
| 4. neur/o | -ectomy | ______ | ______ |
| | -genic | ______ | ______ |
| | -genesis | ______ | ______ |
| 5. oste/o | -rrhaphy | ______ | ______ |
| | -plasty | ______ | ______ |
| | -genesis | ______ | ______ |
| | -ectomy | ______ | ______ |
| | -tomy | ______ | ______ |

| | | | |
|---|---|---|---|
| 6. path/o | -gen | ________ | ________ |
| | -genic | ________ | ________ |
| | -genesis | ________ | ________ |
| 7. psych/o | -genic | ________ | ________ |
| | -genesis | ________ | ________ |
| | -metry | ________ | ________ |
| | -pathy | ________ | ________ |

## EXERCISE 2-7 COMBINING ROOTS AND SUFFIXES ASSOCIATED WITH A MEDICAL PRACTICE OR PRACTITIONER

**Build new words by combining the correct form of each of the roots with the suffixes appearing next to it. Suffixes and their definitions may be found in the Common Suffixes Study Table in this chapter. Then write the meaning of the new word in the space to the right. Refer to a medical dictionary as needed.**

| ROOT | SUFFIX | NEW WORD | MEANING |
|---|---|---|---|
| 1. card/i/o | -logy | ________ | ________ |
| | -logist | ________ | ________ |
| 2. derm/o, dermat/o | -logy | ________ | ________ |
| | -logist | ________ | ________ |
| 3. ger/o/nt/o | -iatrics | ________ | ________ |
| | -logy | ________ | ________ |
| | -logist | ________ | ________ |
| 4. hem/o, hemat/o | -logy | ________ | ________ |
| | -logist | ________ | ________ |
| 5. neur/o | -logy | ________ | ________ |
| | -logist | ________ | ________ |
| 6. oste/o | -logy | ________ | ________ |
| | -logist | ________ | ________ |
| 7. path/o | -logy | ________ | ________ |
| | -logist | ________ | ________ |
| 8. psych/o | -logy | ________ | ________ |
| | -iatry | ________ | ________ |
| | -iatrist | ________ | ________ |

## EXERCISE 2-8 COMBINING ROOTS AND SUFFIXES THAT DENOTE ADJECTIVES

**Build new words by combining the correct form of each of the roots with the suffixes appearing next to it. Suffixes and their definitions may be found in the Common Suffixes Study Table in this chapter. Then write the meaning of the new word in the space to the right. Refer to a medical dictionary as needed.**

| ROOT | SUFFIX | NEW WORD | MEANING |
|---|---|---|---|
| 1. card/i/o | -ac | ____________ | ____________ |
| 2. hem/o, hemat/o | -toxic | ____________ | ____________ |
| 3. derm/o, dermat/o | -al | ____________ | ____________ |
| | -ic | ____________ | ____________ |
| 4. ger/o, geront/o | -iatric | ____________ | ____________ |
| | -al | ____________ | ____________ |
| 5. neur/o | -al | ____________ | ____________ |
| | -ic | ____________ | ____________ |
| 6. spin/o | -al | ____________ | ____________ |
| | -ous | ____________ | ____________ |
| 7. oste/o | -al | ____________ | ____________ |
| | -oid | ____________ | ____________ |

## EXERCISE 2-9 MATCHING SUFFIXES WITH MEANINGS

**Match the suffix in Column 1 with its definition in Column 2.**

| COLUMN 1 | COLUMN 2 |
|---|---|
| 1. __________ -cyte | A. morbid impulse toward a specific object or thought |
| 2. __________ -edema | B. vomiting |
| 3. __________ -emesis | C. a stone, calculus, calcification |
| 4. __________ -sclerosis | D. a condition, a process or state of |
| 5. __________ -tome | E. disease |
| 6. __________ -ism | F. visual examination |
| 7. __________ -lith | G. cell |
| 8. __________ -lysis | H. disintegration |
| 9. __________ -opsy | I. excessive fluid in intracellular tissues |
| 10. __________ -pathy | J. instrument for cutting |
| 11. __________ -phobia | K. level, unchanging |
| 12. __________ -poiesis | L. a narrowing |
| 13. __________ -stomy | M. hardness |
| 14. __________ -stasis | N. permanent opening |
| 15. __________ -stenosis | O. producing |

## EXERCISE 2-10 FILL IN THE BLANK

**For each of the following questions or statements, write the answer in the space provided.**

1. What two suffixes mean "pain?" ____________________
2. *Ang/i/o* is a root meaning "blood vessel." What term means "dilation of a blood vessel?"

   ____________________
3. Angioid means "resembling blood vessels." What part of speech is angioid? ____________________
4. Define angiorrhaphy ____________________
5. What suffix would you add to the root *ang/i/o* to form a term meaning "the act of making a pictorial record of blood vessels?" ____________________

6. What is an angioma? ____________________

7. What does *-plasty* mean? ____________________

8. What term denotes a skin specialist? ____________________

9. Does a gerontologist treat young or old patients? ____________________

10. What is the difference in meaning between *gerontology* and *geriatrics*? ____________________

11. The prefixes *ab-* and *ad-* are opposites; which one means "toward?" ____________________

12. The prefix *pre-* means "before"; what other prefix means the same thing? ____________________

13. Write a brief definition of bradycardia ____________________

14. What does the prefix *extra-* mean in the word extrasensory? ____________________

15. What prefix would you use in a term that means "high blood pressure?" ____________________

16. Given the meaning of *anti-*, what would be the purpose of an anticoagulant?
____________________

17. Given the meaning of the prefix *tri-*, how many cusps does the tricuspid valve have?
____________________

18. What does the prefix *micro-* tell us about the purpose of a microscope? ____________________

19. Write a medical term by combining the prefix *endo-* with the root *card/i/o*, meaning "heart," and the suffix that means "inflammation." Using only your knowledge of these three word parts, write the best definition you can for the term ____________________.

20. The suffix -pnea, meaning "breathing" or "respiration," can follow both tachy- and dys-. Define the terms tachypnea and dyspnea ________________________________________

3

# Organization of the Body

## LEARNING OUTCOMES

***Upon completion of this chapter, you should be able to:***

- Discuss the levels of body organization.
- Describe the anatomic position and cite the directional terms used in relation to the body.
- Name the body planes.
- Name the body cavities.
- Name the divisions of the abdomen and back.
- Pronounce, define, and spell each term introduced in this chapter.

## INTRODUCTION

Learning about how the human body is constructed will help you retain new medical terms by creating a mental picture of where things are. To begin, it is also useful to know the difference between the terms *anatomy* and *physiology*. **Anatomy** comes to us from the Greek word *anatome*, which means "dissection." You may have recognized the word part "tome," which indicates that anatomy has something to do with cutting. **Physiology**, on the other hand, is one of the many "ology" words; in this case, it means study of how the body's parts work together. In short, anatomy reveals the "what it is" and physiology the "how it works."

The "what it is" begins with chemicals that act together to form cells. The cells process the food we eat and the air we breathe. Cells also reproduce themselves, each cell according to the DNA code it contains.

## WORD PARTS RELATED TO BODY ORGANIZATION

Table 3-1 lists many of the word parts that make up terms related to the body as a whole. Not surprisingly, many of them have to do with how the body is divided or where things are located.

## LEVELS OF ORGANIZATION

The body is divided into different levels of organization, starting with the smallest level: cells, tissues, organs, organ (body) systems, and finally organism, which is the body as a whole. Each level is further examined under its own heading (see Figure 3-1).

### Cells

A human body is said to have 10 trillion to 100 trillion cells, depending on whom you ask. Of course, no one has ever actually counted the number of cells in a body, but as all the estimates are in the

**TABLE 3-1 WORD PARTS RELATED TO BODY ORGANIZATION**

| Word Part | Meaning |
|---|---|
| anter/o | front, anterior |
| cerv/o | neck |
| chondr/o | cartilage |
| cyt/o, -cyte | cell |
| dors/o | back |
| gastr/o | stomach, abdomen |
| inguin/o | groin |
| my/o | muscle |
| myel/o | spinal cord |
| neur/o | nerve, neuron |
| poster/o | posterior, back |
| proxim/o | near |
| super/o | superior |
| thorac/o | chest (thorax) |
| trans- | across |

## Word Parts Exercise

After studying Table 3-1, write the meaning of each of the word parts.

| WORD PART | MEANING |
|---|---|
| 1. trans- | 1. ________ |
| 2. dors/o | 2. ________ |
| 3. proxim/o | 3. ________ |
| 4. chondr/o | 4. ________ |
| 5. anter/o | 5. ________ |
| 6. my/o | 6. ________ |
| 7. super/o | 7. ________ |
| 8. cerv/o | 8. ________ |
| 9. inguin/o | 9. ________ |
| 10. myel/o | 10. ________ |

trillions, it's easy to appreciate the body's complexity as a functioning whole. Cells work both individually and together. Although cells differ from one another and consist of different components, they do have some common elements (see Figure 3-2):

- A *cell membrane* that allows certain substances in and out
- A *nucleus* that directs activities within the cell

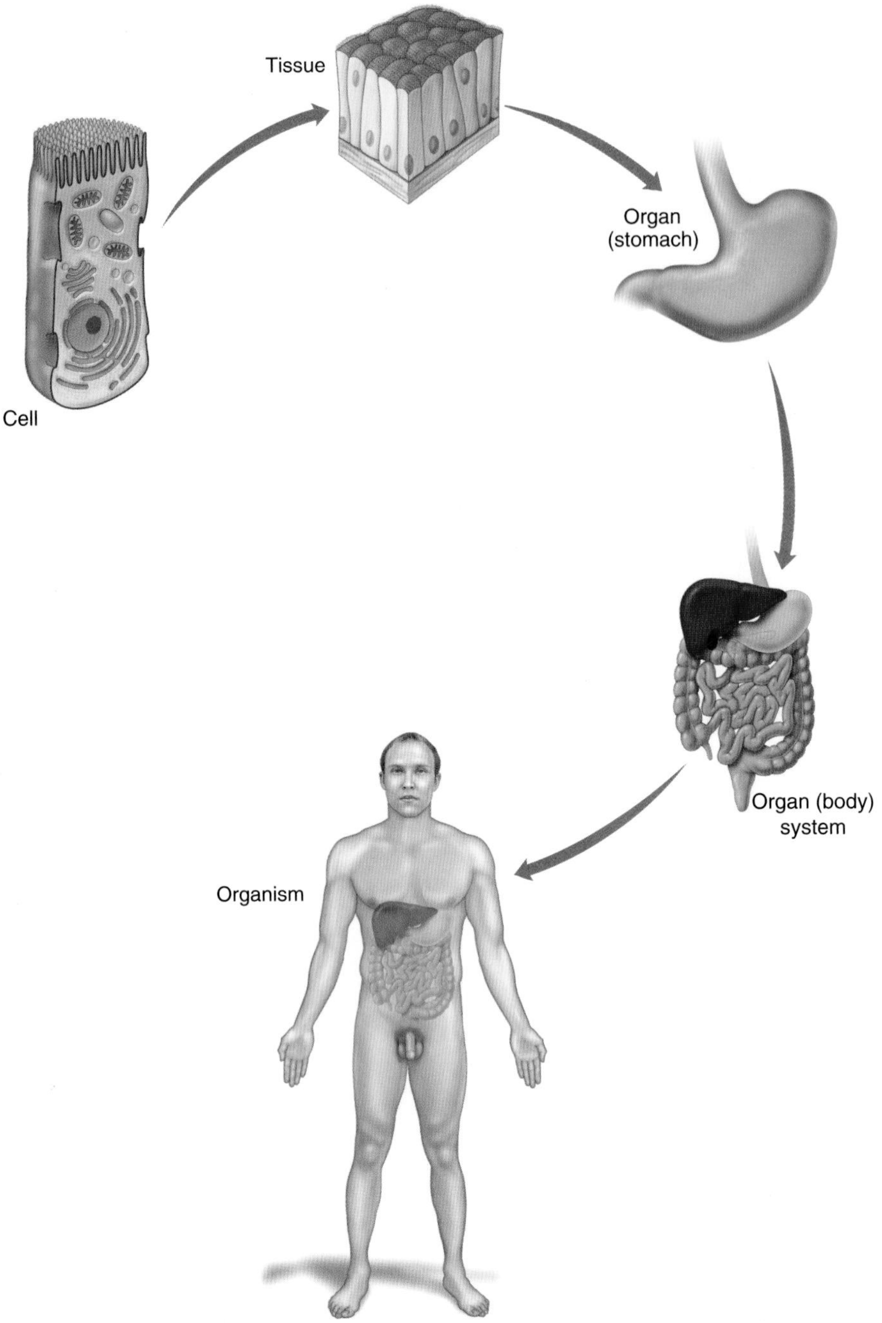


**FIGURE 3-1** The levels of organization in the body beginning with the cell and ending with the organism.



- *Mitochondria* that generate energy for the cell
- *Cytoplasm* that is a watery fluid that fills the spaces outside the nucleus

## Tissues

Cells make up tissues, which are composed of similar cells working together to perform similar tasks. The four types of body tissues are muscle, connective, nerve, and epithelial.

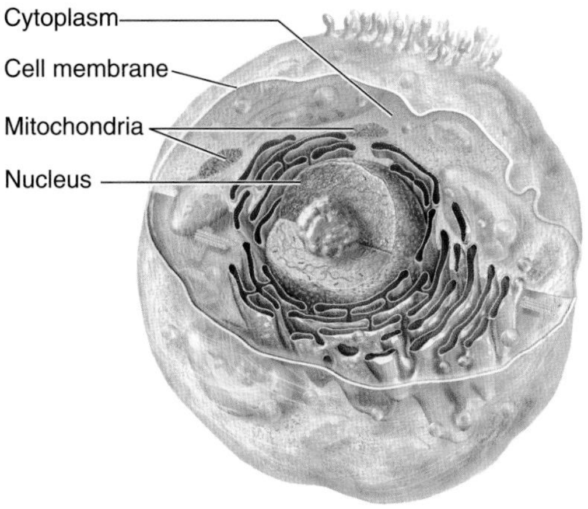


**FIGURE 3-2** Basic structure of a cell. The basic structure of a cell includes the cell membrane, nucleus, mitochondria, and the cytoplasm.

### Organs

Tissues with common functions come together to form the body's organs, which perform specialized functions. Examples of organs are the brain, stomach, and heart.

### Systems

A group of organs forms an organ (body) system, and each system has its own special purpose. Therefore, the rest of this book discusses each system in a chapter of its own.

## NAVIGATING THE BODY

Health care professionals need to be familiar with directional and positioning terms. These terms are frequently used during patient examinations, diagnostic procedures, and treatments.

### Anatomic Position

Directional terms in the field of human anatomy differ from plain language in two ways: first, unlike terms of location, directional terms are language-specific; second, directional terms are specified relative to the anatomic position. In the **anatomic position**, the body is erect and facing forward, and the arms are at the sides with the palms of the hands facing forward (see Figure 3-3). Left and right are from the subject's perspective, not the observer's perspective.

> The inhabitants of Pormpuraaw, a remote Aboriginal community in Australia, have no words for "left" or "right." Instead, they speak of everything in terms of absolute directions (north, south, east, and west). They say things such as, "There's an ant on your southwest leg." To say hello in Pormpuraaw, one asks, "Where are you going?" An appropriate response might be, "A long way to the south-southwest. How about you?" The Pormpuraawans not only know instinctively which direction they are facing, they also spontaneously use their spatial orientation to represent both position and time.

### Directional Terms

Directional terms are adjectives that help describe a complaint, symptom, body part, or process. These terms often have another term that is its opposite, and it is helpful to memorize these terms with their opposite in order to differentiate and understand them. **Superior** means above or nearer to the head. Two

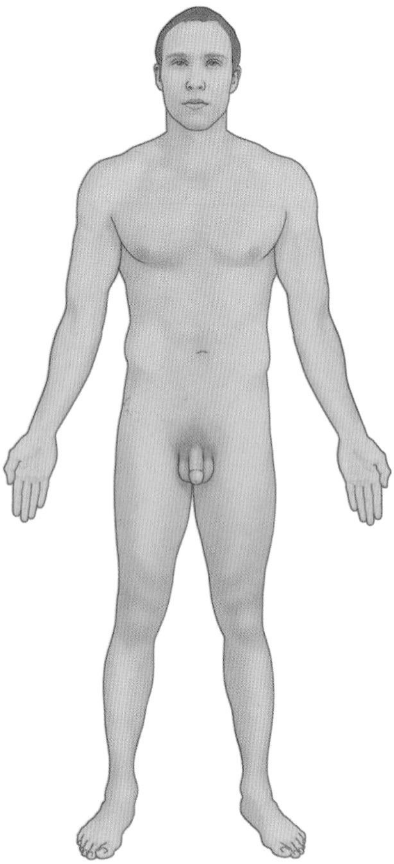

**FIGURE 3-3** Anatomic position. In the anatomic position, the person is standing erect, and palms and body are facing forward.

other words, **cranial** and **cephalic**, also mean "toward the head." For example, "The bruise is superior to the eyebrow." **Inferior** and **caudal** mean below or toward the feet, as in "The mouth is inferior to the nose." **Anterior** is a directional term that relates to the front of the body. An example of the use of *anterior* would be, "The rash covered the entire anterior of the left thigh." **Ventral**, usually used in veterinary anatomy, pertains to the front (anterior) or undersurface of an animal. **Posterior** specifies the back or toward the back of the body. **Dorsal**, generally used in veterinary anatomy, pertains to the back (posterior) or upper surface of an animal. **Medial** means toward the midline of the body, and **lateral** means away from the body's midline or toward the side. You may see the adjective *lateral* used for descriptive purposes as in, "The tumor is located on the lateral wall of the left lung." The final two directional terms are *proximal* and *distal*. **Proximal** refers to something nearer to the body trunk or point of attachment to the body: The shoulder is *proximal* to the elbow. **Distal** means further from the body trunk or point of attachment: The wrist is *distal* to the shoulder and the elbow. See Figure 3-4 for an illustration showing directional terms.

Two terms are used for placing patients in a lying down position. Both are common English words that have been adopted by medical terminology. The two terms are *supine* and *prone*. **Supine** refers to a position in which the patient is lying face up. (It means the same thing in plain English, but it can also mean lazy or simply reluctant to act.) Noticing that the word "up" is included in the first syllable of the word "supine" will help you remember its meaning of "face up" in medical terms.

**Prone** is the opposite of supine and means that the patient is lying face down. Prone, too, means the same thing in plain English with another meaning: "tending toward," as in "Smith is prone to making poor choices." Both supine and prone are frequently used in the operating room and in X-ray reports. For example, "The patient was placed in the supine position." This means that the patient was placed on the operating table on his or her back, lying face up. See Table 3-2 for body position and direction terms.



## Quick Check

**Give a term that has an opposite meaning to the term given.**

1. distal ____________________

2. inferior ____________________

3. anterior ____________________

4. dorsal ____________________

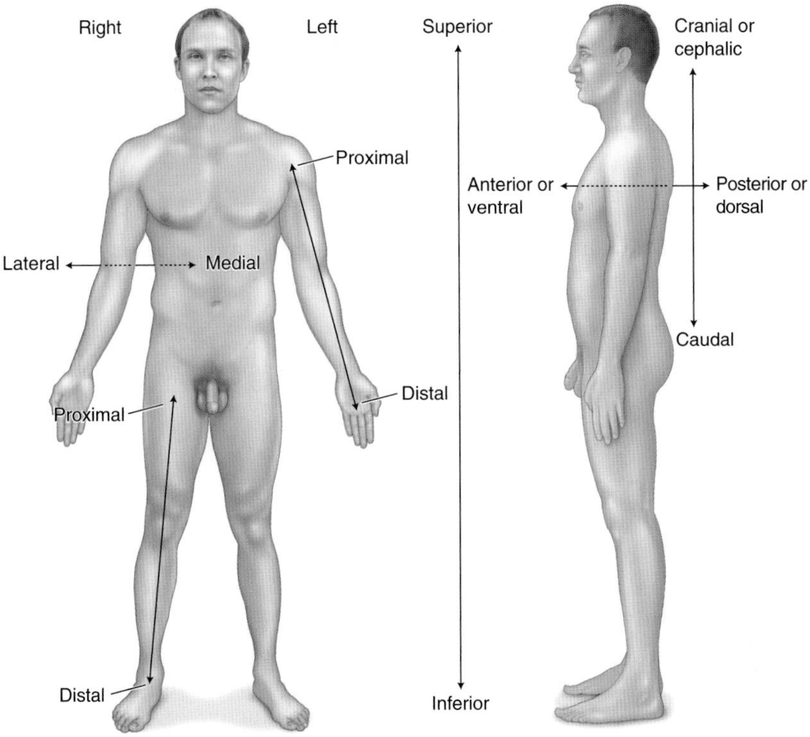


**FIGURE 3-4** Directional terms describe the body part in relationship to another.

**TABLE 3-2 BODY POSITION AND DIRECTIONAL TERMS**

| Term | Direction | Example |
|---|---|---|
| anterior | toward the front | The eyes are on the anterior surface of the face. |
| ventral | toward the belly or undersurface | The nipples were on the ventral body surface. |
| posterior | toward the back | The spine is on the posterior side of the body. |
| dorsal | toward the back or upper surface | The vertebrae are on the dorsal surface. |
| superior | above; toward the head | The neck is superior to the chest. |
| cranial | relating to the head | The brain is in the cranial cavity. |
| cephalic | relating to the head | The neck is cephalic to the hips. |
| inferior | below; toward the soles of the feet | The knee is inferior to the hip; the stomach is inferior to the chest. |
| caudal | pertaining to the tail | The coccyx is caudal to the sacrum. |
| proximal | near the point of attachment to the trunk | The elbow is proximal to the wrist. |
| distal | farther from the point of attachment to the trunk | The fingers are distal to the wrist. |
| lateral | pertaining to the side; away from the middle | The eyes are lateral to the nose. |
| medial | toward the middle of the body | The nose is medial to the eyes. |
| prone | lying flat and face downward | The patient was placed on the operating table in a prone position. |
| supine | lying flat and face upward | The patient was placed on the operating table in a supine position. |

## Body Planes

Body planes are imaginary surfaces within the body (see Figure 3-5). The anatomic position is always their reference point. Three planes are frequently used to locate structural arrangements.

- **Frontal (coronal)**: The frontal (coronal) plane separates the front (anterior) of the body from the back (posterior).
- **Sagittal**: The sagittal plane is any vertical plane that divides the body or organ into unequal left and right sides.
- **Transverse (horizontal)**: This transverse (horizontal) plane separates the body into upper (superior) and lower (inferior) planes, cutting "across" the body.

Aren't some of these terms just plain English? Yes. Alert readers will have noticed that at least some of the adjectives identifying body planes are also present in contexts outside of medicine.

# BODY CAVITIES AND DIVISIONS

A body cavity is defined as a hollow space that contains body organs. The body has several major cavities, including the cranial, spinal, thoracic, and abdominopelvic. The **cranial cavity** houses the brain, and the **spinal cavity** houses the spinal cord.

The **thoracic cavity** contains the lungs, whereas the **abdominopelvic cavity** contains digestive and reproductive organs. The abdominopelvic cavity is divided into a superior **abdominal cavity** and an inferior **pelvic cavity**. The diaphragm is the muscle of breathing known and it physically divides the thoracic and abdominopelvic cavities (see Figure 3-6).

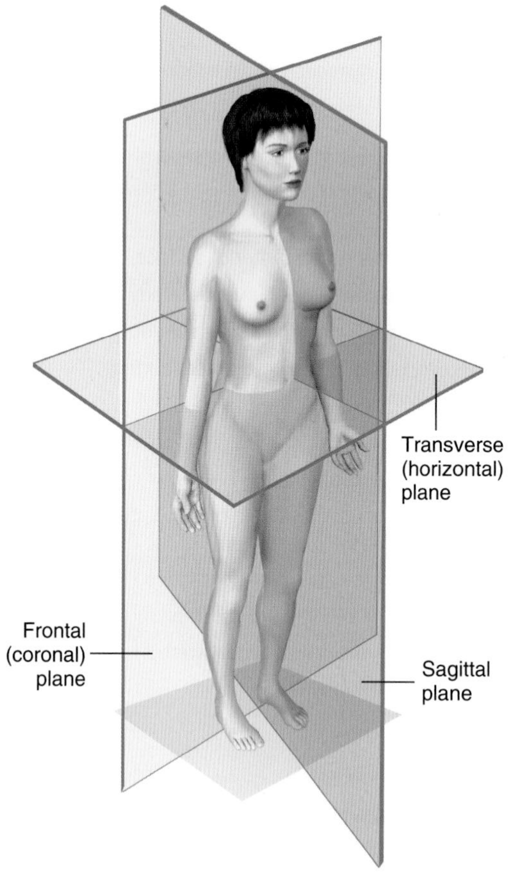


FIGURE 3-5 Body planes divide the body into halves in different ways for reference purposes.

## Divisions of the Abdominopelvic Cavity

A person documenting a physical examination or a surgical procedure needs to describe incisions, procedures, and location of organs. In order to do this effectively, the abdominopelvic cavity is divided into two different ways: either nine regions or four quadrants (see Figure 3-7A, B; Tables 3-3 and 3-4).

### *Nine Regions*

Regions are used to describe the location of underlying organs. Note that in the following list, the number in parentheses refers to two sides within the region, a left and a right, and counts as two regions (see Figure 3-7A and Table 3-3). The regions are named as follows:

- Hypochondriac (2): There are right and left hypochondriac regions. *Chondr-* means "cartilage," and you will recall that the prefix *hypo-* means "below." Hence, these areas are below the cartilage of the ribs on the left and right sides.

- Epigastric: This area is just superior to the stomach. *Epi-* is a prefix that means "beside" or "upon." This area is above the stomach and is situated between the left and right hypochondriac regions.
- Lumbar (2): There are right and left lumbar regions. They are located at waist level on either side of the navel.
- Umbilical: If you look at the nine regions as a tic-tac-toe chart, the umbilical region is the middle section. It contains the umbilicus (navel).
- Hypogastric: This is the bottom square in the middle column of the tic-tac-toe chart, just inferior to the umbilical section.
- Inguinal (2): There are right and left inguinal regions. They lie on either side of the hypogastric section. Inguinal also refers to the "groin" area.

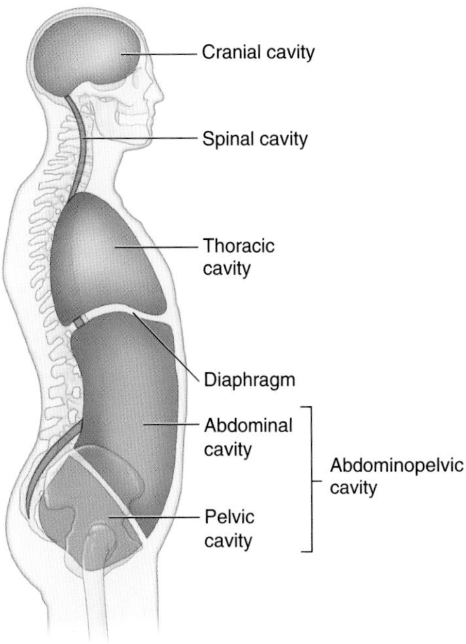


**FIGURE 3-6** The major body cavities shown in lateral view.

Doesn't the word hypochondriac have another definition? Yes, someone with imaginary pains is called a hypochondriac, and the reason for this usage came about because the left side hypochondriac region is roughly where a hypersensitive person might interpret any discomfort as a heart attack.

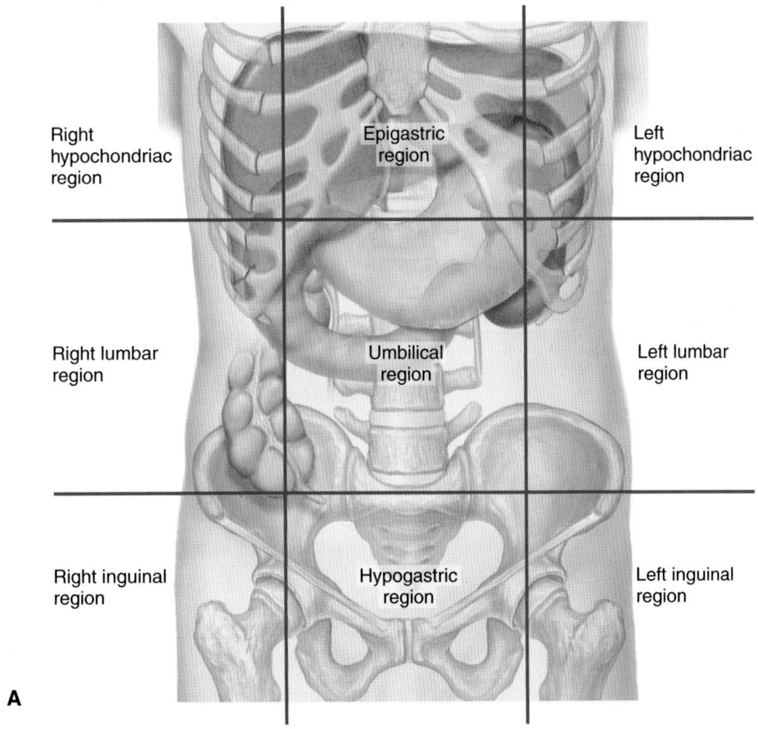


**FIGURE 3-7** Abdominopelvic cavity. **A.** The nine regions of the abdominopelvic cavity.

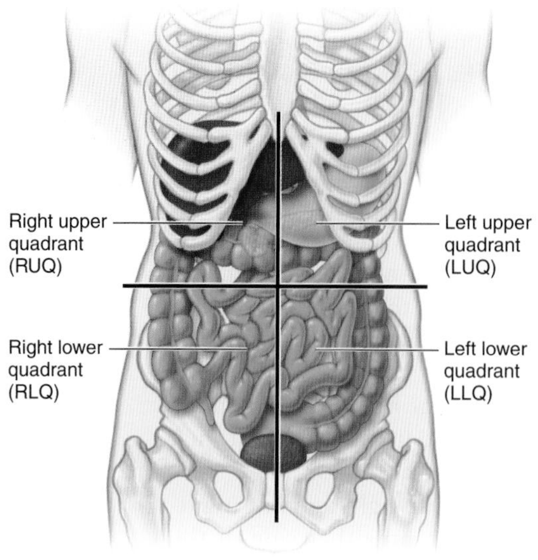


**FIGURE 3-7** **B.** The four quadrants of the abdominopelvic cavity. (*continued*)

### *Four Quadrants*

Four quadrants identify the abdomen (see Figure 3-7B and Table 3-4). The center point is the navel. The quadrants are abbreviated as follows: right upper quadrant (RUQ), left upper quadrant (LUQ), right lower quadrant (RLQ), and left lower quadrant (LLQ).

## Regions of the Spinal Column

The spinal column is a series of vertebrae that extend from the head to the coccyx. The five regions include the cervical (C), thoracic (T), lumbar (L), sacral (S), and coccyx (Co). They are labeled with a capital letter that corresponds to the name of the region (see Figure 3-8; Table 3-5).

The terms for each region describe a part of the back. The cervical section describes the cervix (meaning neck). The thoracic section describes the thorax (meaning chest), the lumbar section describes the lumbus (meaning loin, or part of the side and back between the ribs and the pelvis), the sacral region describes the sacrum (lower back), and the coccygeal region describes the coccyx (tailbone). It is important to recognize which word is the body part and which word is the adjective describing the region in which that body part is located.



**TABLE 3-3** NINE REGIONS OF THE ABDOMEN

| Region | Description |
|---|---|
| left hypochondriac region | left lateral region just below the ribs |
| left lumbar region | left lateral region in the middle row |
| left inguinal region | left lower region of the lower row by the groin |
| epigastric region | middle region in the upper row |
| umbilicus | middle region in the middle row |
| hypogastric region | middle section in the lower row |
| right hypochondriac region | right lateral region just below the ribs |
| right lumbar region | right lateral region in the middle row |
| right inguinal region | right lower region of the lower row by the groin |

**TABLE 3-4 FOUR QUADRANTS OF THE ABDOMEN**

| Term | Organs in Quadrant |
|---|---|
| right upper quadrant (RUQ) | right lobe of liver, gallbladder, portions of the pancreas, small intestines, and colon |
| left upper quadrant (LUQ) | left lobe of liver, spleen, stomach, portions of the pancreas, small intestines, and colon |
| right lower quadrant (RLQ) | contains portions of small intestine and colon, right ovary and uterine tube, appendix, and right ureter |
| left lower quadrant (LLQ) | contains portions of small intestine and colon, left ovary and uterine tube, and left ureter |

Notice that lumbar is used to describe abdominopelvic regions and is also used to describe a section of the back. The lumbar is "the part of the back and sides between the ribs and the pelvis," so it makes sense that it could be used to describe both of these divisions.

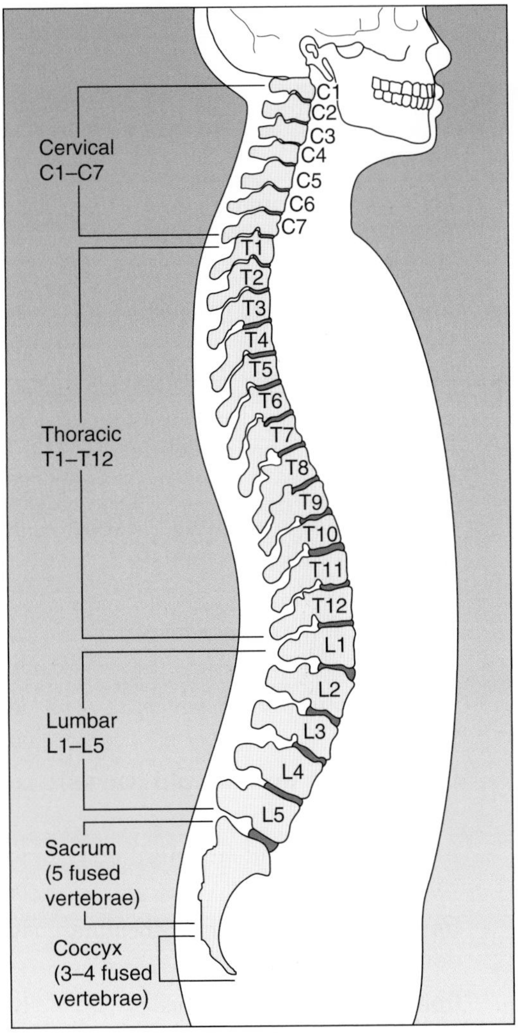


**FIGURE 3-8** The regions of the spinal column show the locations of the vertebrae.

**TABLE 3-5 REGIONS OF THE SPINAL COLUMN**

| Region | Location |
|---|---|
| cervical | neck |
| thoracic | chest |
| lumbar | lower back below waist |
| sacral | lower back |
| coccyx | tailbone |

**Abbreviation Table BODY ORGANIZATION**

| ABBREVIATION | MEANING |
|---|---|
| LLQ | left lower quadrant (of abdomen) |
| LUQ | left upper quadrant (of abdomen) |
| RLQ | right lower quadrant (of abdomen) |
| RUQ | right upper quadrant (of abdomen) |

**Study Table BODY POSITION AND DIRECTIONAL TERMS**

| TERM AND PRONUNCIATION | ANALYSIS | MEANING |
|---|---|---|
| anterior; ventral (an-TEER-ee-er; VEHN-trahl) | Latin word for former; from Latin word *venter* (belly) | toward the front of the body |
| posterior; dorsal (poss-TEE-ree-ohr; dawr-SUHL) | from the Latin word *posterus* (following); from the Latin word *dorsum* (back) | toward the back of the body |
| superior; cephalic (soo-PEER-ee-ohr; se-FAL-ik) | from the Latin word *superus* (above); from the Latin word *cephalicus* (head) | above; toward the head |
| inferior; caudal (ihn-FEER-ee-ohr; KAW-dul) | Latin word for lower; from the Latin word *cauda* (tail of an animal) | below; toward the feet |
| proximal (PROX-ih-mahl) | from the Latin word *proximus* (nearest) | near the point of attachment to the trunk |
| distal (DIS-tahl) | from the Latin word *distantem* (distant) | farther from the point of attachment to the trunk |
| lateral (LAT-eh-rahl) | from the Latin word *lateralis* (lateral) | away from the middle |
| medial (MEE-dee-ahl) | from the Latin word *medialis* (middle) | toward the midline of the body |
| prone (PROWN) | from the Latin word *pronus* (bending down) | lying flat and face down |
| supine (soo-PAHYN) | from the Latin word *supinus* (bending backwards) | lying flat and face up |

**Study Table** BODY CAVITIES AND DIVISIONS

| TERM AND PRONUNCIATION | ANALYSIS | MEANING |
|---|---|---|
| cervical (SUR-vi-kuhl) | from the Latin word *cervix* (neck) | adjective for neck |
| cervix (SUR-viks) | Latin for neck | neck |
| coccygeal (kok-SIJ-ee-uhl) | from the Greek word *kokkyx* (cuckoo) | adjective for tailbone |
| coccyx (KOK-siks) | from the Greek word *kokkyx* (cuckoo) as it resembles the cuckoo's beak | the small bone at the end of the vertebral column; tailbone |
| epigastric (ep-i-GAS-trik) | *epi-* (on); from the Latin *gastricus* (stomach) | area superior to the stomach |
| hypochondriac (hy-poh-KON-dree-ak) | *hypo-* (below); from the Latin *chondriacus* (upper abdomen) | below the ribs; also used as a noun to refer to a person whose illnesses are imaginary |
| hypogastric (hy-poh-GAS-tric) | *hypo-* (below); from the Latin *gastricus* (stomach) | inferior to the stomach |
| inguinal (IN-gwin-uhl) | from the Latin word *inguinalis* (of the groin) | groin |
| lumbar (LUHM-bahr) | from the Latin word *lumbus* (loin) | adjective for lumbus |
| lumbus (LUHM-bus) | Latin for loin | area between the ribs and pelvis |
| sacral (SAY-krahl) | from Latin *os sacrum* (holy bone) | adjective for sacrum |
| sacrum (SAY-krum) | from Latin *os sacrum* (holy bone), as this was often the part of an animal that was offered as a sacrifice | five fused bones of the lower spinal column |
| thoracic (tho-RASS-ik) | from the Latin word *thorax* (breast) | adjective for chest |
| thorax (THOR-ax) | Latin word for breast or chest | chest |
| umbilicus (um-BILL-ih-kuhs) | Latin word for navel or center | navel, belly button |

# END-OF-CHAPTER EXERCISES

## EXERCISE 3-1 MATCHING

**Insert the letter from the right-hand column that matches each numbered item in the left-hand column.**

### A. PLANES OF THE BODY

| | | |
|---|---|---|
| 1. __________ | frontal plane | a. divides the body into upper and lower |
| 2. __________ | sagittal plane | b. divides the body into left and right |
| 3. __________ | transverse plane | c. divides the body into anterior and posterior |

### B. DIRECTIONAL TERMS

| | | |
|---|---|---|
| 1. __________ | superior | a. lying flat and face up |
| 2. __________ | lateral | b. near the point of attachment to the trunk |
| 3. __________ | posterior | c. toward the front; away from the back of the body |
| 4. __________ | medial | d. below; toward the soles of the feet |
| 5. __________ | distal | e. lying flat and face down |
| 6. __________ | prone | f. above; toward the head |
| 7. __________ | supine | g. toward the side; away from the middle |
| 8. __________ | inferior | h. near the back; toward the back of the body |
| 9. __________ | anterior | i. farther from the point of attachment to the trunk |
| 10. __________ | proximal | j. toward the middle of the body |

## EXERCISE 3-2 FILL IN THE BLANK

**Select the correct word from the list to correctly complete the sentence.**

| | | | | |
|---|---|---|---|---|
| anterior | distal | dorsal | inferior | lateral |
| medial | posterior | proximal | superior | ventral |

1. The wrist is ______________ to the elbow.
2. The shoulder is ______________ to the wrist.
3. The lungs are ______________ to the spinal cord.
4. The nose is ______________ to the eyes.

5. The head is __________ to the neck.

6. The ears are __________ to the nose.

7. The shoulder blades are on the __________ side of the body.

8. The chin is __________ to the forehead.

## EXERCISE 3-3 WORD BUILDING

**Add the correct prefix or suffix to the word root to make a new term. Select from the following word parts: *-itis*, *-ic*, *-al*, *hypo-*, *hyper-*, *epi-*, and *trans-*. The first exercise is an example.**

| WORD ROOT | ADD PREFIX OR SUFFIX | MEANING | TERM |
|---|---|---|---|
| 1. gastr/o | *hypo-* <br> *-ic* | below the stomach | *hypogastric* |
| 2. dors/o | __________ | pertaining to the back | __________ |
| 3. chondr/o | __________ | inflammation of the cartilage | __________ |
| 4. thorac/o | __________ | across the chest or thorax | __________ |
| 5. neur/o | __________ | inflammation of a nerve | __________ |
| 6. cardi/o | __________ | pertaining to the region above or upon the heart | __________ |

## EXERCISE 3-4 SHORT ANSWER

**Write the answers to the following questions.**

1. What word describes the position of the ear in relation to the nose? __________

2. What does posterior mean? __________

3. What word describes the position of the elbow in relation to the wrist? __________

4. When the body is in the anatomic position, which direction are the palms of the hands facing? __________

5. What is a synonym for anterior? __________

3 | Organization of the Body

## EXERCISE 3-5 TRUE OR FALSE

**True or False? Circle the correct answer.**

| | | | |
|---|---|---|---|
| 1. | Prone is lying face up. | TRUE | FALSE |
| 2. | The left hypochondriac region is above the left lumbar region. | TRUE | FALSE |
| 3. | The little toe is medial to the big toe. | TRUE | FALSE |
| 4. | The diaphragm is a muscle. | TRUE | FALSE |
| 5. | There are five regions of the spinal column. | TRUE | FALSE |
| 6. | The sacrum is also called the tailbone. | TRUE | FALSE |
| 7. | The sagittal plane divides the body into right and left portions. | TRUE | FALSE |
| 8. | In the anatomic position, the body is horizontal. | TRUE | FALSE |
| 9. | The opposite of lateral is proximal. | TRUE | FALSE |
| 10. | The terms ventral and anterior both mean front. | TRUE | FALSE |

3 | Organization of the Body

# 4 The Integumentary System

## LEARNING OUTCOMES

***Upon completion of this chapter, you should be able to:***

- Name the two main layers of the skin.
- Name the major structures and functions of the integumentary system.
- Pronounce, spell, and define medical terms related to the integumentary system and its disorders.
- Interpret abbreviations associated with the integumentary system.

## INTRODUCTION

The largest organ of the body is the skin, which covers more than 20 square feet on average and weighs about 24 lb. It is the main part of the integumentary system, which also includes hair, nails, sebaceous (oil) glands, and sudoriferous (sweat) glands.

*Integumentum* is Latin for "covering" or "shelter"; thus, the skin, nails, and hair that cover our bodies are called, collectively, the **integumentary system**. The adjective relating to the skin specifically is **cutaneous**.

## WORD PARTS RELATED TO THE INTEGUMENTARY SYSTEM

Word parts related to hair, skin, nails, and color are presented in Table 4-1. It's a good idea to study those word parts, along with the others given in the table, before you go any further. That way, as you go through the text, you can practice deciphering terms using context *and* etymology (study of a word's origin).

**TABLE 4-1 WORD PARTS RELATED TO THE INTEGUMENTARY SYSTEM**

| Word Part | Meaning |
|---|---|
| adip/o | fat |
| cutane/o | skin |
| -cyte, cyt/o | cell |
| derm/o, dermat/o | skin |
| -oma | tumor |
| onych/o | nail |
| pil/o | hair |
| seb/o | sebum (oil; fat) |
| sudor- | sweat |

| WORD PART NAMING A COLOR, POSITION, OR OTHER FEATURE | MEANING |
|---|---|
| albin/o | white |
| cirrh/o | yellow |
| cyan/o | blue |
| epi- | upon |
| erythr/o | red |
| fer/o | to carry |
| ichthy/o | dry, scaly (fishlike) |
| jaund/o | yellow |
| kerat/o | horny tissue or cells |
| melan/o | black |
| myc/o | fungus |
| scler/o | hard |
| sub- | below |
| xanth/o | yellow |
| xer/o | dry |

## Word Parts Exercise

After studying Table 4-1, write the meaning of each of the word parts.

| WORD PART | MEANING |
|---|---|
| 1. dermat/o | 1. ________ |
| 2. myc/o | 2. ________ |
| 3. -cyte, cyt/o | 3. ________ |
| 4. sudor- | 4. ________ |
| 5. erythr/o | 5. ________ |

## Word Parts Exercise *(continued)*

| WORD PART | MEANING |
|---|---|
| 6. xer/o | 6. ______________________ |
| 7. fer/o | 7. ______________________ |
| 8. sub- | 8. ______________________ |
| 9. seb/o | 9. ______________________ |
| 10. epi- | 10. ______________________ |
| 11. albin/o | 11. ______________________ |
| 12. cyan/o | 12. ______________________ |
| 13. ichthy/o | 13. ______________________ |
| 14. cutane/o | 14. ______________________ |
| 15. kerat/o | 15. ______________________ |
| 16. derm/o | 16. ______________________ |
| 17. onych/o | 17. ______________________ |
| 18. melan/o | 18. ______________________ |
| 19. pil/o | 19. ______________________ |
| 20. scler/o | 20. ______________________ |
| 21. cirrh/o, jaund/o, xanth/o | 21. ______________________ |

## STRUCTURE AND FUNCTION

The skin consists of two layers: the **epidermis** and **dermis**. A layer of connective tissue called the **hypodermis** or *subcutaneous layer* lies beneath (deep to) the dermis. Although the hypodermis is not, technically speaking, part of the integumentary system, it is mentioned in this chapter because it connects the dermis to the muscles and tissues beneath it. Also found that deep to the dermis is **adipose** (fat) **tissue** (see Figure 4-1).

The epidermis is the outside layer of skin. It is made up of epithelial tissue, which is also found in other parts of the body covering organs and body cavities. The epidermis protects the body from the outside world, a pretty big job for something only 0.05 mm thick on our eyelids to 1.5 mm thick on the palms of our hands and the soles of our feet. It does not contain blood vessels and is therefore said to be **avascular**, which is also a characteristic of epithelial tissue found elsewhere in the body.

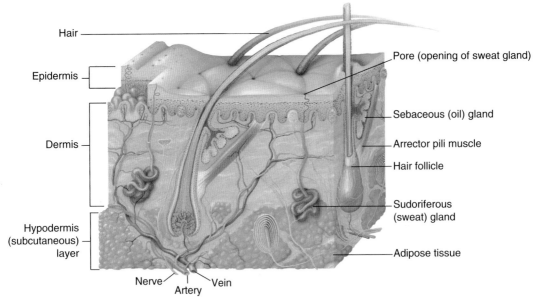

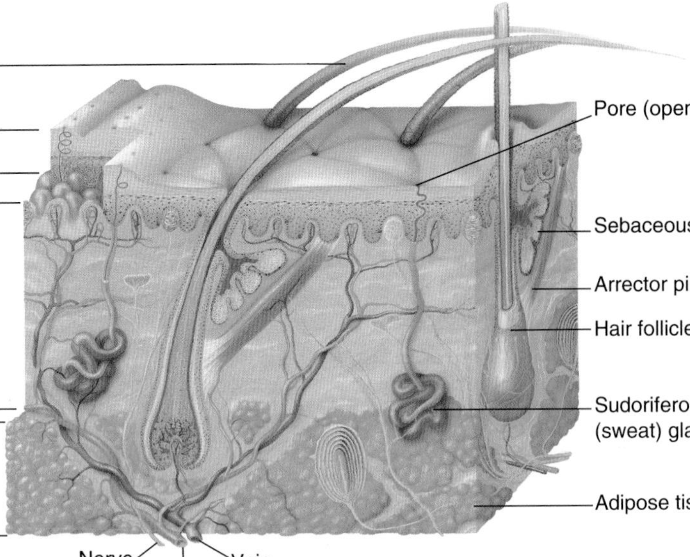


**FIGURE 4-1** The layers of the skin with accessory structures.

## Quick Check

**Fill in the Suffix, and write the resulting word in the Term column. The word that appears in boldface type in the Meaning column is a clue.**

| PREFIX | ROOT | SUFFIX | TERM | MEANING |
|---|---|---|---|---|
| sub- | cutane/o | ________ | ________ | **adjective** meaning "below the skin" |
| no prefix | melan/o | ________ | ________ | a pigment-producing **cell** |
| no prefix | seb/o | ________ | ________ | **adjective** referring to sebum, which may be described as an oil or fat |

Unlike the epidermis, the dermis (sometimes also called the **corium**) contains blood vessels and nerves. So if you get a scratch that hurts and/or bleeds, you will know that you have injured the dermis. The dermis also contains accessory organs, including glands, hair, and nails.

The **sebaceous glands** secrete **sebum**, which is an oily fluid, onto the hair shaft. Sebum moves along the hair shaft toward the surface of the epidermis and lubricates both the skin and hair. The **sudoriferous glands** produce sweat, a watery fluid that evaporates to help cool the body. Sweat reaches the skin surface through an opening called a **pore**. These glands are found over most of the body but are most numerous in the palms of the hands, soles of the feet, forehead, and armpits.

**Hair follicles** produce the hair distributed over much of the body (see Figure 4-1). Hair fibers are composed of a hard protein called **keratin**. Bundles of smooth muscle fibers known as **arrector pili muscles**, pull the hairs erect, causing "goose bumps." Like skin, hair color is determined by the pigment **melanin**, which is a brown–black pigment produced from special cells called **melanocytes**. These melanocytes surround the hair shaft. When a small quantity of melanin is present, the hair color will be light or blonde, and as the quantity of melanin increases, the hair darkens. Gray hair occurs as melanin production decreases with age. In addition to providing color, melanin also protects the skin against ultraviolet (UV) radiation or sunlight.

Like hair, **nails** are also composed of the protein keratin. The **free edge** is the portion of the nail that grows beyond the tips of the fingers or toes. The **lunula** (a Latin word meaning "little moon") is the whitish crescent region of the nail. The **cuticle** is the thin band of tissue that seals the nail to the skin (see Figure 4-2).

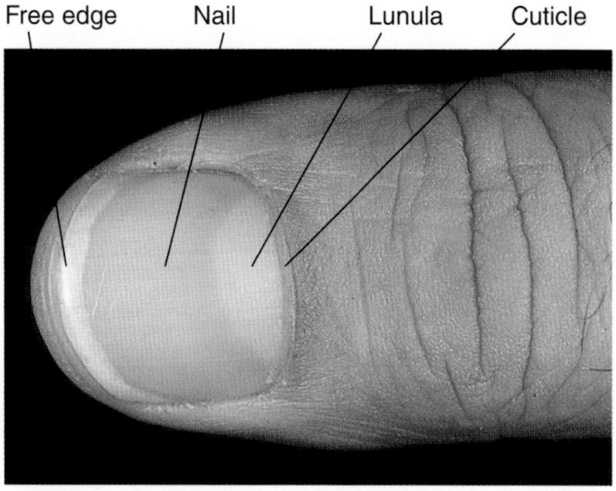


**FIGURE 4-2** Surface view of a nail.

## DISORDERS RELATED TO THE INTEGUMENTARY SYSTEM

Because the skin is visible in its entirety, diagnosing some of its abnormalities is relatively uncomplicated. Moreover, the skin can sometimes provide clues to underlying bodily disorders, which may be signaled by changes in color, by the development of **lesions** (a vague term meaning a wounds or injuries), or by the appearance of other skin rashes.

### Burns

A burn is an injury to the skin caused by heat from any source. The severity of a burn is classified by the depth of the layers of skin involved (see Table 4-2). The body surface area (BSA) is used to express the extent of skin damage.

### Skin Lesions

A lesion may have many different causes and appearances. They may be flat, elevated, or depressed, and each variation has its own medical term (see Figure 4-3).

**Flat lesions:**
- **Macule:** Flat, colored spot <1 cm in diameter. A freckle is an example
- **Plaque:** Flat or lightly raised lesion more than 1 cm in diameter

**Elevated lesions:**
- **Bulla:** Raised, fluid-filled lesion or blister >1 cm in diameter
- **Nodule:** Solid, raised lesion larger than a papule, 0.6 to 2 cm in diameter
- **Papule:** Small, circular, solid elevation of the skin <1 cm in diameter. Warts and pimples are examples
- **Pustule:** Small, circular, pus-filled elevation of the skin, usually <1 cm in diameter
- **Vesicle:** Small, circular, fluid-filled elevation of the skin <1 cm in diameter
- **Wheal:** Smooth, rounded, slightly raised area often associated with itching

**Depressed lesions:**
- **Fissure:** Crack or break in the skin; a slit of any size
- **Ulcer:** An open sore or crater that extends to the dermis resulting from destruction of the skin

**TABLE 4-2** CLASSIFICATION OF BURNS

| Burn Type | Skin Layers Involved |
|---|---|
| first degree | erythema (redness); superficial damage to epidermis; no blisters |
| second degree | blisters; erythema |
| third degree | charring; damage to the epidermis, dermis, hypodermis, muscle, and bone |

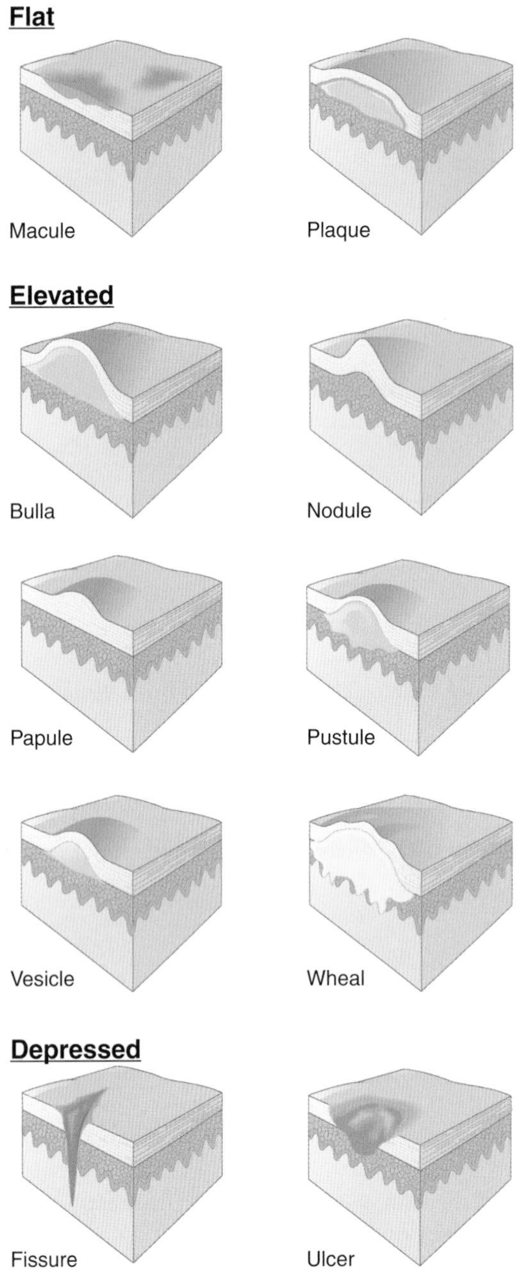


**FIGURE 4-3** Illustrations of some of the more common skin lesions.

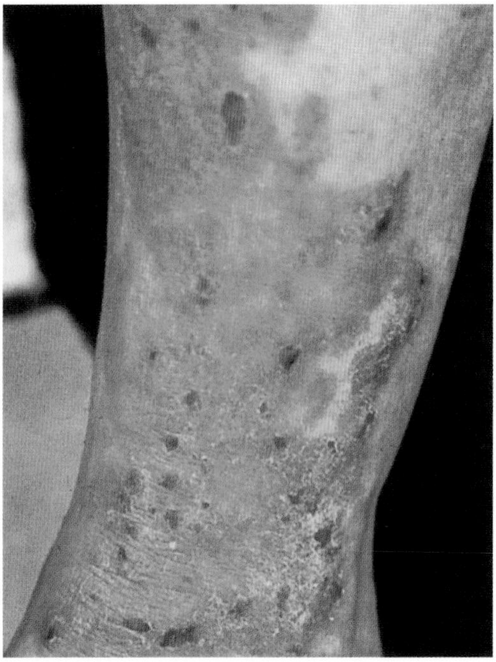

**FIGURE 4-4** Eczema.

## Inflammatory Disorders

Many skin disorders are characterized by inflammation. Inflammation of the skin known as **contact dermatitis** can be caused by exposure to an allergen or by direct contact with a chemical or plant. Poison ivy, for example, may be the diagnosis if the skin is red (**erythematous**), is covered with tiny vesicles, and is itchy. The word **pruritus** is a synonym for itchy. It comes from the Latin verb *prurio*, which means "to itch." There is no corresponding root, although two other terms come from this same verb. They are **pruritic** (relating to pruritus) and **prurigo** (a chronic skin disease marked by a persistent eruption of papules that itch intensely).

**Eczema** is the generic term for inflammation of the skin (see Figure 4-4). **Psoriasis** is an inherited inflammatory condition of the skin (see Figure 4-5). Neither of these terms is derived from actual roots, although the suffix *-iasis* is a common one that, as you may recall from Chapter 2, means condition. **Scleroderma**, as its etymology indicates, is taut, thick, leather-like skin.

## Skin Cancer

Three types of **malignant** (spreading) skin cancers are *basal cell carcinoma*, *squamous cell carcinoma*, and *malignant melanoma* (see Figure 4-6). The term, *malignant*, comes from the Latin *malignans*,

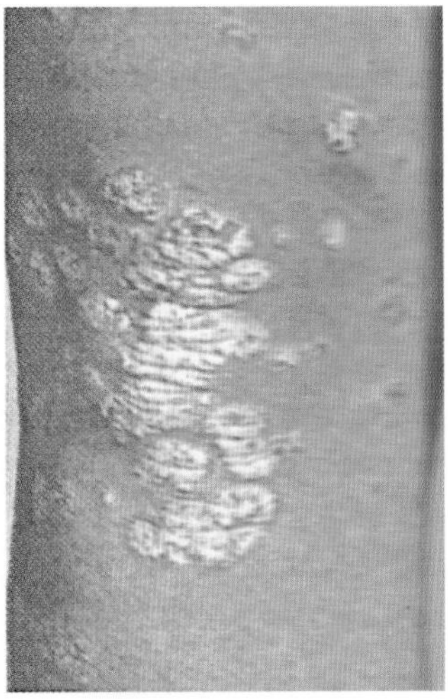

**FIGURE 4-5** Psoriasis.

meaning malicious, and is used to describe an invasive, destructive type of cancer. The suffix *-oma* means tumor. Carcinoma is a cancer derived from epithelial cells and is the most commonly occurring type of cancer. The word carcinoma comes from the Greek words *karkinos* (cancer) and *-oma*. **Malignant melanoma** (also called **melanoma**) is a serious form of skin cancer. Cancer can also be **benign** (nonspreading). *Benign* comes from the Latin *benignus* (kind) and means the cancer is nonmalignant.

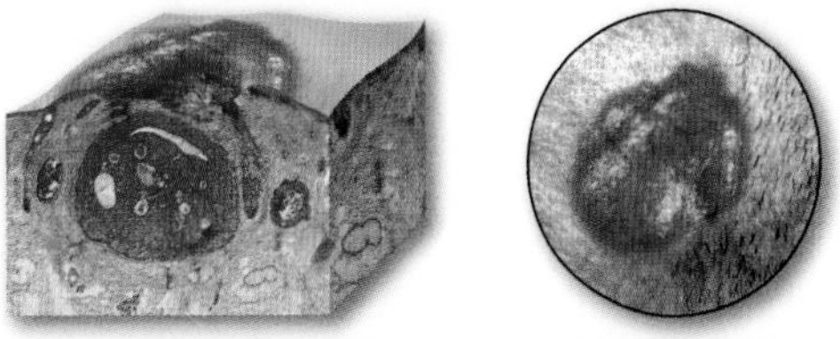

**Basal cell carcinoma**, the most common skin cancer, begins as a papule, enlarges, and develops a central grater. This crater usually only spreads locally.

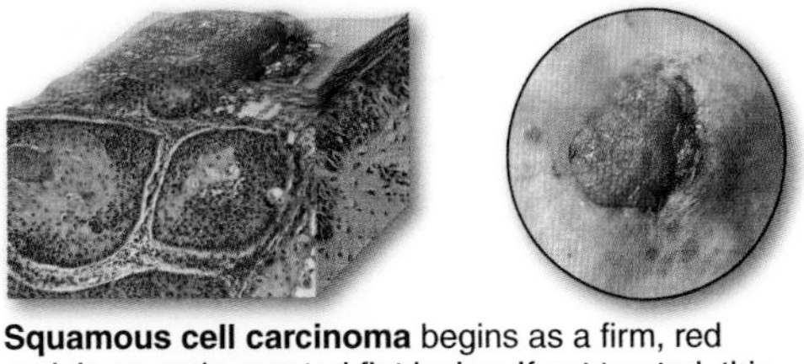

**Squamous cell carcinoma** begins as a firm, red nodule or scaly, crusted flat lesion. If not treated, this cancer can spread.

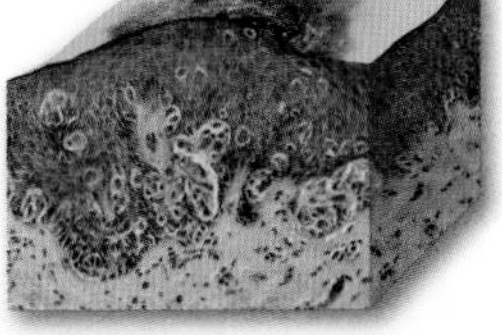

**Malignent melanoma** can arise on normal skin or from an existing mole. If not treated promptly, it can spread downward into other areas of the skin, lymph nodes, or internal organs.

**FIGURE 4-6** Three types of skin cancer.

## Skin Infections

Skin is our protective barrier. When it breaks down, bacteria, viruses, fungi, and parasites have an opportunity to invade our bodies. Many infections, however, can be more annoying than they are serious. The following are examples.

- **Impetigo:** caused by bacteria (*Staphylococcus aureus*) (see Figure 4-7)
- **Scabies:** caused by an egg-laying mite (see Figure 4-8)
- **Tinea:** caused by a fungus (see Figure 4-9)
- **Shingles (herpes zoster):** caused by a virus; symptoms include pain and a vesicular rash that develops along the path of a nerve (see Figure 4-10)

## Other Skin Disorders

Some skin and nail disorders fail to fit previously mentioned categories. They include **decubitus**

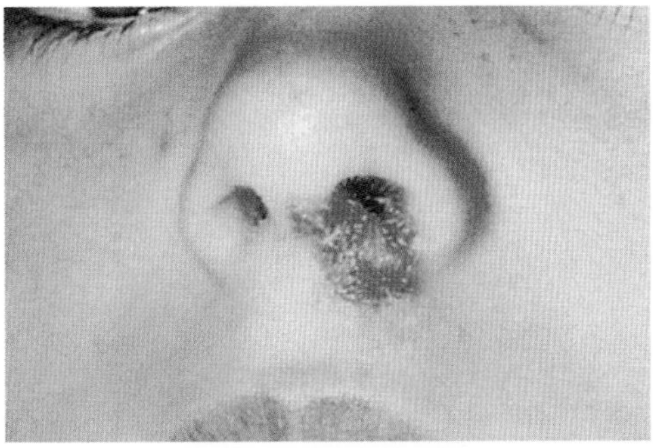

**FIGURE 4-7** Impetigo.

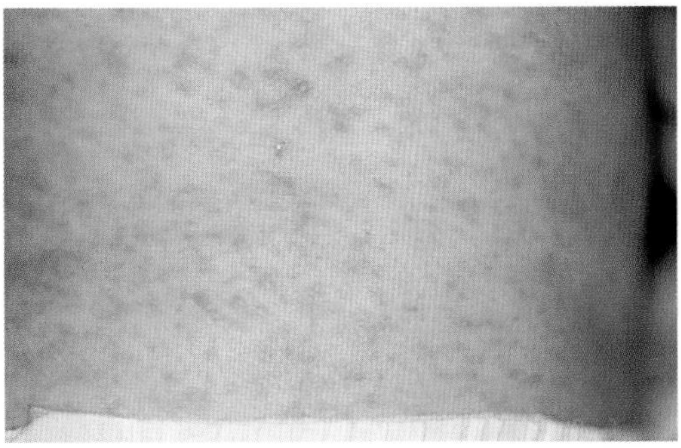

**FIGURE 4-8** Scabies.

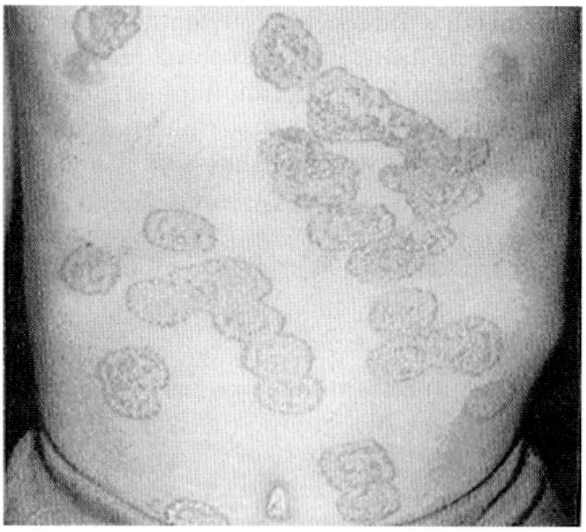

FIGURE 4-9 Tinea (ringworm).

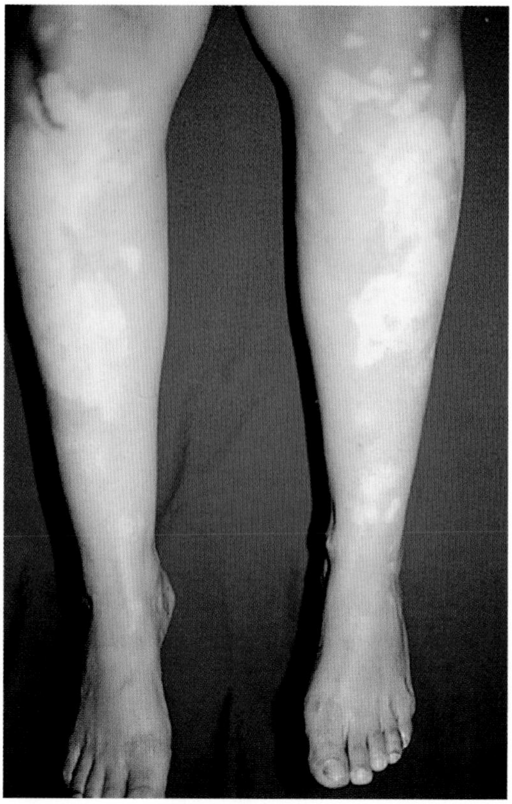

FIGURE 4-11 Vitiligo.

(from a Latin verb that means "to lie down") **ulcers**, also known as *bedsores*; **acne**, a disease of the sebaceous glands common in teens and young adults; **vitiligo**, depigmented blotches or macules that appear on the skin (see Figure 4-11); and **paronychia**, an infection of the skin around the nails (see Figure 4-12).

**Alopecia** is the technical term for baldness. It is not formed from a standard root, although the *-ia* suffix is standard. Other skin conditions include **erythema** (redness) and **ichthyosis** (dryness and scaling of skin that resembles a fish), both of which are formed from standard Greek roots and suffixes. Edema, if you recall from Chapter 2, comes from a Greek word that means *swelling*. It is a standard medical term referring to swelling that occurs anywhere in the body.

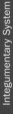

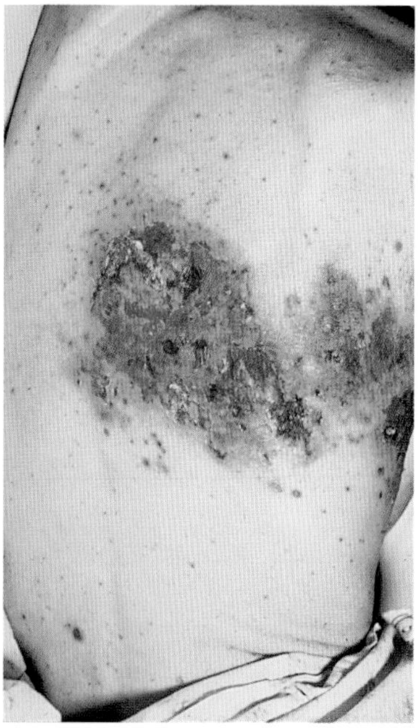

FIGURE 4-10 Shingles (herpes zoster).

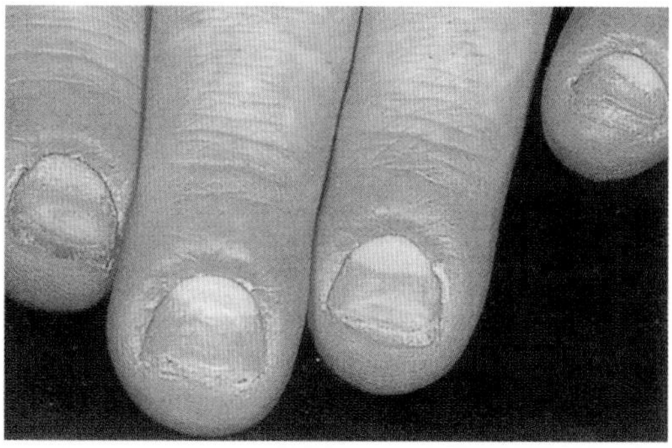

FIGURE 4-12 Paronychia.

## DIAGNOSTIC TESTS, TREATMENTS, AND SURGICAL PROCEDURES

Surgical procedures may be performed on the integumentary system for diagnosis or treatment of abnormal conditions. These procedures may include a **biopsy**, which involves the surgical removal of a small piece of skin for examination, or cryogenic surgery, also called **cryosurgery** or **cryotherapy**. The root *cry/o-* comes from the Greek word *kryos* meaning "cold." In medicine, cryogenic techniques are commonly used to destroy abnormal tissues such as warts, moles, and tumors. Cryogenic surgery often involves the use of liquid nitrogen, which evaporates, or "boils," at −321°F.

In the case of burns and some ulcerated areas, dead tissue prevents new, healthy tissue from growing. In such cases, a surgical procedure known as **debridement** may be used to remove dead tissue. Once again, the standard word parts you learned are absent from this term, which comes from a French adverb meaning "unbridled." That French word describes the purpose of debridement, which is to "unbridle" the body of dead tissue so that new, healthy tissue will be free to replace it.

Nonsurgical treatments include medications applied to the surface of the skin. The term often used to identify this type of treatment is "topical," meaning on top of the skin.

> Doesn't topical mean "relating to a particular topic," such as a topic in the news? Occasionally, the meaning of an English word changes when a segment of the population begins using it to mean something other than its traditional meaning. The word *topical* is such a word. However, its "medical" meaning most likely came first, given that its medical use dates back to the 17th century. Still, dictionaries include the notation *medical* alongside it, probably because English speakers may do a mental double take when encountering its medical use for the first time. Medical terms that fall into this category are identified throughout this book so that, as a medical professional, you will be aware of the possible confusion their use may cause, especially among patients.

Classifications of topical medications are listed as follows:

- **Antibiotics** are used to prevent bacterial infection
- **Antifungals** are used to kill fungi
- **Antipruritics** are used to relieve itching
- **Antiseptics** are used to kill or inhibit bacteria
- **Scabicides** are used to kill scabies mites

Other treatments may include oral or injected medication. An example of an oral medication is a steroid, such as prednisone, which is used to treat many inflammatory skin conditions. Medicines that treat inflammation are called **anti-inflammatory**. Some medications can be given in a **transdermal** manner, which is a method of administering medication through unbroken skin by a patch or ointment.

Surgical options include **dermatoplasty** (plastic surgery repair for the skin), and **incision and drainage** (**I&D**) that involves cutting a wound open and allowing it to drain.

Nail treatments include **onychectomy**, the surgical removal of a nail, and **onychotomy**, an incision into a nail.

> An antipruritic is used to relieve itching. Another medication that is easily confused with this is an antipyretic, which is used to reduce fever. Antipruritic and antipyretic are easy to mix up, but have very different purposes.

## PRACTICE AND PRACTITIONERS

The physician who specializes in the diagnosis and treatment of skin disorders is called a **dermatologist** (dermato + log + ist). The study of the skin and its related conditions is called **dermatology** (dermato + logy).

## Abbreviation Table THE INTEGUMENTARY SYSTEM

| ABBREVIATION | MEANING |
|---|---|
| BSA | body surface area |
| I&D | incision and drainage |
| SLE | systemic lupus erythematosus |
| UV | ultraviolet |

## Study Table THE INTEGUMENTARY SYSTEM

| TERM AND PRONUNCIATION | ANALYSIS | MEANING |
|---|---|---|
| **Structure and Function** | | |
| adipose tissue (AD-ih-pohs TISH-yoo) | from the Latin word *adeps* (fat) | fatty tissue |
| arrector pili muscles (uh-REK-tor PYE-lye MUS-elz) | from the Latin meaning "that which raises" + *pilus* (hair) + *musculus* (muscle) | bundles of smooth muscle fibers attached to hair follicles that cause the hairs to stand on end causing characteristic "goose bumps" |
| avascular (ay-VAS-kyuh-lahr) | *a-* (without); from the Latin word *vasculum* (small vessel) | without blood vessels |
| corium (KO-ree-uhm) | Latin for skin | synonym for dermis |
| cutaneous (cue-TAYN-ee-uhs) | from the Latin word *cutis* (skin) | adjective referring to the skin |
| cuticle (CUE-tih-kuhl) | from the Latin word *cutis* (skin) | the thin band of tissue that seals the nail to the skin |
| dermis (DUR-mis) | from the Greek word *derma* (skin) | inner layer of skin |
| epidermis (ep-ih-DUR-mis) | *epi-* (upon); *dermis* (skin) | outer layer of the skin |
| free edge (FREE EJ) | from German *frei* (free) | distal region at which the nail ends |
| hair follicles (HAIR FAWL-ik-uhlz) | from the Latin word *folliculus* (a small sac) | small sacs in the skin from which hair grows |
| hypodermis (high-poh-DER-mis) | from the Greek word *hypo* (under); *dermis* (skin) | layer immediately beneath the epidermis; also called the subcutaneous layer |
| integumentary system (in-teg-yoo-MEN-tuh-ree SIS-tem) | from the Latin word *integumentum* (a covering) | the membrane covering the body, including the epidermis, dermis, hair, nails, and glands |
| keratin (KERR-uh-tin) | from the Greek word *keras* (horn) | protein that forms hair, nails, and the tough outer layer of skin |

**Study Table** THE INTEGUMENTARY SYSTEM *(continued)*

| TERM AND PRONUNCIATION | ANALYSIS | MEANING |
|---|---|---|
| lunula (LOO-new-luh) | from the Latin word *luna* (moon) | white, crescent-shaped area of a nail |
| melanin (MEL-uh-nihn) | from the Greek word *melas* (black) | dark pigment present in skin and other parts of the body |
| melanocytes (muh-LAN-uh-sites) | from the Greek word *melas* (black); *-cyte* (cell) | cells that produce melanin |
| nail (NAILS) | from Old English *naegel* (nail) | translucent plates covering the distal ends of the fingers and toes |
| pore (POR) | from the Greek word *poros* passageway) | an opening |
| sebaceous glands (se-BAY-shus GLANDZ) | from the Latin word *sebum* (tallow and by extension, grease, oil, fat) | oil-producing glands |
| sebum (SEE-bum) | Latin for tallow or grease | oily secretion |
| subcutaneous (sub-ku-TAY-nee-us) | *sub-* (beneath); *cutane* (skin); *-ous* (adjective suffix) | beneath the skin |
| sudoriferous glands (soo-doe-RIFF-uh-russ GLANDZ) | from two Latin words: *sudor* (sweat) and *fero* (to carry) | sweat-producing glands |
| **Disorders** | | |
| abscess (AB-sehs) | from the Latin word *abscessus* (a going away) | localized collection of pus in any body part; frequently associated with swelling and inflammation |
| acne (ak-nee) | from modern Latin from Greek *aknas*, a misreading of *akmas* (highest point or peak) | inflammatory papular and pustular eruption of the skin |
| albinism (al-BY-nih-zum) | from the Latin word *albus* (white) and *-ism* (condition) | partial or total absence of pigment of the skin, hair, and eyes |
| alopecia (al-oh-PEE-shee-uh) | from the Greek word *alopekia* (literally, fox mange) | partial or complete loss of hair; baldness |
| benign (buh-NINE) | from the Latin word *benignus* (kind) | nonmalignant type of tumor |
| bulla (BUHL-uh) | Latin for bubble | raised, fluid-filled lesion >1 cm in diameter |
| carcinoma (kahr-suh-NOH-muh) | from the Greek words *karkinos* (cancer) and *–oma* (tumor) | malignant neoplasm derived from epithelial cells |

*(continued)*

**Study Table** THE INTEGUMENTARY SYSTEM (*continued*)

| TERM AND PRONUNCIATION | ANALYSIS | MEANING |
|---|---|---|
| comedo (KOM-eh-do) | Latin for glutton | blackhead; dilated hair follicle filled with bacteria; primary lesion in acne |
| contact dermatitis (KON-takt dur-muh-TY-tiss) | *dermat/o* (skin); *-itis* (inflammation) | inflammation of the skin |
| cyanosis (SY-uh-no-siss) | *cyan/o* (blue); *-osis* (abnormal condition) | abnormal condition signaled by bluish discoloration of tissue |
| cyst (sist) | from the Greek word *kystis* (bladder) | closed sac or pouch in or under the skin that contains fluid or solid material |
| decubitus ulcers (dih-KYOO-bi-tuhs UHL-serz) | from the Latin word *decumbere* (to lie down); from the Latin word *ulcus* (sore) | chronic ulcers that appear in pressure areas over a bony prominence in immobilized patients |
| dermatomycosis (DUR-matt-oh-MI-ko-sis) | *dermat/o* (skin); *myc/o* (fungus); *-osis* (abnormal condition) | fungal infection of the skin |
| diaphoresis (dy-ah-for-EE-sis) | Greek for perspiration | synonym for perspiration |
| ecchymosis (ek-ee-MOH-sis) | *ec-* (out); from *chymos* (Greek word for juice); *-osis* (abnormal condition) | a purple patch more than 3 mm in diameter caused by blood under the skin; see also petechiae |
| eczema (EK-zee-ma) | from the Greek word *eczeo* (boil over) | inflammatory condition of the skin characterized by erythema (redness), vesicles, and crusting with scales |
| epidermitis (epp-ih-dur-MY-tiss) | *epi-* (upon); *-dermis* (skin); *-itis* (inflammation) | inflammation of the epidermis |
| erythema (ehr-ih-THEE-ma) | Greek for flush | abnormal redness of the skin |
| erythematous (err-ih-THEE-muh-tus) | from the Greek word *erythema* (flush) | relating to or marked by erythema |
| excoriation (ex-COR-ee-ay-shun) | from the Latin verb *excorio* (to skin) | scratch mark; linear break (caused most often from scratching) in the skin surface |
| fissure (FISH-er) | from the Latin word *fissura* (cleft) | a break in the skin |
| hemangioma (hee-man-jee-OH-ma) | *hem/o* (blood); *angi/o* (vessel); *-oma* (tumor) | benign tumor of blood vessels; birthmark |

**Study Table** THE INTEGUMENTARY SYSTEM (*continued*)

| TERM AND PRONUNCIATION | ANALYSIS | MEANING |
|---|---|---|
| herpes zoster (HER-peez ZAHS-tuhr) | from the Greek word *herpo* (to creep) | viral infection producing the eruption of highly painful vesicles that may follow a nerve path; also called *shingles* |
| hyperhidrosis (hyper-HY-droh-sis) | *hyper-* (above normal); *hidr* (sweat); *-osis* (condition) | profuse sweating; increased or excessive perspiration; may be caused by heat, menopause, or infection |
| ichthyosis (ik-thee-OH-sis) | *ichthy/o* (fishlike); *-osis* (abnormal condition) | abnormally dry skin; scaly; resembling fish skin |
| impetigo (im-peh-TYE-goh) | from the Latin verb *impeto* (attack) | inflammatory skin disease with pustules that rupture and become crusted |
| keloid (KEE-loid) | from the Greek word *kelis* (tumor) and *-oid* (like) | overgrowth of scar tissue |
| lesions (LEE-zhunz) | from the Latin verb *laedo* (to injure) | wound, injury, or pathologic change in body tissue |
| macule (MAK-yul) | from the Latin word *macula* (spot) | flat, discolored area that is flush with the skin; birthmark or freckle |
| malignant (muh-LIG-nuhnt) | from the Latin word *malignans* (malicious) | locally invasive and destructive growth |
| malignant melanoma (muh-LIG-nuhnt (mel-uh-NO-muh) | from the Latin word *malignans* (malicious) + *melan/o* (black); *-oma* (tumor) | tumor of the melanocytes; skin cancer characterized by dark-pigmented, irregular-shaped lesion; another name for *melanoma* |
| melanoma (mel-uh-NO-muh) | *melan/o* (black); *-oma* (tumor) | tumor of the melanocytes; skin cancer characterized by dark-pigmented, irregular-shaped lesion; another name for *malignant melanoma* |
| nevus (NEE-vuhs) | Latin for birthmark | mole; pigmented skin blemish that is usually benign but may become cancerous |
| nodule (NOD-yul) | from the Latin word *nodus* (knot) | a small node or circumscribed swelling |
| onychomalacia (ON-ih-ko-muh-LAY-shee-uh) | *onych/o* (nail); *-malacia* (softening) | softening of the nails |

(*continued*)

**Study Table** THE INTEGUMENTARY SYSTEM (*continued*)

| TERM AND PRONUNCIATION | ANALYSIS | MEANING |
|---|---|---|
| onychopathy (on-ih-KOP-uh-thee) | *onych/o* (nail); *-pathy* (disease) | any disease of the nails |
| papule (pap-yul) | from the Latin word *papula* (pimple) | small, circumscribed solid elevation of the skin |
| paronychia (pahr-oh-NIK-ee-uh) | *para-* (alongside); *onych/o* (nail); *-ia* (condition) | infection around a nail |
| petechiae (peh-TEE-kee-ee) | from the Italian word *petecchia* (small hemorrhagic spots) | tiny hemorrhagic spots on the skin <3 mm in diameter; see also ecchymosis |
| plaque (PLAK) | from the French from the Dutch word *plak* (plate) | flat or slightly raised lesion >1 cm in diameter |
| polyp (PAHL-ip) | from the Latin word *polypus* (a growth on a stem) | a mass of tissue that bulges outward from the skin's surface on a stem or stalk of mucous membrane |
| prurigo (proo-RYE-goh) | from the Latin verb *prurio* (to itch) | a chronic disease of the skin marked by a persistent eruption of papules that itch intensely |
| pruritic (proo-RIT-ik) | from the Latin verb *prurio* (to itch) | relating to pruritus (itching) |
| pruritus (pru-RYE-tis) | from the Latin verb *prurio* (to itch) | itching |
| psoriasis (soh-RYE-ih-sis) | Greek for being itchy | chronic skin disease characterized by itchy, red, silvery-scaled patches |
| pustule (PUST-yul) | from the Latin word *pustula* (pimple) | small (up to 1 cm in diameter) circumscribed elevation of the skin containing pus |
| scabies (SKAY-beez) | from the Latin verb *scabo* (to scratch) | contagious infection caused by a mite |
| scleroderma (sklehr-oh-DER-muh) | *scler/o* (hardness); *-derma* (skin) | chronic disease characterized by thickening and hardening of the skin |
| shingles (SHING-elz) | from the Latin word *cingulum* (girdle) | viral infection producing the eruption of highly painful vesicles that may follow a nerve path; another name for *herpes zoster* |
| systemic lupus erythematosus (SLE) (sis-TEM-ik LOO-pus err-ih-THEE-muh-tus) | from the Latin word *lupus* (wolf) | inflammatory disease characterized by scaly red patches on the skin, especially the face, and affecting connective tissue in organs |

**Study Table** THE INTEGUMENTARY SYSTEM (*continued*)

| TERM AND PRONUNCIATION | ANALYSIS | MEANING |
|---|---|---|
| tinea (TIN-ee-uh) | Latin for worm | any fungal infection of the skin (tinea barbae = beard; tinea capitis = head; tinea pedis = athlete's foot) |
| ulcer (UL-ser) | from the Latin word *ulcus* (a sore) | an open sore or lesion of the skin; a lesion through the skin or a mucous membrane resulting from loss of tissue |
| urticaria (ur-tih-KAR-ee-uh) | from the Latin word *uro* (to burn) | hives; allergic reaction of the skin characterized by eruption of pale red elevated patches |
| verruca (ve-ROO-kuh) | Latin for wart | wart; caused by a virus |
| vesicle (VES-ih-kal) | from the Latin word *vesicula* (blister) | small, fluid-filled, raised lesion; a blister |
| vitiligo (vit-il-EYE-go) | from the Latin word *vitium* (blemish) | localized loss of skin pigmentation characterized by milk-white patches |
| wheal (WHEEL) | from the Old English verb *hwelian* (to form pus) | smooth, rounded, slightly elevated area often associated with itching |
| **Diagnostic Tests, Treatments, and Surgical Procedures** | | |
| antibiotics (an-tee-BYE-ah-tiks) | *anti-* (against); *biotic* (organism) | agents that kill bacteria |
| antifungals (an-tee-FUNG-ulz) | *anti-* (against); *fungal* (fungus) | agents that kill fungi |
| anti-inflammatory (an-tee-ihn-FLAM-ah-tor-ee) | *anti-* (against); *inflammatory* (inflammation) | agent that reduces inflammation |
| antipruritics (an-tee-pryu-RIH-tiks) | *anti-* (against); *pruritic* (itching) | agents that reduce itching |
| antipyretics (an-tee-PYE-reh-tiks) | *anti-* (against); *pyretic* (burning) | agents that reduce fever |
| antiseptic (an-tih-sep-tik) | *anti-* (against); *septic* (poison) | agent that inhibits the growth of infectious agents |
| biopsy (BUY-op-see) | *bi-* (from the Greek combining form of *bio* [life]); *-opsis* (sight) | process of removing tissue for diagnostic examination |
| cryosurgery (kry-oh-SUR-juh-ree) | *cryo-* (cold); surgery (common English word) | an operation using freezing temperature to destroy tissue |
| cryotherapy (kry-oh-THER-uh-pee) | *cryo-* (cold); *therapia* (Latin word for service done to the sick) | the use of cold in the treatment of a disease |

(*continued*)

**Study Table** THE INTEGUMENTARY SYSTEM (*continued*)

| TERM AND PRONUNCIATION | ANALYSIS | MEANING |
|---|---|---|
| debridement (deh-BREED-ment) | *de-* (removal); *bridement* (from the word *bridle*, the part of the riding harness by which a rider controls the horse) | removal of necrotic or dead tissue from a wound or burn |
| dermatoplasty (dur-MAT-oh-plass-tee) | *dermat/o* (skin); *-plasty* (surgical repair) | plastic surgery repair performed on the skin |
| incision and drainage (I&D) | from the Latin *incidere* (cut into) | cutting open of a wound or lesion, such as an abscess, and letting out or draining the contents, such as pus |
| onychectomy (on-ih-KEK-toh-mee) | *onych/o* (nail); *-ectomy* (excision) | surgical removal of a nail |
| onychotomy (on-ih-KOT-oh-mee) | *onych/o* (nail); *-tomy* (incision) | incision into a nail |
| scabicides (SKAY-bih-sides) | *scabies* (see above); *-cide* (destruction) | agents lethal to mites |
| transdermal (trans-DUR-muhl) | *trans-* (across); *derm/o* (skin); *-al* (adjective suffix) | a method of administering medication through the unbroken skin via patch or ointment |
| **Practice and Practitioners** | | |
| dermatologist (dur-MUH-tol-uh-jist) | *dermat/o-* (skin); *-logist* (specialty of) | physician who specializes in dermatology |
| dermatology (dur-MUH-tol-uh-jee) | *dermat/o-* (skin); *-logy* (study of) | study of the skin and diseases of the skin |

## END-OF-CHAPTER EXERCISES

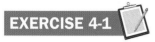

### EXERCISE 4-1 LABELING: SKIN

**Using the following list, choose the correct terms to label the diagram correctly.**

| | | |
|---|---|---|
| adipose tissue | arrector pili muscle | artery |
| dermis | epidermis | hair |
| hair follicle | hypodermis (subcutaneous) layer | nerve |
| pore (opening of sweat gland) | sebaceous (oil) gland | sudoriferous (sweat) gland |
| vein | | |

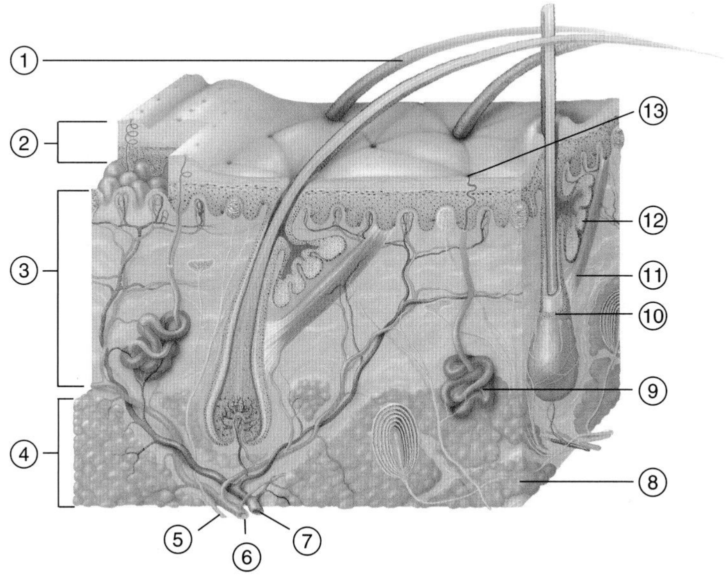


1. ____________________
2. ____________________
3. ____________________
4. ____________________
5. ____________________
6. ____________________
7. ____________________
8. ____________________
9. ____________________
10. ____________________
11. ____________________
12. ____________________
13. ____________________



### EXERCISE 4-2 WORD PARTS

**Break each of the following terms into its word parts: prefix, root, or suffix. Give the meaning of each word part and then define the term.**

**EXAMPLE** transdermal

prefix: trans-, across

root: derm, skin

suffix: al, adjective suffix

definition: a method of administering medication through unbroken skin

1. avascular

   prefix: ______________________________

   root: ______________________________

   definition: ______________________________

2. *epidermis*

   prefix: ______________________________

   root: ______________________________

   definition: ______________________________

3. *melanocyte*

   root: ______________________________

   suffix: ______________________________

   definition: ______________________________

4. *scabicide*

   root: ______________________________

   suffix: ______________________________

   definition: ______________________________

5. *dermatomycosis*

   root: ______________________________

   root: ______________________________

   suffix: ______________________________

   definition: ______________________________

6. *onychectomy*

   root: ______________________________

   suffix: ______________________________

   definition: ______________________________

7. ecchymosis

   prefix: ______________________________

   root: ______________________________

   suffix: ______________________________

   definition: ______________________________

8. antiseptic

   prefix: ______________________________

   root: ______________________________

   definition: ______________________________

## EXERCISE 4-3 WORD BUILDING

**Use the word parts listed to build the terms defined.**

| | | | | |
|---|---|---|---|---|
| dermat/o | -ia | ichthy | -logy | sub- |
| -oma | -plasty | -malacia | -tomy | para- |
| -osis | hem/o | hyper- | -itis | |
| cutaneous | angi/o | hidr | onych/o | |

1. ________________ plastic surgery repair performed on the skin
2. ________________ benign tumor of blood vessels
3. ________________ inflammation of the skin
4. ________________ beneath the skin
5. ________________ incision into a nail
6. ________________ the study of the skin and diseases of the skin
7. ________________ softening of the nails
8. ________________ infection around a nail
9. ________________ dry, scaly, fishlike skin
10. ________________ profuse sweating; increased perspiration

## EXERCISE 4-4 MATCHING

**Match the term with its definition.**

| | | |
|---|---|---|
| 1. __________ | nevus | a. birthmark |
| 2. __________ | verruca | b. thickened scar |
| 3. __________ | macule | c. blackhead |
| 4. __________ | alopecia | d. mole |
| 5. __________ | keloid | e. wart |
| 6. __________ | comedo | f. baldness |
| 7. __________ | diaphoresis | g. profuse sweating; increased perspiration |
| 8. __________ | erythema | h. abrasion of upper skin layers |
| 9. __________ | excoriation | i. flat, discolored spot |
| 10. __________ | hemangioma | j. redness of the skin |
| 11. __________ | cyst | k. localized collection of pus in any part of the body |
| 12. __________ | abcess | l. a closed sac or pouch in or under the skin that contains fluid or solid material |

## EXERCISE 4-5 MULTIPLE CHOICE

**Choose the correct answer for the following multiple-choice questions.**

1. If **myc/o** is the root for fungus, what is the term that means "condition of the nail caused by fungus"?
   a. mycosis
   b. onychomycosis
   c. trichomycosis
   d. onychomalacia

2. If **ichthy** is the root word for dry, fishlike, what is the term for a condition of being extremely dry?
   a. ichthyioma
   b. ichthyosis
   c. ichthyema
   d. ichthiitis

3. The term to describe a lesion of the skin containing pus is
   a. verruca
   b. pustule
   c. bulla
   d. macule

4. A large blister filled with fluid is called a ____________________.
   a. hemangioma
   b. furuncle
   c. cutis
   d. bulla

5. The medical term for natural or abnormal baldness that may be total or partial is ____________________.
   a. dermoplasty
   b. alopecia
   c. urticaria
   d. transdermal

6. The term that best describes the thin band of tissue that seals the nail to the skin is ____________________.
   a. corium
   b. follicle
   c. cuticle
   d. epidermis

7. The term that best describes the cell that produces the pigment that provides color to the skin and hair is ____________________.
   a. keratocyte
   b. melanocyte
   c. erythrocyte
   d. leukocyte

8. Which term describes a fungal infection of the skin?
   a. analgesic
   b. dermatomycosis
   c. dermatitis
   d. abscess

9. A viral infection that produces the eruption of highly painful vesicles that may follow a nerve path is ____________________.
   a. shingles
   b. verruca
   c. herpes zoster
   d. a and c

10. An antipruritic reduces ____________________.
    a. fever
    b. infection
    c. inflammation
    d. itching

11. An antibiotic kills ____________________.
    a. fungi
    b. viruses
    c. scabies
    d. bacteria

12. The term *cyst* comes from the Greek word *kystis* meaning ____________________.
    a. pus
    b. bladder
    c. hill
    d. bump

13. Corium is a synonym for ____________________.
    a. cuticle
    b. dermis
    c. nail
    d. lunula

14. Diaphoresis is a synonym for ____________________.
    a. perspiration
    b. exhalation
    c. excretion
    d. inhalation

15. A macule is a ____________________.
    a. small node
    b. scratch mark
    c. flat, discolored area that is flush with the skin
    d. fluid-containing sac beneath the skin

## EXERCISE 4-6 FILL IN THE BLANK

**Fill in the blank with the correct answer.**

1. A firm scar that forms in the healing of a sore or wound is a(n) ____________________.
2. A ____________________ is a small slit or crack-like lesion.
3. ____________________ is a condition with a bluish discoloration of tissue.
4. A chronic disease characterized by thickening and hardening of the skin is called ____________________.
5. Absence or loss of hair is a condition called ____________________.
6. Partial or complete absence of pigment of the skin, hair, and eyes is termed ____________________.
7. A loss of skin pigmentation with milk-white skin patches is a condition known as ____________________.
8. ____________________, or hives, is an allergic reaction of the skin characterized by pale red eruptions.
9. The removal of a small piece of living tissue for examination under a microscope is called a(n) ____________________.
10. A(n) ____________________ is a mass of tissue that bulges outward and grows on a stem or stalk.

## EXERCISE 4-7 ABBREVIATIONS

**Write out the term for the following abbreviations.**

1. ________________________________ BSA
2. ________________________________ I&D

**Write the abbreviation for the following terms.**

3. ______________ systemic lupus erythematosus
4. ______________ ultraviolet

## EXERCISE 4-8 SPELLING

**Select the correct spelling of the medical term.**

1. ____________________ is the surgical removal of a nail.
   a. Onychectomie
   b. Onichektomy
   c. Onchyectomy
   d. Onychectomy

2. ____________________ plantaris is commonly known as a plantar wart.
   a. Verrooca
   b. Veruca
   c. Verucca
   d. Verruca

3. A ____________________ is a smooth, rounded, slightly elevated area often associated with itching.
   a. wheel
   b. weal
   c. wheal
   d. weel

4. ____________________ is characterized by eruption of pale red elevated patches.
   a. Urticaria
   b. Uticaria
   c. Uticarria
   d. Urtikaria

5. ____________________ is an inflammatory condition of the skin characterized by erythema, vesicles, and crusting with scales.
   a. Excema
   b. Ecksema
   c. Exzema
   d. Eczema

6. The removal of necrotic (dead) tissue from a wound or burn is called ____________________.
   a. debreedment
   b. dibreedment
   c. debridement
   d. dibridement

7. A chronic skin disease characterized by itchy, silvery-scaled patches is ____________________.
   a. soriasis
   b. psoriasis
   c. psorasis
   d. soariasis

8. A ____________________ is a specialist who diagnoses and treats skin diseases.
   a. dermotologist
   b. dermatologyst
   c. dermatolocist
   d. dermatologist

9. The adjective meaning *itchy* is ____________________.
   a. pruritic
   b. puritic
   c. pyretic
   d. pruitic

10. An ____________________ is an abnormal redness of the skin.
   a. erythema
   b. erathema
   c. airethema
   d. erethema

## EXERCISE 4-9 CASE STUDY

**Read the case and write a definition for each underlined term in the appropriate space. Think about some of the statements the dermatologist believes are important enough to include in the report. For example, who diagnosed what? What do pets and children have to do with a diagnosis?**

**CHIEF COMPLAINT:** Rash on the face

**PRESENT ILLNESS:** A 29-year-old white female states that last week she started having some itching on her forehead. She went to the doctor who prescribed erythromycin, an (1) antibiotic. Two days later, the rash covered her entire face. The patient was diagnosed with (2) impetigo and was admitted to the hospital for treatment.

**CONSULTATION:** Dr. Smith, a (3) dermatologist, saw the patient. The chart was reviewed, and the patient was examined. The patient is married and has no children and no pets. She developed (4) dermatitis on her forehead 2 weeks ago that has spread to her entire face. The rash has become more (5) erythematous, and she now has (6) pustules on her forehead, nose, and cheeks. Facial (7) edema persists, and she is almost unable to open her eyes. She has been given additional antibiotics and an (8) antipruritic medication. She developed (9) pruritus on her feet, which was thought to be a reaction to the antibiotic, so the medication was changed to another antibiotic.

**IMPRESSION:** Impetigo; allergic response to erythromycin. Patient responds to change in antibiotic. Continue with current antibiotic regimen and continue to monitor patient. Thank you for allowing me to participate in this interesting case. I will follow patient and provide additional suggestions if warranted.

*Dr. Smith*

| **Term** | **Definition** |
| --- | --- |
| 1. ________________ | ________________________________________ |
| 2. ________________ | ________________________________________ |
| 3. ________________ | ________________________________________ |
| 4. ________________ | ________________________________________ |
| 5. ________________ | ________________________________________ |

6. ______________ ______________________________________________

7. ______________ ______________________________________________

8. ______________ ______________________________________________

9. ______________ ______________________________________________

10. Why did Dr. Smith ask about children and pets? ______________________________

______________________________________________________________________

5

# The Skeletal System

## LEARNING OUTCOMES

***Upon completion of this chapter, you should be able to:***

- Name the major structures and functions of the skeletal system.
- Differentiate between the axial and appendicular skeleton.
- State the medical terms that name the three types of joints.
- Pronounce, spell, and define medical terms related to the skeletal system and its disorders.
- Interpret abbreviations associated with the skeletal system.

## INTRODUCTION

Our skeletons form the basic structures of our bodies, much like the framework of concrete and steel does in a tall building. Buildings constructed in earthquake zones are designed to move and sway so they won't fall down when the earth moves beneath them. We look upon such buildings as marvels of modern engineering, perhaps without giving a thought to the human skeleton, which allows us to walk, run, talk, gesture, throw things, and even draw up plans for tall buildings.

## WORD PARTS RELATED TO THE SKELETAL SYSTEM

Many terms having to do with the skeletal system are made up of the word parts listed in **Table 5-1**. Other word parts you have already learned are also used to make up some terms in this chapter. Prefixes you learned in Chapter 2, such as dia- (through), epi- (outside), endo- (inside), and peri- (around), for example, will be evident in terms introduced under the "Structure and Function" heading. Important word parts to know for this chapter are related to the Greek words, *osteon* for bone and *mys* for muscle. It is also important to know that not every term has a root. The reason is simple: we borrow freely from Greek and Latin, and if you stop to think about that practice, you will realize that every word or word fragment we use is—in a narrow sense at least—a potential root. In other words, prefixes and suffixes can sometimes form the central idea of a term.

Isn't it true that some people have more than 206 bones? The response 206 was deemed correct on a Jeopardy television program, so it must be true! All joking aside, the exact number of bones can vary slightly from one person to another because some people have extra ribs, vertebrae, or sesamoid bones that develop around joints.

| TABLE 5-1 WORD PARTS RELATED TO THE SKELETAL SYSTEM | |
|---|---|
| **Word Part** | **Meaning** |
| -algia | pain |
| amphi- | both sides |
| ankyl/o | stiff, fused, closed |
| arthr/o | joint |
| brachi/o | arm |
| calcane/o | calcaneus, heel bone |
| carp/o | wrist |
| cervic/o | neck |
| chondr/o | cartilage |
| cost/o | rib |
| crani/o | cranium |
| dactyl/o | finger, toe |
| -ectomy | surgical removal |
| electr/o | electricity |
| femur/o | femur, thighbone |
| -gram | written record of |
| humer/o | humerus, upper arm bone |
| -itis | inflammation |
| kinesi/o | movement |
| -kinesia | movement |
| kyph/o | hump |
| -logy | study of |
| lord/o | swayback, curve |
| lumb/o | lower back |
| -malacia | softening |
| muscul/o | muscle |
| my/o | muscle |
| myel/o | bone marrow |
| -oma | tumor |
| orth/o | correct, straight |
| os/te/o | bone |
| ped/o | foot, child |
| pelv/o | pelvis |
| phalang/o | bones of fingers and toes |
| -physis | growth |
| -plasty | surgical repair |
| -porosis | porous |
| -scopy | to visually examine |
| spondyl/o | vertebrae |
| syn- | joined together |
| thorac/o | thorax, chest |
| vertebr/o | vertebrae |
| zygo- | joined (yoked) together |

## Word Parts Exercise

After studying Table 5-1, write the meaning of each of the word parts.

| WORD PART | MEANING |
|---|---|
| 1. lord/o | 1. ________________ |
| 2. zygo- | 2. ________________ |
| 3. carp/o | 3. ________________ |
| 4. ped/o | 4. ________________ |
| 5. os/te/o | 5. ________________ |
| 6. phalang/o | 6. ________________ |
| 7. -algia | 7. ________________ |
| 8. crani/o | 8. ________________ |
| 9. syn- | 9. ________________ |
| 10. -itis | 10. ________________ |
| 11. my/o, muscul/o | 11. ________________ |
| 12. -scopy | 12. ________________ |
| 13. kinesi/o | 13. ________________ |
| 14. orth/o | 14. ________________ |
| 15. femur/o | 15. ________________ |
| 16. -malacia | 16. ________________ |
| 17. -plasty | 17. ________________ |
| 18. arthr/o | 18. ________________ |
| 19. pelv/o | 19. ________________ |
| 20. -physis | 20. ________________ |
| 21. brachi/o | 21. ________________ |
| 22. dactyl/o | 22. ________________ |

## Word Parts Exercise (continued)

| | |
|---|---|
| 23. cost/o | 23. ______________________ |
| 24. myel/o | 24. ______________________ |
| 25. electr/o | 25. ______________________ |
| 26. thorac/o | 26. ______________________ |
| 27. humer/o | 27. ______________________ |
| 28. -porosis | 28. ______________________ |
| 29. ankyl/o | 29. ______________________ |
| 30. spondyl/o, vertebr/o | 30. ______________________ |
| 31. -gram | 31. ______________________ |
| 32. -kinesia | 32. ______________________ |
| 33. amphi- | 33. ______________________ |
| 34. calcane/o | 34. ______________________ |
| 35. kyph/o | 35. ______________________ |
| 36. cervic/o | 36. ______________________ |
| 37. -logy | 37. ______________________ |
| 38. chondr/o | 38. ______________________ |
| 39. lumb/o | 39. ______________________ |
| 40. -ectomy | 40. ______________________ |
| 41. -oma | 41. ______________________ |

## STRUCTURE AND FUNCTION

The human skeleton begins to form about 6 weeks after fertilization and continues to grow and develop until the person is around 25 years old. Its approximately 206 bones have many functions.

The skeleton serves as a rigid but articulating (movable at joints) framework for muscles and other tissues. It also protects our vital organs by forming a shield against jarring and bumps. Its less obvious jobs are to store minerals and to make blood cells.

The skeleton is divided into two parts: the **axial skeleton** and **appendicular skeleton** (see Figure 5-1). The words axial and appendicular are adjective forms of the words axis and appendix. Axis is the Latin word for "axle," but has become a common English word meaning an imaginary straight line, such as the one between the north and south poles of the earth. The axial skeleton has an axis running from the middle of the top of your head to the bottom of your spine. The axial skeleton therefore includes the bones on this axis: the skull, chest, and spinal column.

The appendicular skeleton comprises the arms and legs, along with the shoulder and pelvic bones. Although the appendicular skeleton has nothing to do with the body's "appendix," those two body parts do have a common classic word origin: the Latin word *appendix* refers to something attached to something else. Thus, the appendicular skeleton is attached to the axial skeleton, and the appendix is attached to the large intestine.

The skeletal system depends on *ligaments*, *tendons*, and *joints* to allow for movement. Ligament comes from the Latin word *ligamentum*, meaning "a band" or "banding." **Ligaments** are bands of tissue that connect two bones together. Tendon comes from a different Latin word, the verb *tendere*, which means to stretch, which is what tendons do. **Tendons** attach muscles to bone. The difference between these two connective tissues is that ligaments connect two bones, whereas tendons connect a muscle to a bone. Strictly speaking, of course, these two terms belong to the muscular system, but they are mentioned here because their function is essential to the skeleton.

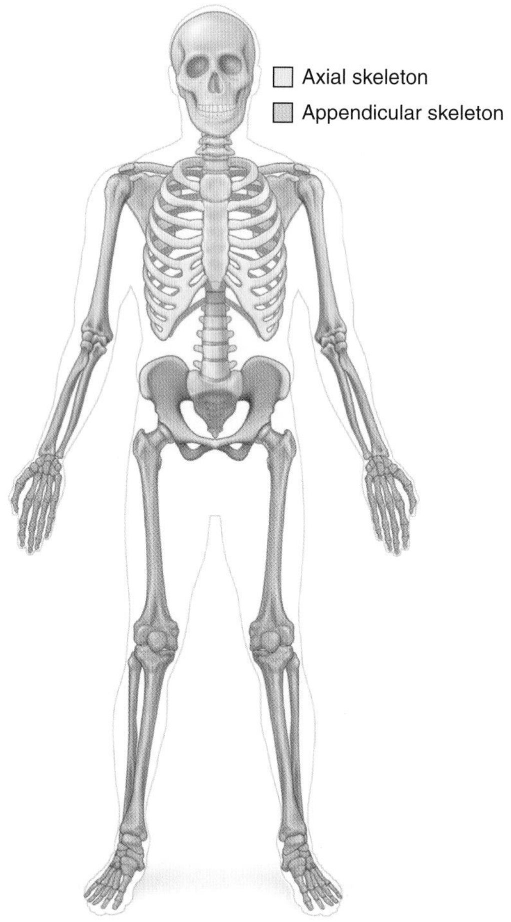


**FIGURE 5-1** Axial and appendicular skeletons. The axial skeleton is shown in yellow, and the appendicular skeleton is shown in gray.

**Joints**, also called *articulations*, are the places where bones come together. They are not separate structures or tissues.

**Ossification** is bone formation and it begins early in fetal development when the skeleton is composed mostly of cartilage. During the second and third months of fetal development, cartilage hardens and turns into bone. Bone is made up of **osseous tissue**, a form of connective tissue with mature bone cells called **osteocytes**.

The bones of the skeleton are of different shapes, sizes, and makeup. They may be essentially flat, such as those found in the cranium and ribs. They may also be short, such as those in the wrist and ankles, or long, such as those found in the arms, legs, hands, and feet.

Long bones have subparts that are named. The term **diaphysis** is the shaft of a long bone, and the term **epiphysis** is the name given to each end of a long bone. The **epiphyseal plate** is the growth area of a long bone. The term for the inside of the diaphysis is **medullary cavity**. Because it is a cavity, it is hollow, and *medullary* means that the cavity contains marrow. *Marrow* is the tissue that produces blood cells.

**Compact bone** is hard, dense bone and makes up the diaphysis. **Spongy bone** is mesh-like bone tissue and is found in the epiphyses.

Most bone surfaces are covered with a membrane called the **periosteum**. The inner surface of the medullary cavity is lined with a thin layer of cells called the **endosteum** (see Figure 5-2).

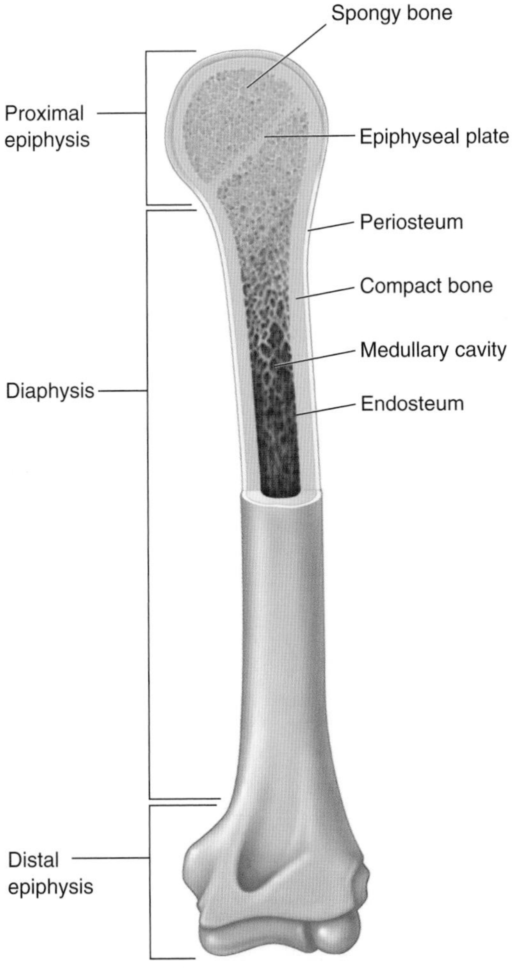


**FIGURE 5-2** Parts of a long bone.

By now, you are probably familiar with the prefixes *peri-* and *endo-*. But if you didn't automatically identify those prefixes, as meaning around and inside, you may benefit from a review of Chapter 2, Table 2-8.

## The Axial Skeleton

The axial skeleton is composed of the bones of the **cranium** (head), thorax, and **vertebral column** (series of vertebrae from the cranium to the coccyx). Cranial bones enclose and protect the brain. The six main cranial bones include the **frontal bone**; two **parietal bones**, one on each side; two **temporal bones**, on the sides of the head; and the **occipital bone** (see Figure 5-3).

The main facial bones are the *nasal bone*, *zygomatic bones*, the *maxilla*, and the *mandible*. The **nasal bone** forms the bridge of the nose, and the two **zygomatic bones** form the cheeks. The **maxilla** is the immovable upper jawbone, and the **mandible** is the movable lower jawbone.

The cranial bones are joined by **cranial sutures**, which are fibrous membranes that join them. These include the *coronal suture*, *squamous suture*, and *lambdoid suture*.

> Isn't *maxilla* Latin for jawbone? Yes. So where does the word mandible come from if we already have a Latin word for jawbone? Mandible comes from the Latin word *mandibula*, which means "to chew," and the mandible moves while chewing.

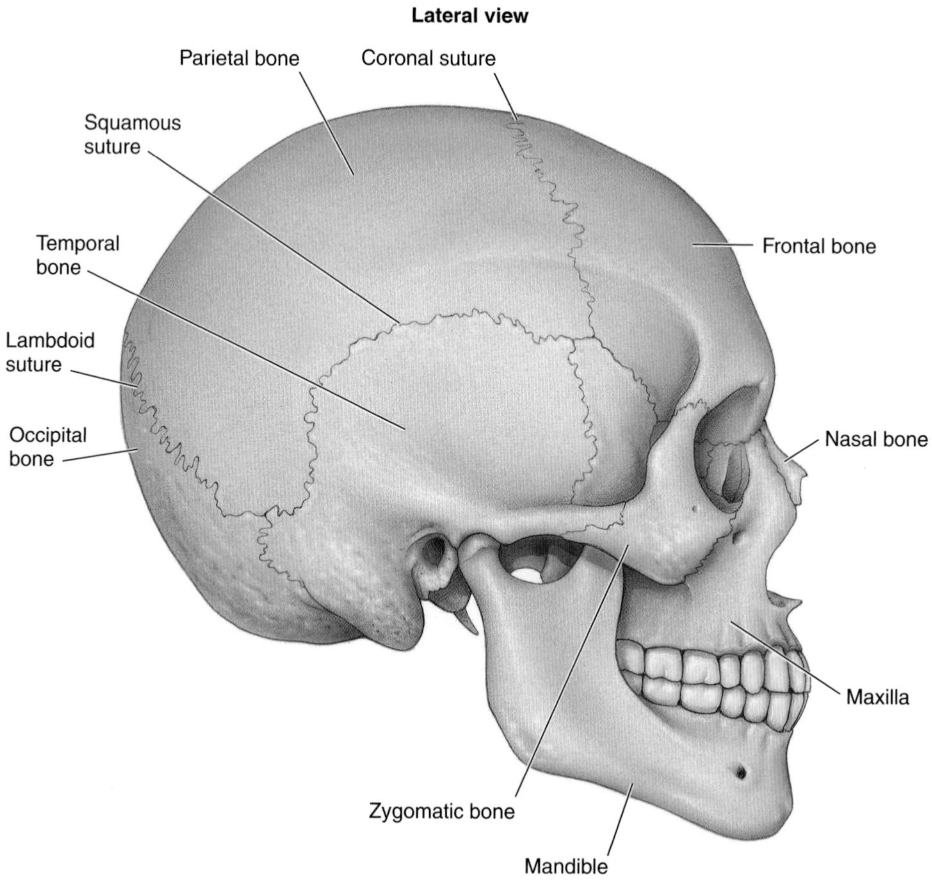


**FIGURE 5-3** The bones of the cranium, face, and the associated sutures.

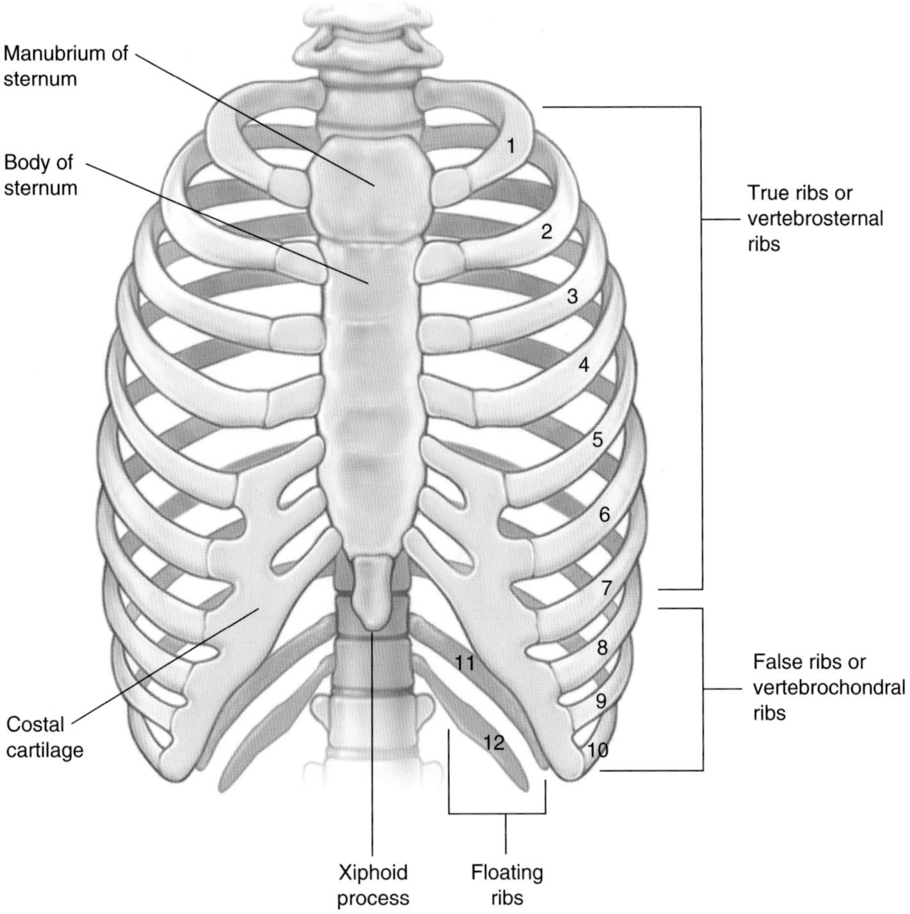


**FIGURE 5-4** The thoracic cage.

The skeleton of the **thorax** (*thorax*, breastplate) is known as the **thoracic cage**. The thoracic cage includes the 12 thoracic vertebrae, 12 ribs, costal (rib) cartilages, and the sternum. Parts of the flat **sternum** are the manubrium, body, and xiphoid process. The major organs inside the thoracic cage are the heart and lungs (see Figure 5-4).

Rib pairs are attached to their correspondingly numbered **vertebrae** (back bones). Ribs 1 to 7 are called *true ribs* or *vertebrosternal ribs* because their cartilages attach directly to the sternum. Ribs 8 to 12 are the five lower ribs that do not attach directly to the sternum. Ribs 8 to 10 are called *false ribs* or *vertebrochondral* ribs. The last two rib pairs (11 and 12) "float," which means that they are attached only to the vertebrae (see Figure 5-4).

The spinal column includes five sections of vertebrae (*vertebra*, singular). The naming of a vertebra consists of a prefix letter (C for cervical, T for thoracic, and L for lumbar), followed by a number indicating the placement on the column. There are 7 cervical vertebrae, 12 thoracic vertebrae, and 5 lumbar vertebrae. At the base of the spinal column are the sacrum and coccyx. The **sacrum** is formed by five fused sacral vertebrae, and the **coccyx** contains three to five fused coccygeal vertebrae (see Figure 5-5).

Isn't the cervix part of the female reproductive system? The word *cervix* is Latin for "neck." The words cervix and cervical refer not only to the "neck" of the uterus, part of the female reproductive system (see Chapter 15), but also to the neck to which the head is attached.

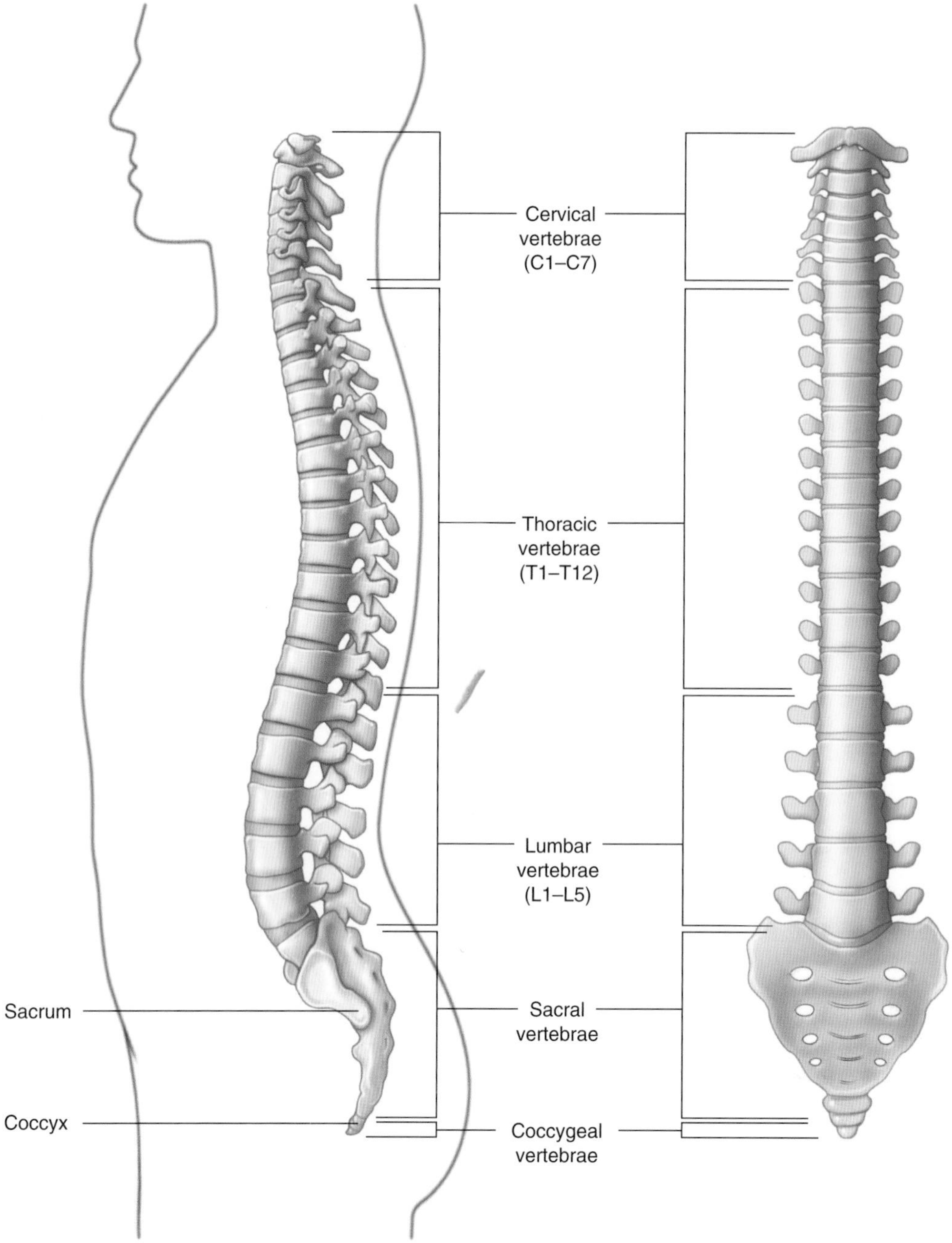


**FIGURE 5-5** The vertebral column in sagittal (anteroposterior) and anterior views.

The sacrum is joined to the hip bones and, therefore, is part of the pelvic girdle, which is part of the appendicular skeleton. Although the sacrum is not part of the axial skeleton, it is mentioned here because of its association with the vertebral column.

## The Appendicular Skeleton

As mentioned previously, the appendicular skeleton consists of the body's appendages (upper limbs and lower limbs) and the areas to which these appendages are attached: the shoulder and pelvic girdles. An upper limb is also called an *upper extremity*, and a lower limb is also called a *lower extremity*. Shoulder bones, although associated with the chest, are part of the appendicular skeleton. The main bones of the *shoulder girdle* are the **clavicle** (collarbone) and the **scapula** (shoulder blade) (see Figure 5-6).

The long arm bone extending from the shoulder and ending at the elbow is called the **humerus**, not because it is the "funny bone" but because *humerus* is the Latin word for "shoulder." However, there is a connection with the word "humorous." The phrase "funny bone" was most probably coined as a joke because the ulnar nerve, which causes the pins-and-needles sensation when it is struck, is located where the humerus joins the elbow (see Figures 5-6 **and** 5-7).

The forearm consists of the **ulna** and **radius**, which extend from the elbow to the wrist (see Figure 5-7). The wrist includes eight bones, arranged in two rows, called **carpal bones** (*karpos*, wrist). These bones are the *scaphoid*, *lunate*, *triquetrum*, *pisiform*, *trapezium*, *trapezoid*, *capitate*, and *hamate*. The five **metacarpals** are the hand bones that lie "beyond" the carpal bones, connecting the wrist to the fingers. The 14 **phalanges** are the bones that make up the fingers. The term *phalanges* is the plural form of *phalanx*, which is Greek for "line of soldiers." The bones of the wrist and hand are shown in Figure 5-8.

The pelvic girdle, so named because it surrounds and protects the pelvic organs, consists of the two hip bones (right and left), joined anteriorly at the pubic symphysis and posteriorly at the sacrum. The **hip bone**, also called the *os coxae*, is a fusion of three bones: the **ilium**, the **ischium**, and the **pubis**.

The **femur**, Latin for "thigh," is a long bone that extends from the hip to the knee, and the **tibia** and **fibula** are long bones that extend from the knee to the ankle. The femur attaches to the hip bone at the *acetabulum* (see Figures 5-9 and 5-10). The tibia, Latin for "shin," is the shin bone or heavy bone of the leg; the fibula, from the Latin word *figibula*, meaning "fastener," does not bear the body's weight, but together with the tibia, it is connected to the **talus** (ankle bone) (see Figure 5-11). The **patella** (kneecap) is a "floating" bone that is imbedded in the tendon of the thigh muscle. It offers protection to the knee joint (see Figure 5-10).

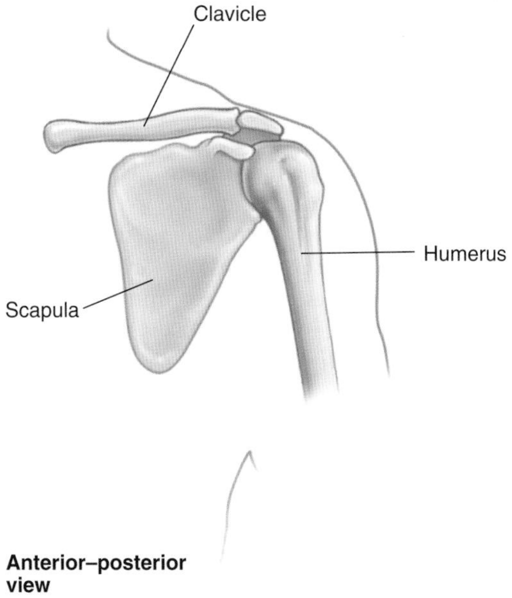


**FIGURE 5-6** The bones of the shoulder girdle show the articulation with the humerus.

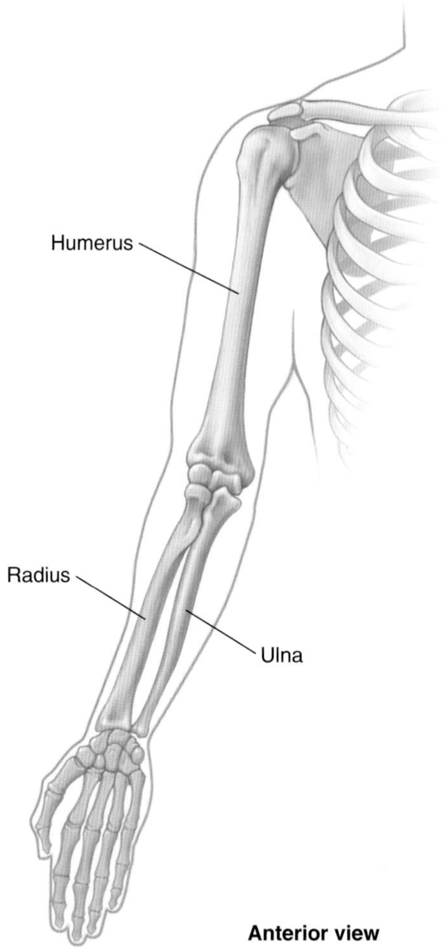


**FIGURE 5-7** Bones of the upper limb. The arm contains the humerus, and the forearm is made up of the radius and ulna.

*Tarsus* (from the Greek *tarsos*, meaning "a flat surface") is sometimes used as a technical name for the ankle. The seven **tarsal bones** of the ankle and the five **metatarsals** of the foot correspond with the carpal bones and metacarpals of the wrist and hand. The tarsal bones are the *talus*; *calcaneus*; *navicular*; *medial*, *lateral*, *and intermediate cuneiforms*; and *cuboid*. Just like the fingers, the bones making up the toes are also called **phalanges**. The bony protrusion at the distal end of the fibula is called the **lateral malleolus**; the bony process on the tibia is the **medial malleolus**. The heel bone, or **calcaneus**, is the largest bone in the foot. Figure 5-11 shows the bones of the ankle and foot.

## Joints

A **joint**, or *articulation*, is the place where bones come together. Some joints, such as the knee and elbow, are highly movable, and some have little or no movement. A joint with no movement is called a **synarthrosis**. Any of the suture joints in the cranium would be a good example of a synarthrosis. A joint with little movement is called an **amphiarthrosis**. The vertebral bodies within the vertebral column are examples of amphiarthroses. A joint that is freely movable is called a **diarthrosis** or a **synovial joint**. Examples of diarthroses are the shoulder, knee, and ankle.

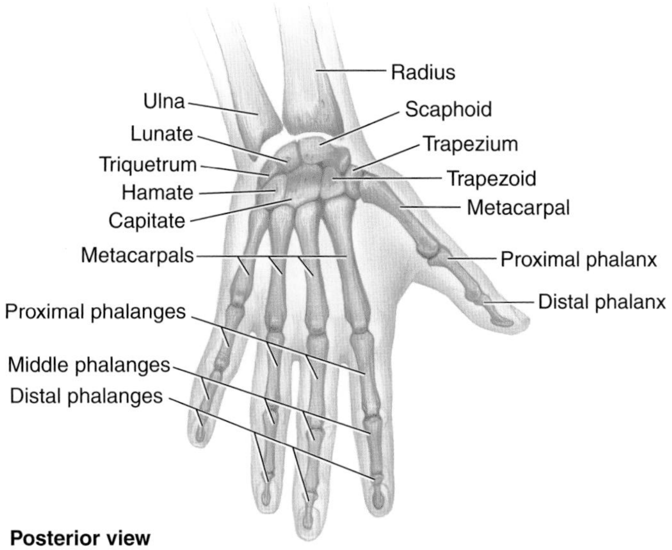


**FIGURE 5-8** Wrist and hand bones. Eight carpal bones form the wrist. Five metacarpals and 14 phalanges form the hand. The pisiform is not visible in this view.

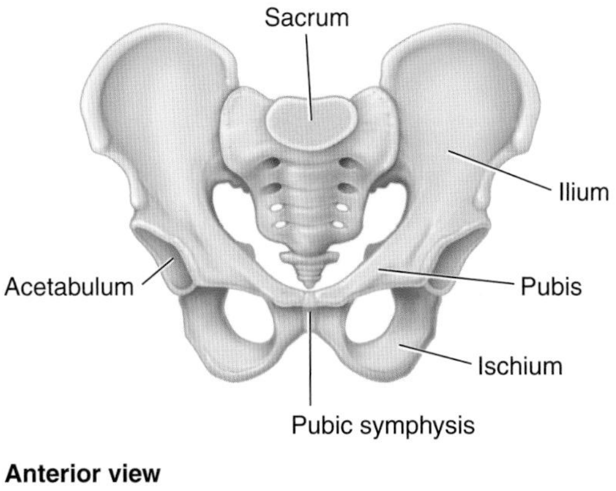


**FIGURE 5-9** The bones of the pelvic girdle.

The spaces within each synovial joint are filled with a viscous liquid called **synovial fluid**. Although the spaces in even a large joint are so tiny that less than 1/100th of an ounce of synovial fluid is needed to fill it, the fluid is needed to lubricate the joint as it moves and to cushion it against shock. Synovial joints permit a variety of movements and are further classified based on *how* they move. The knee and elbow joints, for example, are "hinge joints" that allow *flexion* (decreasing the angle at a joint causing bending of the limb) and *extension* (increasing the angle at a joint causing straightening of the limb). The "ball-and-socket joint" of the shoulder provides the greatest range of motion (ROM) including rotation.

**Cartilage**, a precursor of bone tissue, is classified as connective tissue, but it is mentioned here because cartilage enables movement in the synovial joints.

**Bursae** (*bursa*, singular) are found wherever tendons or ligaments impinge on other tissues. Bursae are spaces within connective tissue filled with synovial fluid.

Figure 5-12 shows the various movements at synovial joints, and Table 5-2 describes their various movements.

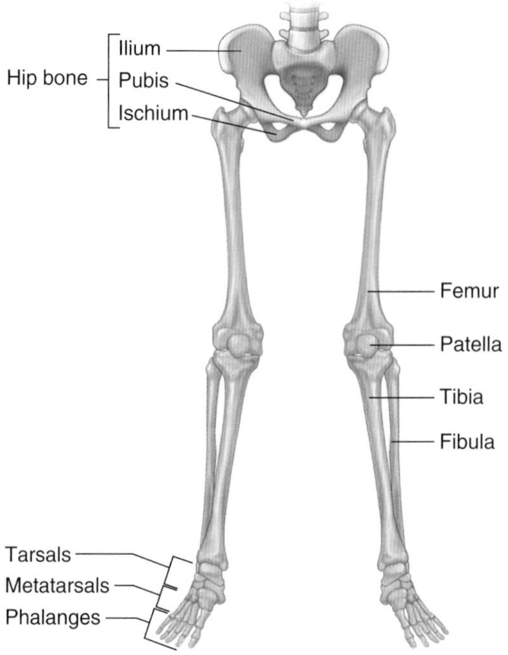


**FIGURE 5-10** Bones of the pelvic girdle and lower limb.

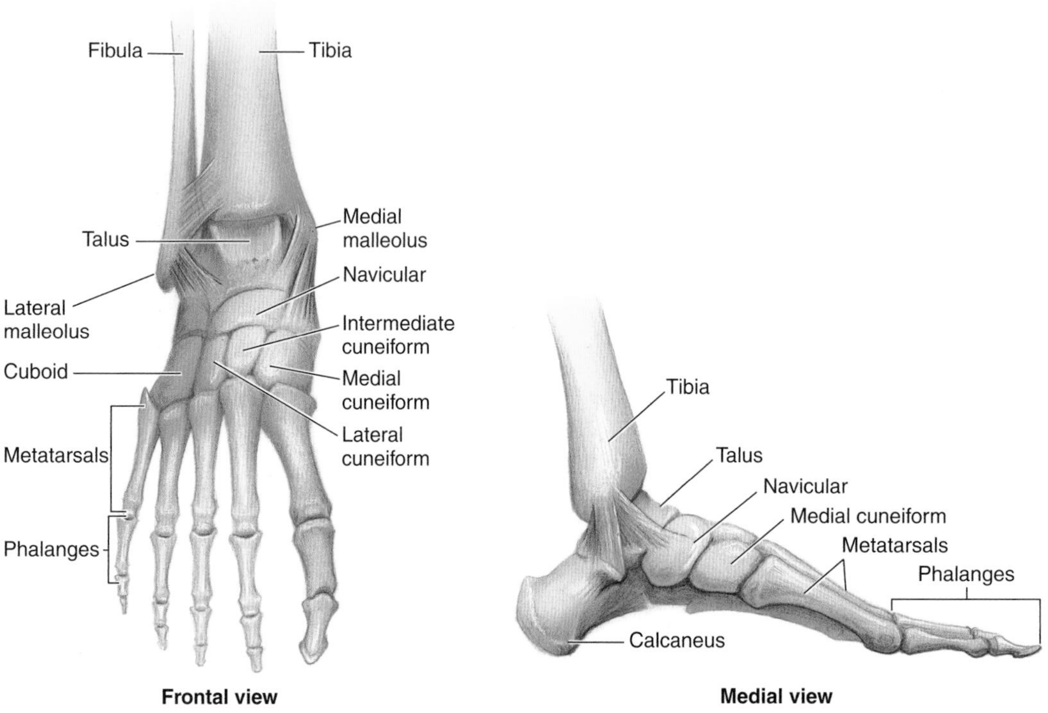


**FIGURE 5-11** Bones of the ankle and foot.

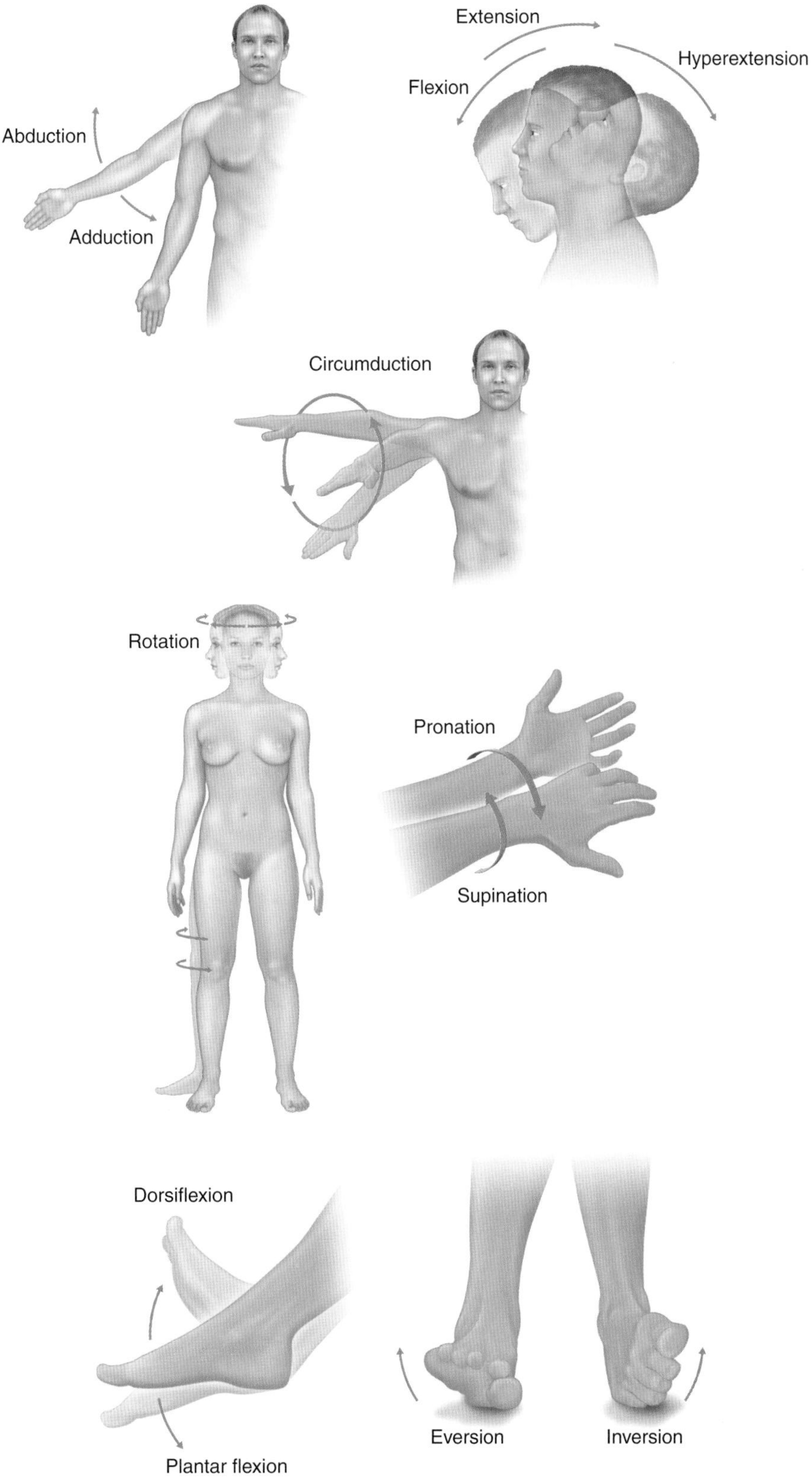


**FIGURE 5-12** Movements at joints.

## Quick Check

**Fill in the blank with the correct answer.**

1. Osseous tissue consists of special mature bone cells called ______________.
2. A diarthrosis is a joint that has free movement. It is also called a ______________ joint.
3. The facial bones include the nasal bone, the two zygomatic bones, the maxilla, and the ______________.

## DISORDERS RELATED TO THE SKELETAL SYSTEM

A **sprain** is a tear in a ligament or the fibrous tissue that connects bones. A **fracture** (Fx) is a broken bone. However, all fractures are not the same. Some are simple breaks, and some are not. If the fracture is a **simple fracture** (**closed fracture**), there is no open skin. If the broken bone protrudes through the skin, it is called a **compound fracture** (**open fracture**).

**COMMON TYPES OF FRACTURES**

| Fracture | Description | Example |
|---|---|---|
| Simple (closed) | break in which there is no open skin | 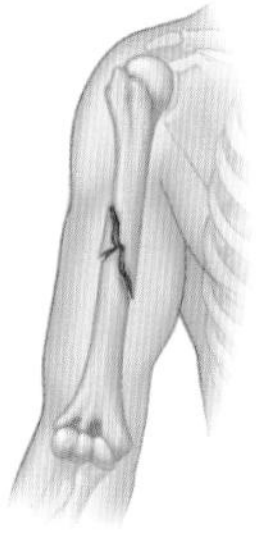 simple (closed) |
| Compound (open) | broken bone protrudes through the skin | 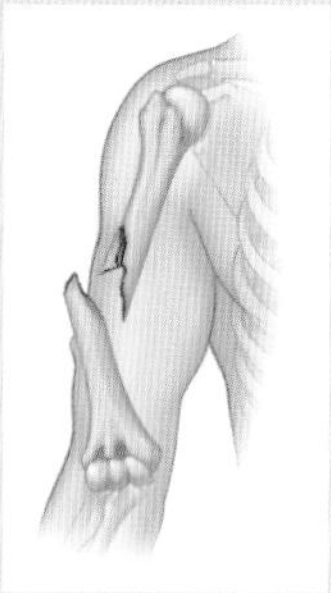 compound (open) |

COMMON TYPES OF FRACTURES (*CONTINUED*)

| Fracture | Description | Example |
|---|---|---|
| Comminuted | break in which the bone is crushed or splintered | 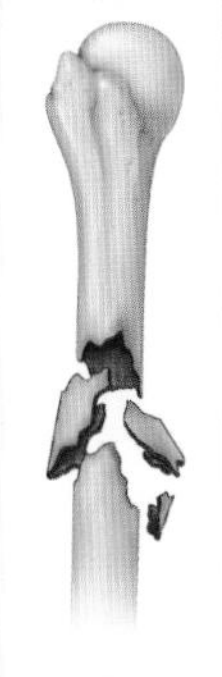 **comminuted** |
| Spiral | break is S-shaped, usually caused by a twisting injury | 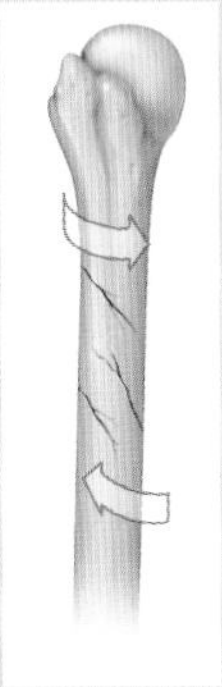 **spiral** |
| Transverse | break is straight across the shaft of the bone, at a right angle to the long axis | 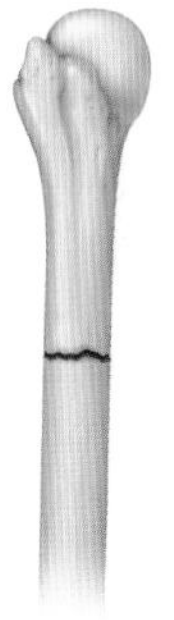 **transverse** |
| Greenstick | Incomplete break in which the bone bends | 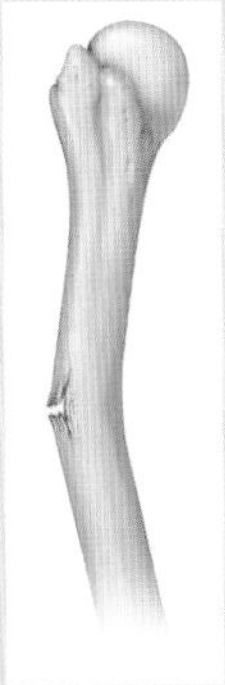 **greenstick** |

**TABLE 5-2 MOVEMENTS OF SYNOVIAL JOINTS**

| Movement | Description |
|---|---|
| abduction | movement away from the midline of the body |
| adduction | movement toward the midline of the body |
| flexion | decreasing the angle of a joint; movement that bends a limb |
| extension | increasing the angles of a joint; movement that straightens a limb |
| hyperextension | excessive extension beyond the anatomic position |
| circumduction | movement in a circular direction from a central point |
| rotation | turning a body part on its own axis |
| pronation | turning the palm posteriorly |
| supination | turning the palm anteriorly |
| dorsiflexion | bending the sole foot upward toward the shin |
| plantar flexion | bending the sole of the foot downward or pointing the toes downward |
| eversion | turning the sole of the foot outward |
| inversion | turning the sole of the foot inward |

Bone disorders arising from disease include conditions such as **osteomyelitis**, an inflammation caused by bacteria. **Osteoporosis** is a bone disorder characterized by a decrease in bone density and mass. Two other bone disorders are **rickets**, causing bowed legs in children, and **osteomalacia**, which is bone softening in adulthood. These two conditions result from vitamin deficiency and lack of calcium absorption. **Neoplasms** or tumors of the bone may be primary or secondary (from other sites in the body). **Osteosarcoma** is a tumor of the bone. **Chondrosarcoma** is a tumor that arises in cartilage.

Joint disorders include **arthritis**, a general term used to denote joint inflammation. General wear and tear on joints results in **osteoarthritis**. **Rheumatoid arthritis** (RA) also results in inflammation, but has a different cause than osteoarthritis. RA is attributed to an immunologic abnormality that results in inflammation with subsequent tissue destruction (see Figure 5-13).

The spine has a number of conditions that affect it. A disc that protrudes into the vertebral canal and puts pressure on the spinal nerve is called a **herniated disc**. Compression fractures of the vertebrae may produce **kyphosis** (humpback) and loss of height. **Lordosis** is an abnormal curvature in the lumbar region. **Scoliosis** is a sideways curvature of the spine that may occur in any region of the spine (see Figure 5-14).

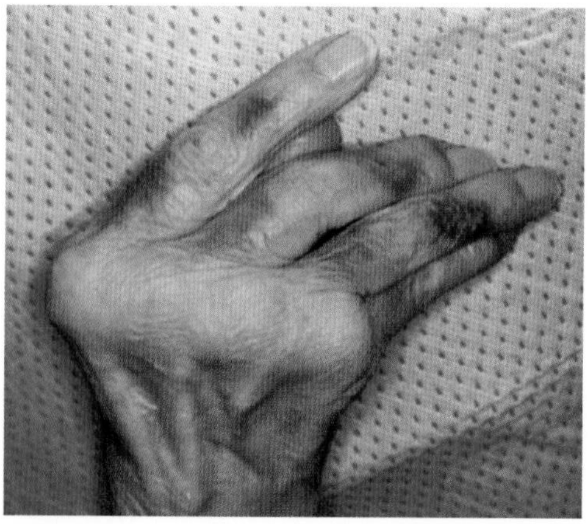

**FIGURE 5-13** Advanced rheumatoid arthritis. These hands show joint swelling and finger deformity.

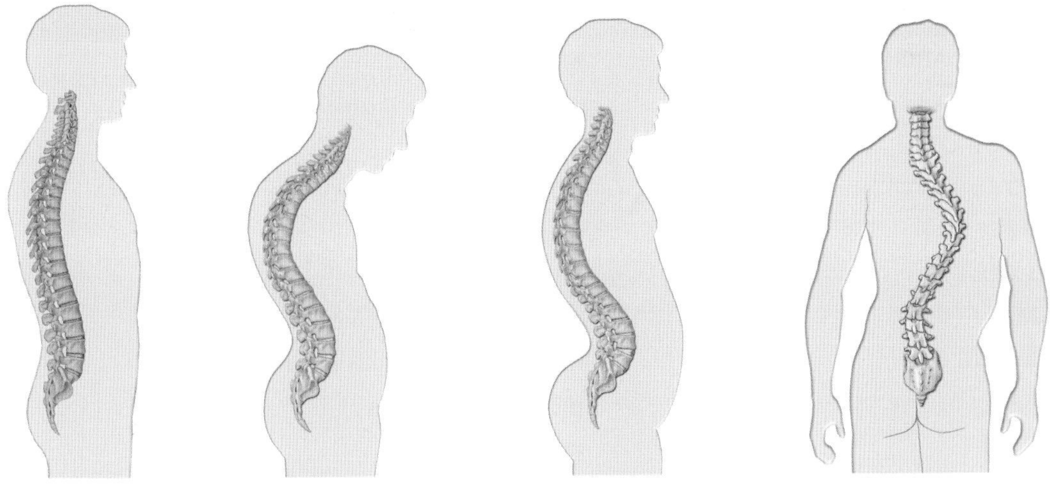


**FIGURE 5-14** Abnormal curvatures of the spine can cause pain and disfigurement.

## DIAGNOSTIC TESTS, TREATMENTS, AND SURGICAL PROCEDURES

Treatment of a fracture consists of **reduction** (realignment) of the broken bone. In some cases, **traction** (Tx) (using elastics or pulley and weights to maintain alignment) may be needed. Casts and splints are used to immobilize a broken bone during the healing process.

Symptomatic treatments (just treating the symptoms but not the problem) are also common with skeletal system conditions. For osteoarthritis, treatment may include medication for pain and inflammation and/or physical therapy. For conditions like RA, treatments consist of medication, rest, and physical therapy. Another option is **arthrocentesis**, which drains fluid and relieves the pressure in the joint.

## PRACTICE AND PRACTITIONERS

A number of specialists work in the branch of **orthopedics** (*orthopedic medicine*), all of them engaged in the diagnosis and treatment of patients with musculoskeletal disorders. **Orthopedic surgeons** coordinate patient care with **physical therapists** (professionals who treat disorders with physical methods), **occupational therapists** (professionals who rehabilitate through performance of activities of daily living), **kinesiologists** (professionals who aid by studying body movements), or other practitioners in sports medicine. A **rheumatologist** is a physician who specializes in the treatment of joint disorders and arthritic conditions.

What is the difference between occupational therapy and physical therapy? The goal of occupational therapy is for the individual to be able to take care of themselves and complete activities of daily living, such as getting in and out of the car, getting dressed, or being able to push a grocery cart in the store. This type of therapy is common for people who recently had surgery, such as total hip replacement (THR) or total knee arthroplasty (TKA), or after something like a stroke. Physical therapy focuses on muscle groups to help the individual improve strength, balance, and ROM. Physical therapy is common after sports injuries, like an anterior cruciate ligament (ACL) tear.

## Abbreviation Table THE SKELETAL SYSTEM

| ABBREVIATION | MEANING |
|---|---|
| ACL | anterior cruciate ligament |
| C (C1–C7) | cervical |
| CT | computed tomography |
| Fx | fracture |
| L (L1–L5) | lumbar |
| MRI | magnetic resonance imaging |
| NSAID | nonsteroidal anti-inflammatory drug |
| RA | rheumatoid arthritis |
| ROM | range of motion |
| S | sacral |
| T (T1–T12) | thoracic |
| THR | total hip replacement |
| TKA | total knee arthroplasty |
| TKR | total knee replacement |
| Tx | traction |

## Study Table THE SKELETAL SYSTEM

| TERM AND PRONUNCIATION | ANALYSIS | MEANING |
|---|---|---|
| **Structure and Function** | | |
| amphiarthrosis (AM-fee-ar-THRO-sihs) | *amphi-* (both sides); *arthr/o* (joint); *-osis* (abnormal condition) | joint with little movement |
| appendicular skeleton (APP-ehn-DIHK-yu-lahr SKEL-uh-tun) | adjective referring to something that is added or attached | bones of the limbs, including the shoulder girdle and pelvic girdle |
| axial skeleton (AX-ee-uhl SKEL-uh-tun) | adjective form of axis, a common English word | articulated bones of the head, vertebral column, and thorax |
| brachial (BRAY-kee-uhl) | *brachi/o* (arm); *-al* (adjective suffix) | having to do with an arm |
| bursae (BUR-see; *bursa*, singular) | a Latin word meaning "purse" | saclike connective structure found in some joints that contains synovial fluid; protects moving parts from friction |
| calcaneus (kal-KAY-nee-uhs) | Latin word for heel | the heel bone |
| carpal (KAR-pahl) bones | adjective form of carpus (wrist) | wrist bones |
| cartilage (CAR-tih-lij) | from the Latin word *cartilagin* (gristle) | dense, flexible connective tissue |

**Study Table** THE SKELETAL SYSTEM (*continued*)

| TERM AND PRONUNCIATION | ANALYSIS | MEANING |
|---|---|---|
| cervical (SUR-vih-kuhl) | *cervic/o* (neck); *-al* (adjective suffix) | adjective describing the vertebrae (C1–C7) in the neck region; also used in connection with the uterus, which is part of the female reproductive system |
| cervix (SUR-vix) | Latin word for neck | neck (also the neck of the uterus) |
| clavicle (KLAV-ih-cuhl); the adjective is clavicular (kla-VIK-yu-luhr) | from the Latin word *clavicula* (a small key) | the collarbone |
| coccyx (KOK-six); the adjective is coccygeal (kok-SIH-jee-uhl) | from the Greek word *kokkyx* (cuckoo) | the tailbone, made up of the four fused vertebrae at the base of the spinal column |
| compact (KOM-pakt) bone | common English word | type of dense bone |
| cranial bones (KRAY-nee-uhl) | *crani/o* from the Greek word *kranion* (skull); *-al* (adjective form) | collectively, and along with other minor bones, the frontal bone, two parietal bones, two temporal bones, and the occipital bone |
| cranial sutures (KRAY-nee-uhl SOO-churz) | from the Latin word *sutura* (seam) | fibrous membrane forming an immovable joint that joins the skull bones |
| cranium (KRAY-nee-um) | from medieval Latin, *kranion* (skull) | the bones of the head |
| diaphysis (dye-AFF-ih-sihs) | a Greek word (growing between) | shaft of the long bone |
| diarthrosis (dy-ar-THRO-sihs) | a Greek word (articulation) | synonym for synovial joint |
| endosteum (ehn-DOST-ee-um) | *endo-* (inside); *oste/o* (Greek word for bone) | inner membrane layer of the bone |
| epiphyseal (ep-ih-FIZ-ee-ul) plate | relating to an epiphysis (bone end) | disk of cartilage between the metaphysis and epiphysis of an immature long bone; growth plate |
| epiphysis (eh-PIFF-ih-sihs) | *epi-* (upon); *-physis* (growth) | end of the long bone (proximal, distal) |
| extension (ehx-TEN-shun) | a common English word | to straighten a joint |
| femur (FEE-muhr) | a Latin word (thigh) | thighbone |
| fibula (FIHB-yu-lah) | a Latin word (clasp) | the lateral leg bone |
| flexion (FLEHX-shun) | from the Latin verb *flecto* (bend) | bending a joint |

(*continued*)

**Study Table** THE SKELETAL SYSTEM (*continued*)

| TERM AND PRONUNCIATION | ANALYSIS | MEANING |
|---|---|---|
| frontal bone (FRUN-tuhl) | frontal (adjective form of English noun: front) | one of the six main cranial bones |
| hip bone | from the Old English, *hype* | large flat bone formed by the fusion of the ilium, ischium, and pubis |
| humerus (HUE-muh-ruhs) | Latin for shoulder | the long bone extending from the shoulder to the elbow |
| ilium (IL-ee-uhm) | Latin for flank | one of the three bones fused together to form the hip bone |
| ischium (IS-kee-uhm) | Latin for hip | one of the three bones fused together to form the hip bone |
| joint | from the Latin word *iunctus* (connected, associated) | place where two bones come together |
| lateral malleolus (LAT-er-ul mahl-ee-OHL-us) | from the Latin words, *lateralis* (side) and *malleus* (hammer) | projection on the lateral side of the lower end of the fibula |
| ligaments (LIG-uh-ments) | from the Latin word *ligamentum* (a tie or binding) | tissue that connects two bones |
| lumbar (LUM-bar) | from the Latin word *lumbus* (loin); *-ar* (adjective suffix) | adjective describing the vertebrae (L1–L5) in the lower vertebral column |
| mandible (MAN-dih-buhl); the adjective is mandibular (man-DIB-yu-luhr) | from the Latin verb *mandere* (to chew) | the lower jawbone |
| maxilla (MAX-ih-luh); the adjective is maxillary (MAX-ih-lahr-ee) | Latin for jawbone | the bone above the upper teeth |
| medial malleolus (mee-DEE-ul mahl-ee-OHL-us) | from the Latin words *medialis* (middle) and *malleus* (hammer) | projection on the medial side of the lower end of the tibia |
| medulla (MUH-duhl-uh) | Latin for marrow | soft, marrow-like structure |
| medullary cavity (MED-yul-her-ee) | an adjective form of *medulla* (Latin for marrow) | bone marrow cavity |
| metacarpals (MEHT-uh-KAR-puhl) | *meta-* (beyond); carp from *carpus* (wrist); *-al* (adjective suffix) | the five bones extending from the wrist to the first knuckle in each hand |
| metatarsals (MEH-tah-TAHR-sahlz) | *meta-* (beyond); tarsal from *tarsos* (flat surface); *-al* (adjective suffix) | the bones between the tarsals and the phalanges (toes) of the foot |
| nasal bone (NAY-zuhl) | *nas/o* (nose); *-al* (adjective suffix) | a facial bone (nose) |

**Study Table** THE SKELETAL SYSTEM (*continued*)

| TERM AND PRONUNCIATION | ANALYSIS | MEANING |
|---|---|---|
| occipital bone (ox-SIP-it-uhl) | *occiput* (Latin for back of the head); *-al* (adjective suffix) | one of the six main cranial bones |
| os coxae (OSS COX-ay) | *os* (Latin for bone); *coxae* (Latin: genitive case for hip) | hip bone |
| osseous tissue (OSS-ee-us) | from the Latin word *osseus* (bony); *-ous* (adjective suffix) | bone tissue |
| ossification (OSS-ihf-ih-KAY-shun) | *os* (bone); *facio* (Latin verb for make) | bone formation |
| osteocytes (OSS-tee-oh-syt) | *oste/o* (bone); *-cyte* (cell) | mature bone cells |
| osteogenesis (oss-tee-oh-JENN-uh-sis) | *oste/o* (bone); *-genesis* (origin) | formation of bone |
| parietal bones (puh-RY-uh-tuhl) | from a Latin word *paries* (wall) and *-al* (adjective suffix) | two of the six main cranial bones |
| patella (pah-TELL-ah) | Latin for small plate | kneecap |
| pectoral girdle (pek-TOR-uhl) | from *pectus*, a Latin word (chest); *-al* (adjective suffix) | the shoulder girdle |
| periosteum (pair-ee-OST-ee-um) | *peri-* (around); *oste/o* (bone) | membrane that surrounds the outside of the bone |
| phalanges (FAY-lanj-es) | plural of the Greek word *phalanx* (a column of soldiers) | fingers (singular form is phalanx) |
| pubis (PYU-bihs) | short for "os pubis"; from the Latin word *pubertas* (grown up) | one of the three bones fused together to form the hip bone |
| radius (RAY-dee-uhs); the adjective is radial (RAY-dee-uhl) | a Latin word (a rod or a spoke of a wheel) | one of the two bones (the other is the ulna) extending from the elbow to the wrist |
| sacrum (SAK-rum); the adjective is sacral (SAK-ruhl) | short for "os sacrum," a Latin word meaning "sacred" | bone formed from five vertebrae fused together near the base of the vertebral column |
| scapula (SKAP-yu-luh); plural is scapulae (SKAP-yu-lay); the adjectival form is scapular (SKAP-yu-luhr) | Latin for shoulder blade | the shoulder blade |
| spongy (SPUN-jee) bone | common English words | type of bone tissue |
| sternum (STUR-nuhm) | from the Greek word *sternon* (chest) | the breastbone; parts include the manubrium, body, and xiphoid process |
| synarthrosis (syn-AR-thr-oh-sihs) | *syn-* (together); *arthr/o* (joint); *-osis* (condition) | joint with no movement |
| synovial (sy-NOH-vee-ahl) joint | *syn-* (together); Latin *ovum* (egg); *-al* (adjective suffix) | freely movable joint; diarthrosis |

*(continued)*

**Study Table** THE SKELETAL SYSTEM (*continued*)

| TERM AND PRONUNCIATION | ANALYSIS | MEANING |
|---|---|---|
| talus (TAY-luhs) | Latin for ankle | the bone in the ankle that articulates with the tibia and fibula |
| tarsal (TAR-sahl) bones | from the Greek word *tarsos* (a flat surface, sole of the foot) | the bones of the sole of the foot |
| tarsus (TAR-suhs) | from the Greek word *tarsos* (a flat surface) | ankle |
| tendons (TEN-duhnz) | from the Latin verb *tendere* (to stretch) | connective tissue that connects muscle to bone |
| temporal bones (TEMP-uh-ruhl) | from the Latin *tempus* (time, temple) | two of the six main cranial bones; located on the side of the head near the ears |
| thoracic (tho-RASS-ik) cage | from the Greek word *thorax* (breastplate, the chest) | skeleton of the thoracic consisting of the thoracic vertebrae, ribs, costal (rib) cartilages, and sternum |
| thorax (THOR-ax) | from the Greek word *thorax* (breastplate, the chest) | chest |
| tibia (TIH-bee-ah); the adjective form is tibial (TIH-bee-al) | Latin for flute | shin bone |
| ulna (ULL-nah); the adjective is ulnar (ULL-nahr) | Latin for forearm | one of the two bones (the other is the radius) extending from the elbow to the wrist |
| vertebrae (VUR-tuh-bray); singular is vertebrae (VUR-tuh-bruh) | from the Latin verb *verto* (to turn) | one of the 33 segments making up the vertebral column |
| vertebral (VER-te-brul) column | from the Latin verb *verto* (to turn) | series of vertebrae extending from the cranium (head) to the coccyx (tailbone) |
| xiphoid process (ZEYE-foyd) | from the Greek word *xipho* (sword), *-oid* (resemblance to) | bony, dagger-like structure at the lower end of the sternum |
| zygomatic bones (ZI-go-MAT-ik) | from the Greek word *zygoma* (bolt or bar); *-tic* (adjective suffix) | a facial bone (cheek, one of two) |
| **Disorders** | | |
| arthralgia (ar-THRAL-jee-uh) | *arthr/o* (joint); *-algia* (pain) | pain in a joint |
| arthritis (ar-THRY-tuhs) | *arthr/o* (joint); *-itis* (inflammation) | inflammation of a joint |

**Study Table** THE SKELETAL SYSTEM (*continued*)

| TERM AND PRONUNCIATION | ANALYSIS | MEANING |
|---|---|---|
| arthrochondritis (ARTH-roh-konn-DRY-tihs) | *arthr/o* (joint); *chondr/o* (cartilage); *-itis* (inflammation) | inflammation of joint cartilage |
| arthropathy (ar-THROP-ah- thee) | *arthr/o* (joint); *-pathy* (disease or disorder) | any disorder of a joint |
| arthrosis (ar-THROW-sihs) | *arthr/o* (joint); *-osis* (abnormal condition of) | degenerative joint changes |
| brachialgia (BRAY-kee-AL-jee-uh) | *brachi/o* (arm); *-algia* (pain) | pain in the arm |
| bursitis (burr-SY-tihs) | *burs/o* (bursa); *-itis* (inflammation) | inflammation of a bursa |
| carpal tunnel syndrome (KAR-puhl TUN-uhl SINN-druhm) | *carp/o* (wrist); *-al* (adjective suffix); *syn-* (together); from the Greek *dromos* (a running) | condition characterized by wrist pain, caused by chronic entrapment of the median nerve within the carpal tunnel |
| chondromalacia (konn-droh-muh-LAY-she-uh) | *chondr/o* (cartilage); *-malacia* (softening) | softening of cartilage |
| chondropathy (kon-DROP-ah-thee) | *chondr/o* (cartilage); *-pathy* (disease or disorder) | disease of cartilage |
| chondrosarcoma (KONN-droh-sar-KOH-ma) | *chondr/o* (cartilage); *sarc/o* (flesh); *-oma* (tumor) | malignant tumor arising from the cartilage |
| closed fracture (FRAK-chur) | from the Latin word *fractura* (a break) | break in the bone in which the skin is intact at the site; also called simple fracture |
| compound fracture (KOM-pound FRAK-chur) | from the Latin word *fractura* (a break) | break in the bone where the bone comes through the skin; also called open fracture |
| costalgia (koss-TAL-jee-uh) | *cost/o* (rib); *-algia* (pain) | rib pain |
| costochondritis (KOSS-toh-kon-DRY-tihs) | *cost/o* (rib); *chondr/o* (cartilage); *-itis* (inflammation) | inflammation of rib cartilage |
| dactylalgia (DAKK-tihl-AL-jee-uh) | *dactyl/o* (finger, toe); *-algia* (pain) | pain in the fingers |
| dactylodynia (DAKK-tihl-oh-DINN-ee-uh) | *dactyl/o* (finger, toe); *-dynia* (pain) | pain in the fingers |
| fracture (FRAK-chur) | from the Latin word *fractura* (break) | break in a bone |
| herniated disc (HER-nee-ay-ted disk) | from the Latin word *hernia* (rupture); *disc/o* (disk) | protrusion of a fragmented intervertebral disc in the intervertebral foramen with potential compression of a nerve |
| kyphosis (ky-FOH-sis) | *kyph/o* (humped); *-sis* (condition) | humpback; anteriorly concave curvature of the thoracic and sacral region of the spine |

*(continued)*

**Study Table** THE SKELETAL SYSTEM (*continued*)

| TERM AND PRONUNCIATION | ANALYSIS | MEANING |
|---|---|---|
| lordosis (lohr-DOH-sis) | from the Greek word *lordosis* (a bending backwards) | swayback; abnormal anteriorly convex curvature of the lumbar part of the spine |
| megadactyly (meg-uh-DAKK-tuh-lee) | *mega- (enlargement); dactyl/o* (finger, toe) | enlargement of one or more fingers or toes |
| neoplasms (NEE-oh-plazumz) | *neo-* (new); *plasma* (thing formed) | abnormal tissue that grows rapidly |
| open fracture | *open* (exposed) | bone break in which the skin is lacerated and there is an open wound; also called compound fracture |
| ostealgia (oss-tee-AL-jee-uh) | *oste/o* (bone); *-algia* (pain) | pain in a bone; also called osteodynia |
| osteitis (oss-tee-EYE-tihs) | *oste/o* (bone); *-itis* (inflammation) | inflammation of bone |
| osteochondritis (OSS-tee-oh-konn-DRY-tihs) | *oste/o* (bone); *chondr/o* (cartilage); *-itis* (inflammation) | inflammation of bone and associated cartilage |
| osteodynia(oss-tee-oh-DINN-ee-uh) | *oste/o* (bone); *-dynia* (pain) | pain in a bone; also called ostealgia |
| osteomalacia (OSS-tee-oh-muh-LAY-she-uh) | *oste/o* (bone); *-malacia* (softening) | softening of bone |
| osteomyelitis (OSS-tee-oh-my-eh-LY-tihs) | *oste/o* (bone); *myel/o* (marrow); *-itis* (inflammation) | inflammation of bone marrow |
| osteopenia (oss-tee-oh-PEEN-ee-uh) | *oste/o* (bone); *-penia* (deficiency) | abnormally low bone density |
| osteoporosis (OSS-tee-oh-puh-RO-sihs) | *oste/o* (bone); *por/o* (porous); *-sis* (condition) | atrophy and thinning of bone tissue |
| osteosarcoma (OSS-tee-oh-sar-KOH-ma) | *oste/o* (bone); *sarc/o* (flesh-like); *-oma* (tumor) | highly malignant tumor of the bone |
| rheumatoid arthritis (ROO-mah-toid ar-THRY-tuhs) | from the Greek word *rheuma* (flux); *-oid* (resemblance of) | systemic autoimmune disease occurring more often in women that affects the connective tissue; involves many joints, especially those of the hands and feet |
| rickets (RIH-kehts) | common English word; might be an alteration of the Greek word *rhakhitis* | disease due to vitamin D deficiency characterized by deficient calcification and soft bones associated with skeletal deformities |
| scoliosis (skohl-ee-OH-sis) | *scoli/o* (twisted); *-sis* (condition) | lateral curvature of the spine; S-shaped curvature |

**Study Table** THE SKELETAL SYSTEM (*continued*)

| TERM AND PRONUNCIATION | ANALYSIS | MEANING |
| --- | --- | --- |
| simple fracture (FRAK-chur) | from the Latin word *fractura* (a break) | break in the bone in which the skin is intact at the site; also called closed fracture |
| sprain (SPRAYN) | common English word; unknown origin | injury to a ligament |
| syndrome (SIN-drum) | *syn-* (together); from the Greek *dromos* (running) | collection of signs and symptoms occurring together and characterizing a medical condition |
| **Diagnostic Tests, Treatments, and Surgical Procedures** | | |
| analgesics (an-al-GEE-ziks) | *an-* (absence); from the Greek word *gesis* (sensation) | medication used to relieve pain |
| anti-inflammatory (AN-ty-in-FLAMM-ah-tohr-ee) | *anti-* (against); inflammatory (common English word) | medication used to reduce inflammation (e.g., used to reduce joint inflammation in arthritis) |
| arthrectomy (ar-THREK-tuh-mee) | *arthr/o* (joint); *-ectomy* (surgical removal) | excision of a joint |
| arthrocentesis (arth-roh-senn-TEE-sihs) | *arthr/o* (joint); *-centesis* (surgical puncture for aspiration) | removing fluid from a joint through a needle puncture |
| arthrogram (ARTH-roh-gram) | *arthr/o* (joint); *-gram* (record or picture) | imaging of a joint after injecting a contrast dye to aid visualization |
| arthrometry (arth-ROM-uh-tree) | *arthr/o* (joint); *-metry* (process of measuring) | measurement of the amount of movement in a joint |
| arthroplasty (ARTH-roh-plass-tee) | *arthr/o* (joint); *-plasty* (surgical repair) | surgical repair of a joint |
| arthroscope (ARTH-roh-skope) | *arthr/o* (joint); *-scope* (instrument for viewing) | device used in arthroscopy |
| arthroscopy (ahr-THRAW-skoh-pee) | *arthr/o* (joint); *-scopy* (use of instrument for viewing) | examination of the interior of a joint |
| arthrotomy (ar-THRAWT-uh-mee) | *arthr/o* (joint); *-tomy* (cutting operation) | surgical incision into a joint |
| carpectomy (kar-PEK-tuh-me) | *carp/o* (wrist); *-ectomy* (surgical removal) | excision of part of the wrist |
| chondroplasty (KONN-droh-plass-tee) | *chondr/o* (cartilage); *-plasty* (surgical repair) | surgical repair of cartilage |
| computed tomography (CT) scan | from the Greek *tomos* (slice, section) and *graphy* (image) | noninvasive imaging test; imaging anatomical information from a cross-sectional plane of the body |
| costectomy (koss-TEK-tuh-mee) | *cost/o* (rib); *-ectomy* (surgical removal) | excision of a rib |

(*continued*)

**Study Table** THE SKELETAL SYSTEM (*continued*)

| TERM AND PRONUNCIATION | ANALYSIS | MEANING |
|---|---|---|
| magnetic resonance imaging (MRI) | from Latin *resonantia* (echo) | a diagnostic radiograph in which the magnetic nuclei of a patient are aligned in a magnetic field; these signals are converted into tomographic images |
| myelogram (MY-el-loh-gram) | *myel/o* (bone marrow); *-gram* (record or picture) | X-ray of the spinal column using contrast medium |
| narcotic (nahr-KAH-tik) | *narc/o* (sleep) | drug derived from opium with potent analgesic effects; potential effects of dependency through prolonged use |
| nonsteroidal anti-inflammatory drug (NSAID) | from the Greek *stereos* (solid lipid) | medication that exerts analgesic and anti-inflammatory actions |
| ostectomy (oss-TECK-tuh-mee) | *oste/o* (bone); *-ectomy* (surgical removal) | surgical removal of bone |
| osteoplasty (OSS-tee-oh-plass-tee) | *oste/o* (bone); *-plasty* (surgical repair) | surgical repair of bone |
| osteorrhaphy (OSS-tee-oh-raff-ee) | *oste/o* (bone); *-rrhaphy* (surgical suturing) | suturing together the parts of a broken bone |
| osteotomy (oss-tee-AW-tuh-mee) | *oste/o* (bone); *-tomy* (cutting operation) | surgical cutting of bone |
| reduction (ree-DUK-shun) | common English word | correcting a fracture by realigning the bone pieces |
| traction (TRAK-shun) | common English word | using elastics or pulley and weights to maintain alignment; a pulling or dragging force exerted on a limb in a distal direction |
| vertebrectomy (ver-tuh-BREKK-tuh-mee) | from the Latin word *verto* (to turn); *-ectomy* (surgical removal) | excision (resectioning) of a vertebra |
| **Practice and Practitioners** | | |
| kinesiologist (ki-nee-see-ol-UH-jist) | *kinesis* (Greek for movement); *-logist* (one who studies a certain field) | practitioner who studies movement and the involved structures |
| occupational therapist (ok-YOU-pey-shun-uhl THER-uh-pist) | *occupationem* (Latin for business); *therapia* (Latin for curing the sick) | practitioner who works to increase independent function through therapy |

**Study Table** THE SKELETAL SYSTEM (*continued*)

| TERM AND PRONUNCIATION | ANALYSIS | MEANING |
|---|---|---|
| orthopedics (or-thoh-PEE-diks) | *orth/o* (straight or correct); *ped-* (child); *-ic* (adjective suffix) | the medical specialty concerned with the development, preservation, restoration, and function of the musculoskeletal system |
| orthopedic surgeon (or-thoh-PEE-dik SUR-juhn) | *orth/o* (straight or correct); *ped-* (child); *-ic* (adjective suffix) | a physician in the field of orthopedics (can be MD or DO) |
| physical therapist (FIZ-i-kul THER-uh-pist) | *physicalis* (Latin for nature); *therapia* (Latin for curing the sick) | practitioner who works to restore correct muscle movement and ability |
| rheumatologist (ROO-mah-tah-lo-gist) | *rheumat/o* (flux); *-logist* (one who studies a certain field) | physician who treats joint and connective tissue disorders such as arthritis |
| rheumatology (ROO-mah-tah-lo-gee) | *rheumat/o* (flux); *-logy* (the study of) | field of specialty that deals with joints and connective tissue disorders |

## END-OF-CHAPTER EXERCISES

### EXERCISE 5-1 LABELING: SKELETON

**Using the following list, choose the correct terms to label the diagram correctly.**

| | | | | |
|---|---|---|---|---|
| calcaneus | femur | metacarpals | phalanges | sternum |
| carpal bones | fibula | metatarsals | radius | tarsal bones |
| clavicle | humerus | patella | ribs | tibia |
| costal cartilage | ilium | pubis | sacrum | ulna |
| cranium | mandible | phalanges | scapula | vertebral column |
| facial bones | | | | |

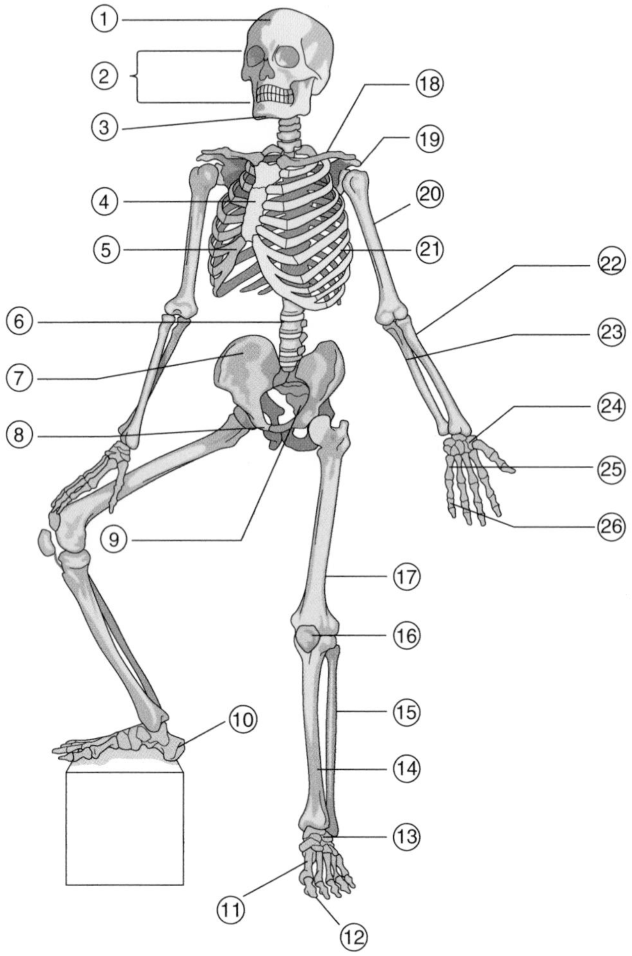


| | | | | |
|---|---|---|---|---|
| 1. ____________ | 7. ____________ | 13. ____________ | 19. ____________ | 25. ____________ |
| 2. ____________ | 8. ____________ | 14. ____________ | 20. ____________ | 26. ____________ |
| 3. ____________ | 9. ____________ | 15. ____________ | 21. ____________ | |
| 4. ____________ | 10. ____________ | 16. ____________ | 22. ____________ | |
| 5. ____________ | 11. ____________ | 17. ____________ | 23. ____________ | |
| 6. ____________ | 12. ____________ | 18. ____________ | 24. ____________ | |

## EXERCISE 5-2 LABELING: LONG BONE

**Using the following list, choose the correct terms to label the diagram correctly.**

| | | |
|---|---|---|
| compact bone | endosteum | periosteum |
| diaphysis | epiphyseal plate | proximal epiphysis |
| distal epiphysis | medullary cavity | spongy bone |

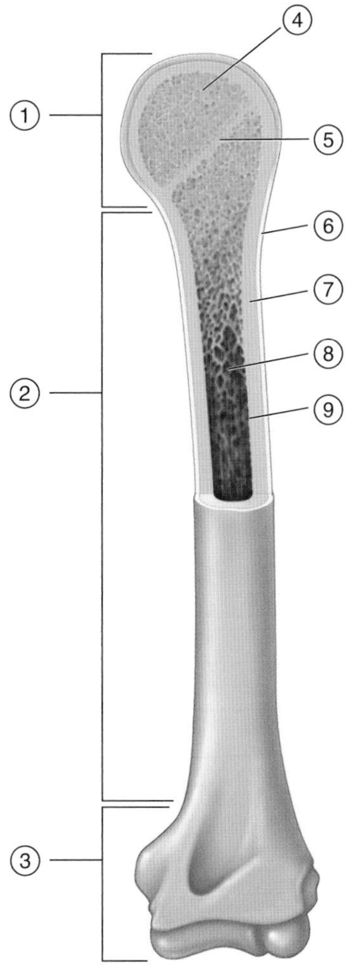


| | | |
|---|---|---|
| 1. ____________ | 4. ____________ | 7. ____________ |
| 2. ____________ | 5. ____________ | 8. ____________ |
| 3. ____________ | 6. ____________ | 9. ____________ |

## EXERCISE 5-3 WORD PARTS

**Break each of the following terms into its word parts: prefix, root, or suffix. Give the meaning of each word part and then define the term.**

1. *osteorraphy*

 root: ______________________________

 suffix: ______________________________

 definition: ______________________________

2. *arthrocentesis*

 root: ______________________________

 suffix: ______________________________

 definition: ______________________________

3. *brachialgia*

 root: ______________________________

 suffix: ______________________________

 definition: ______________________________

4. *osteochondritis*

 root: ______________________________

 root: ______________________________

 suffix: ______________________________

 definition: ______________________________

5. *carpectomy*

 root: ______________________________

 suffix: ______________________________

 definition: ______________________________

6. *chondrosarcoma*

 root: ______________________________

 root: ______________________________

 suffix: ______________________________

 definition: ______________________________

7. *dactylomegaly*

root: ____________________

suffix: ____________________

definition: ____________________

## EXERCISE 5-4 WORD BUILDING

**Use the word parts listed to build the terms defined.**

| | | | | |
|---|---|---|---|---|
| -algia | -dynia | -itis | myel/o | sarc/o |
| arthr/o | -ectomy | kinesi/o | -oma | -scopy |
| cardi/o | electr/o | -logy | oste/o | |
| chondr/o | -gram | -malacia | -plasty | |
| cost/o | inter- | my/o | -porosis | |

1. ____________________ inflammation of the bone and bone marrow
2. ____________________ visual examination of a joint
3. ____________________ abnormal softening of cartilage
4. ____________________ imaging of a joint
5. ____________________ pain in a joint
6. ____________________ the study of movement of body parts
7. ____________________ surgical repair of cartilage
8. ____________________ pertaining to the area between the ribs
9. ____________________ inflammation of the bone
10. ____________________ a highly malignant tumor of the bone
11. ____________________ surgical repair of a joint
12. ____________________ X-ray of the spine
13. ____________________ inflammation of the cartilage
14. ____________________ bones with diminished density; porous
15. ____________________ pain in the ribs

## EXERCISE 5-5 MATCHING

**Match the term in the first column with its definition in the second column.**

| | | |
|---|---|---|
| 1. ________________ | abduction | a. backward bending of hand or foot |
| 2. ________________ | rotation | b. bending the foot toward the ground |
| 3. ________________ | plantar flexion | c. straightening a limb |
| 4. ________________ | extension | d. motion around a central axis |
| 5. ________________ | dorsiflexion | e. motion away from the body |
| 6. ________________ | flexion | f. bending motion |
| 7. ________________ | adduction | g. motion toward the body |

## EXERCISE 5-6 MULTIPLE CHOICE

**Choose the correct answer for the following multiple choice questions.**

1. The formation of a bone is called ________________.
   a. osteoporosis
   b. osteology
   c. orthogenesis
   d. osteogenesis

2. The bony structure that forms the upper part of the sternum is the ________________.
   a. manubrium
   b. mandible
   c. temporomadibular joint
   d. maxilla

3. An abnormal outward curvature of the thoracic spine is called ________________.
   a. spondylosis
   b. lumbago
   c. lordosis
   d. kyphosis

4. The cartilaginous lower portion of the sternum is called the ________________.
   a. xiphoid process
   b. sacroiliac
   c. olecranon process
   d. pelvic girdle

5. The collar bone is the ________________.
   a. ischium
   b. ulna
   c. clavicle
   d. zygomatic

6. The bones of the hands are the ________________.
   a. tarsals
   b. metacarpals
   c. metatarsals
   d. calcaneus

7. The bones of the fingers and toes are the ________________.
   a. metatarsals
   b. carpal
   c. phalanges
   d. fibulas

8. The heel bone is the ________________.
   a. ilium
   b. zygomatic
   c. ulna
   d. calcaneus

9. The bones of the spine are the ________________.
   a. vertebrae
   b. temporals
   c. maxilla
   d. scapula

10. The shoulder blade is the ________________.
    a. scapula
    b. sternum
    c. maxilla
    d. scoliosis

11. Which term does not belong with the others?
    a. scoliosis
    b. rickets
    c. RA
    d. diaphysis

12. Which term does not belong with the others?
    a. humerus
    b. fibula
    c. radius
    d. ulna

13. Which term does not belong with the others?
    a. deltoid muscle
    b. patella
    c. sternum
    d. carpal bone

14. Which term does not belong with the others?
    a. sclerosis
    b. kyphosis
    c. scoliosis
    d. lordosis

15. Which term does not belong with the others?
    a. cervical
    b. parietal
    c. thoracic
    d. lumbar

## EXERCISE 5-7 FILL IN THE BLANK

**Fill in the blank with the correct answer.**

1. The word that means "inflammation of a joint" is ________________.
2. Aspiration of fluid from a joint by a needle puncture is a(n) ________________.
3. The physician who treats disorders of the skeletal system is called a(n) ________________.
4. A break in the bone where the bone comes through the skin is called an open fracture or a ________________ fracture.
5. Bone marrow can be found in the ________________ cavity.
6. A(n) ________________ connects tissue to bone.
7. A(n) ________________ is the protrusion of a fragmented intervertebral disc in the intervertebral foramen and can cause compression of a nerve.

## EXERCISE 5-8 ABBREVIATIONS

**Write out the term for the following abbreviations.**

1. ____________________________ ACL
2. ____________________________ CT
3. ____________________________ C1
4. ____________________________ TKA
5. ____________________________ L5
6. ____________________________ RA
7. ____________________________ NSAID
8. ____________________________ MRI

**Write the abbreviation for the following terms.**

9. ________________ total hip replacement

10. ________________ fracture

11. ________________ traction

12. ________________ range of motion

13. ________________ thoracic vertebra 12

14. ________________ total knee replacement

15. ________________ magnetic resonance imaging

## EXERCISE 5-9 SPELLING

**Select the correct spelling of the medical term.**

1. A practitioner who studies movement and the involved structures is a ________________.
   a. kinesiologist
   b. kinisiologist
   c. kynesiologist
   d. kiniseologist

2. Suturing together the parts of a broken bone is called ________________.
   a. osteorhaphy
   b. osteorrhaphy
   c. osteorafy
   d. osteoraphy

3. The measurement of the amount of movement in a joint is ________________.
   a. athrometery
   b. arthrometry
   c. athrometry
   d. arthrometery

4. ________________ are used to relieve pain.
   a. Analjesics
   b. Analgisics
   c. Analgezics
   d. Analgesics

5. RA stands for ________________.
   a. rhumatoid arthritis
   b. rhuematoid arthritis
   c. rheumatoid arthritis
   d. rheumitoid arthritis

6. ________________ is an adjective which means having to do with an arm.
   a. Brakial
   b. Breakial
   c. Braychial
   d. Brachial

7. ________________ is a condition where the bone tissue atrophies and thins.
   a. Osteoporosis
   b. Ostioporosis
   c. Osteopourosis
   d. Osteoporosys

8. The long bone that extends from the shoulder to the elbow and is Latin for "shoulder" is the ________________.
   a. humerous
   b. humeres
   c. humerus
   d. humeris

9. The posterior part of the hip bone is the ________________.
   a. ischium
   b. ishium
   c. ichium
   d. ischiem

10. Another name for the kneecap is the ________________.
    a. patela
    b. patella
    c. pattela
    d. pattella

## EXERCISE 5-10 CASE STUDY

The underlined medical terms refer to a physician, a condition, or a treatment. Replace the underlined terms with a description.

Mrs. Smith, an 82-year-old woman, was out walking her dog on a cold day. She slipped on a patch of ice, fell, and incurred painful injuries. In the emergency room, Dr. Farley Burrows, an orthopedic surgeon (1), examined her. Mrs. Smith had limited ROM (2) in her right wrist and was experiencing pain in her left hip. Dr. Burrows ordered x-rays, which revealed a comminuted fracture (3) in the wrist and compression fracture (4) in the hip. He then performed a reduction (5) of the wrist bone and ordered that Mrs. Smith be admitted to the hospital and placed in traction (6) to maintain realignment of her hip.

**Write your descriptions of each of the underlined terms or phrases in the spaces.**

1. ______________________________

2. ______________________________

3. ______________________________

4. ______________________________

5. ______________________________

6. ______________________________

# The Muscular System

6

## LEARNING OUTCOMES

***Upon completion of this chapter, you should be able to:***

- Name the three types of muscle tissue.
- Define terms related to muscle names and functions.
- Describe the types of muscle movement.
- Pronounce, spell, and define medical terms related to the muscular system and its disorders.
- Interpret abbreviations associated with the muscular system.

## INTRODUCTION

In the preceding chapter, you learned that there are approximately 206 bones in the human body. The total number of muscles is harder to calculate because of the various ways to distinguish them. But it is safe to say that there are approximately three times as many muscles as there are bones. Moreover, muscles make up about half of our total body weight.

We normally think of muscles as necessary for lifting objects, running, jumping, throwing a ball, or swinging a golf club. Even though that is true, muscles are also needed for seeing, talking, eating, digesting, breathing, smiling, frowning, blinking, and so on. And let's not forget the muscle that pumps blood through our bodies (the heart), which is discussed in Chapter 10. This is because while the heart's structure is a muscle, its function is better related to the cardiovascular system than to the muscular system.

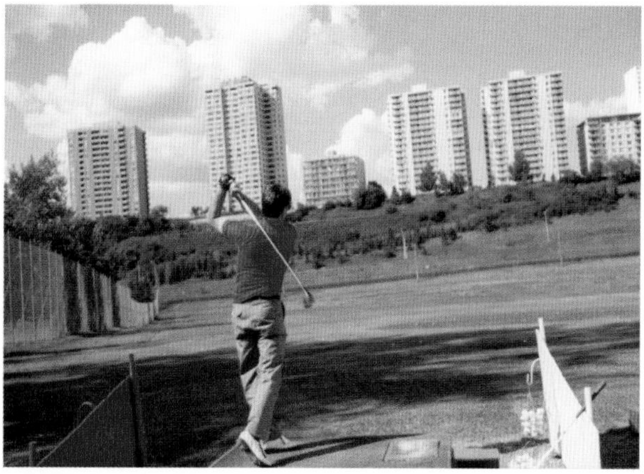

## WORD PARTS RELATED TO THE MUSCULAR SYSTEM

The parts presented in Table 6-1 are often found in terms related to the muscular system. The two main word parts are my/o and muscul/o, which both mean muscle. Other word roots refer to the movement of muscles such as kine- and kinesi/o.

**TABLE 6-1** COMMON WORD PARTS RELATED TO THE MUSCULAR SYSTEM

| Word Part | Meaning |
|---|---|
| fasci/o | fibrous membrane |
| fibr/o | fiber |
| hemi- | half |
| kine-, kinesi/o | movement |
| ligament/o | ligament |
| muscul/o | muscle |
| my/o | muscle |
| para- | alongside, near |
| -paresis | partial or incomplete paralysis |
| -plegia | paralysis |
| quadri- | four |
| sthen/o | strength |
| tend/o, tendin/o | tendon |
| ton/o | tone |

### Word Parts Exercise

After studying Table 6-1, write the meaning of each of the word parts.

| WORD PART | MEANING |
|---|---|
| 1. ligament/o | 1. ______ |
| 2. tend/o, tendin/o | 2. ______ |
| 3. ton/o | 3. ______ |
| 4. -plegia | 4. ______ |
| 5. muscul/o | 5. ______ |
| 6. kine-, kinesi/o | 6. ______ |
| 7. -paresis | 7. ______ |
| 8. sthen/o | 8. ______ |
| 9. my/o | 9. ______ |
| 10. quadri- | 10. ______ |

*(continued)*

## Word Parts Exercise (continued)

| WORD PART | MEANING |
|---|---|
| 11. fasci/o | 11. ____________ |
| 12. fibr/o | 12. ____________ |
| 13. hemi- | 13. ____________ |
| 14. para- | 14. ____________ |

# STRUCTURE AND FUNCTION



Muscles can be characterized by their location, cell characteristics (striated or nonstriated), and control of movement (voluntary or involuntary). The three types of muscle tissue are skeletal, smooth, and cardiac (see Figure 6-1).

## Skeletal Muscle

Of the three types, **skeletal muscle** is the largest group, comprising more than 600 separate muscles. Skeletal muscle is so named because it attaches muscles to bone. These voluntary muscles are made up of **muscle fibers**, the name for *muscle cells* in muscle tissue with a rich blood vessel network. A bundle of muscle fibers is called **fascicle**. **Fascia** encloses muscle and groups of muscles. **Tendons** are made of connective tissue that connects muscle to bone (see Figure 6-2). **Ligaments** are bands of fibrous connective tissue that connect bones to bones or bones to other structures and offer support to muscles.

| Comparison of the different types of muscle | | | |
|---|---|---|---|
| | Skeletal | Smooth | Cardiac |
| Location | Attached to bones | Wall of hollow organs, vessels, respiratory passageways | Wall of heart |
| Cell characteristics | 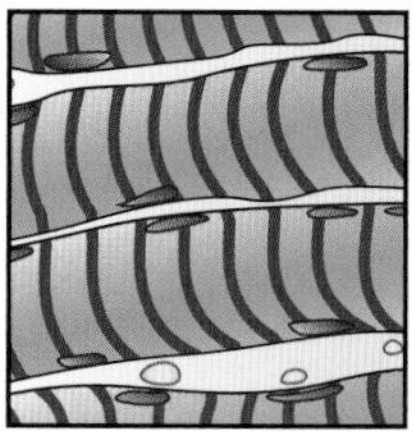 Long and cylindrical, multinucleated, heavily striated | 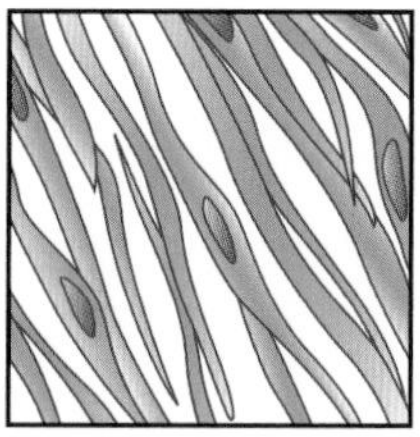 Tapered at each end, single nucleus, nonstriated | 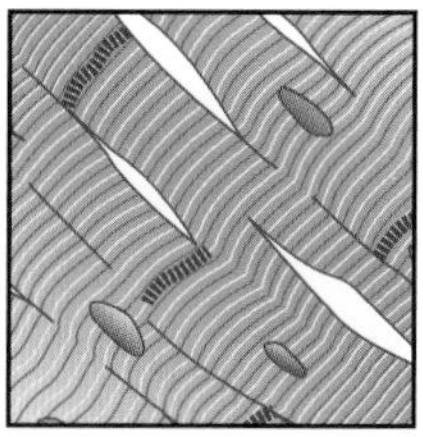 Branching networks, single nucleus, lightly striated |
| Control | Voluntary | Involuntary | Involuntary |

**FIGURE 6-1** A comparison of the three types of muscle tissue.

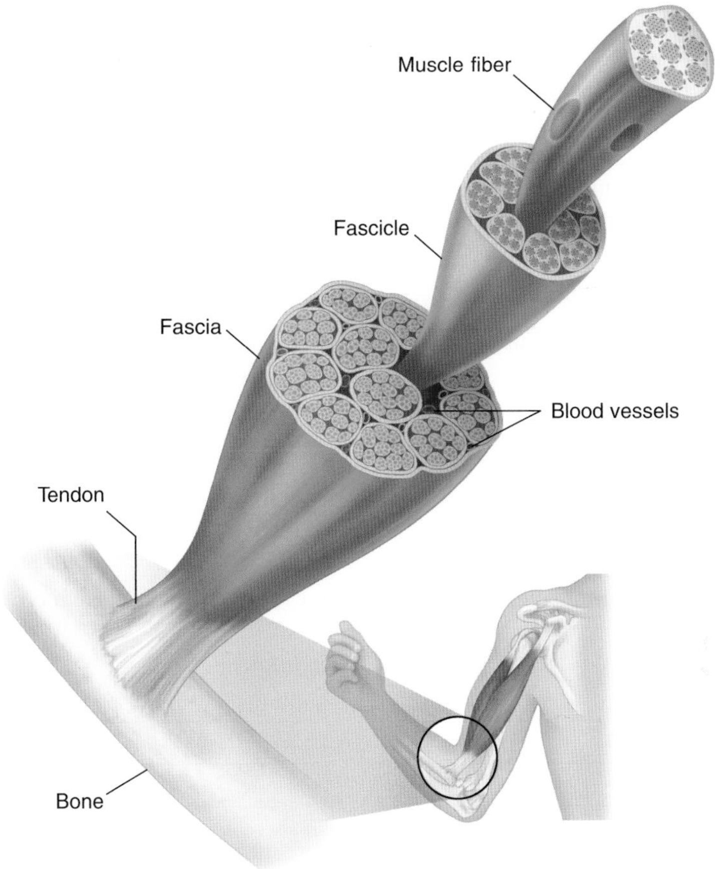


**FIGURE 6-2** Components of skeletal muscle tissue. Tendons attach skeletal muscles to bone.

Contractions of skeletal muscles pull on bones at joints to produce movement. The muscle that is responsible for the main movement is considered the **prime mover** or **agonist**. The muscle that opposes the movement is the **antagonist.** For example, in the arm, the biceps brachii (anterior arm muscle) is the prime mover, and the triceps brachii (posterior arm muscle) is its antagonist. After contracting, muscle tension lessens, and muscles then relax (see Figure 6-3). Review **Table 5-2** in the previous chapter, which describes muscle movements at a joint.

Skeletal muscle is also known as **striated muscle** because the dark and light bands in the muscle fibers create a striated (striped) appearance. Skeletal muscle is unlike smooth or cardiac muscle because skeletal muscle is voluntary. It also produces heat, which is generated by rapid, small contractions (shivering), and these muscles maintain posture.

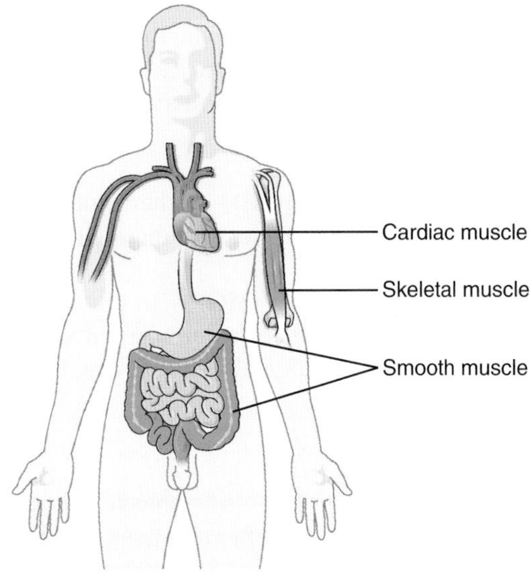


**FIGURE 6-3** The three types of muscle tissue and their locations.

## Smooth Muscle

**Smooth muscle**, which acts involuntarily, lines blood vessels, respiratory passageways, the digestive tract, and walls of hollow internal organs (see Figure 6-3). In blood vessels, smooth muscle contractions regulate the diameter of the vessels to help control blood flow. In respiratory passageways, smooth muscle regulates air flow; and in the digestive tract, smooth muscle contracts to move substances through passageways with wavelike motions. Smooth muscle is also known as **nonstriated muscle** because it lacks the striped appearance that skeletal muscle has.

## Cardiac Muscle

**Cardiac muscle**, also known as heart muscle, forms the wall of the heart (see Figure 6-3). It acts involuntarily and has a lightly striated appearance. Cardiac muscle is responsible for the heart's pumping action. This subject is discussed in detail in Chapter 10.



### Quick Check

Name the three types of muscle tissue and give an example of where each type may be located.

| MUSCLE TISSUE TYPE | LOCATION |
|---|---|
| 1. ______________________ | ______________________ |
| 2. ______________________ | ______________________ |
| 3. ______________________ | ______________________ |

# DISORDERS RELATED TO THE MUSCULAR SYSTEM

Disorders of the muscular system often involve other systems. However, the terms introduced in the following discussion are specific to the muscular system only.

Most muscle disorders are caused by physical trauma, such as those occurring in sports or accidents. Others are chronic and are listed first.

## Chronic Disorders

**Muscular dystrophy (MD)** is a hereditary, progressive degenerative disorder that causes skeletal muscle weakness. The most common childhood MD is **Duchenne dystrophy**, which affects only males.

**Myasthenia gravis (MG)** is an immunologic disorder characterized by fluctuating weakness, especially of the facial and external eye muscles. Signs and symptoms can include drooping eyelids, double vision, difficulty talking, and **dysphagia** (difficulty swallowing).

Two words that students commonly mix up are dysphagia and dysphasia. Considering the words are only one letter apart, it's easy to do. The root word of dysphagia is the Greek word ***phage***, meaning "eater." So dysphagia is difficulty swallowing. The root word of dysphasia is the Greek word ***phase***, meaning "to speak." So dysphasia is difficulty speaking.

**Fibromyalgia** is a disorder characterized by widespread aching and stiffness of muscles and soft tissues, fatigue, tenderness, and sleep disorders. The cause of fibromyalgia is unknown, and it may coexist with other chronic diseases.

**Amyotrophic lateral sclerosis** (ALS), also called *Lou Gehrig's disease*, is considered a neurologic disease that affects the nerves and nervous system, but its signs and symptoms are seen in the muscles. It is a fatal, progressive degeneration of the nerve tracts of the spinal cord leading to muscular **atrophy**, which is muscle shrinking and wasting.

## Cumulative Trauma and Sports Injuries

Cumulative trauma disorders (CTDs) are often caused by repetitive, work-related motions that damage muscles, tendons, joints, or nerves. A common one is **carpal tunnel syndrome**, which is a painful condition of the hand and fingers caused by compression of the median nerve in the wrist (see Figure 6-4).

The rotator cuff of the shoulder is formed by four muscles and reinforcing tendons of the shoulder joint. When these muscles become inflamed and swollen from overuse, a **rotator cuff injury** occurs.

**Epicondylitis** is an inflammation of an epicondyle, a bony projection on the distal humerus. When the lateral epicondyle is affected, it is termed "tennis elbow" because it is common in tennis players. When the medial epicondyle is affected, it is known as "golfer's elbow" because it is common in golfers (see Figure 6-5).



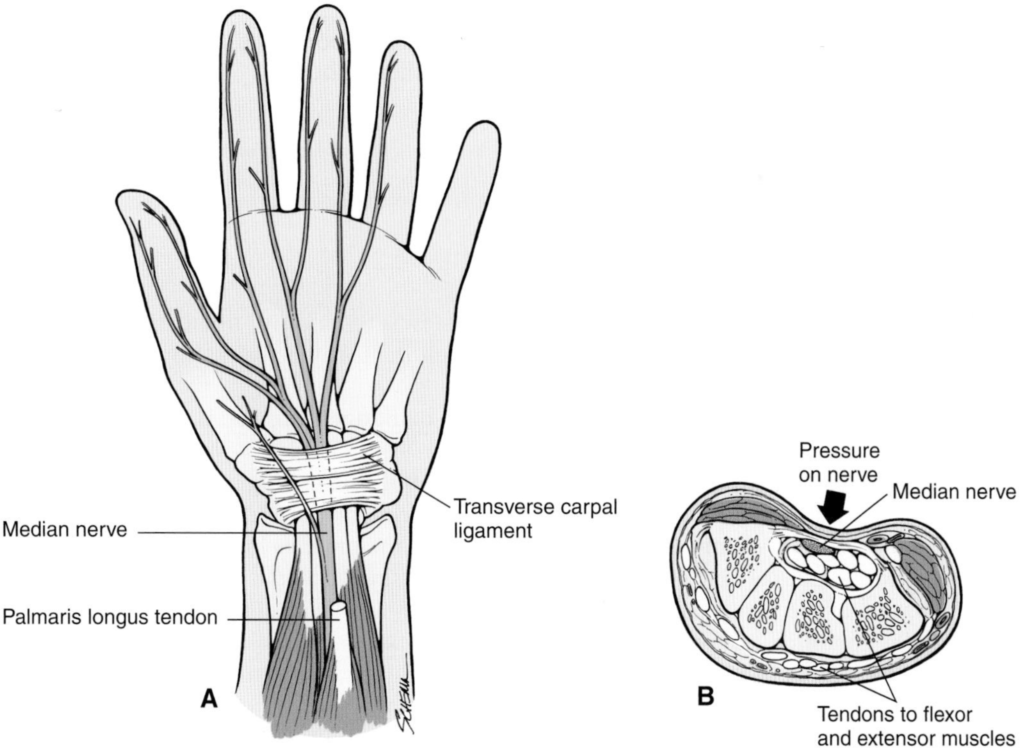


**FIGURE 6-4** Carpal tunnel syndrome. **A.** Pressure on the median nerve as it passes through the carpal (wrist) bones causes numbness and weakness in the areas of the hand supplied by the nerve. **B.** Cross-section of the wrist shows compressing of the median nerve.

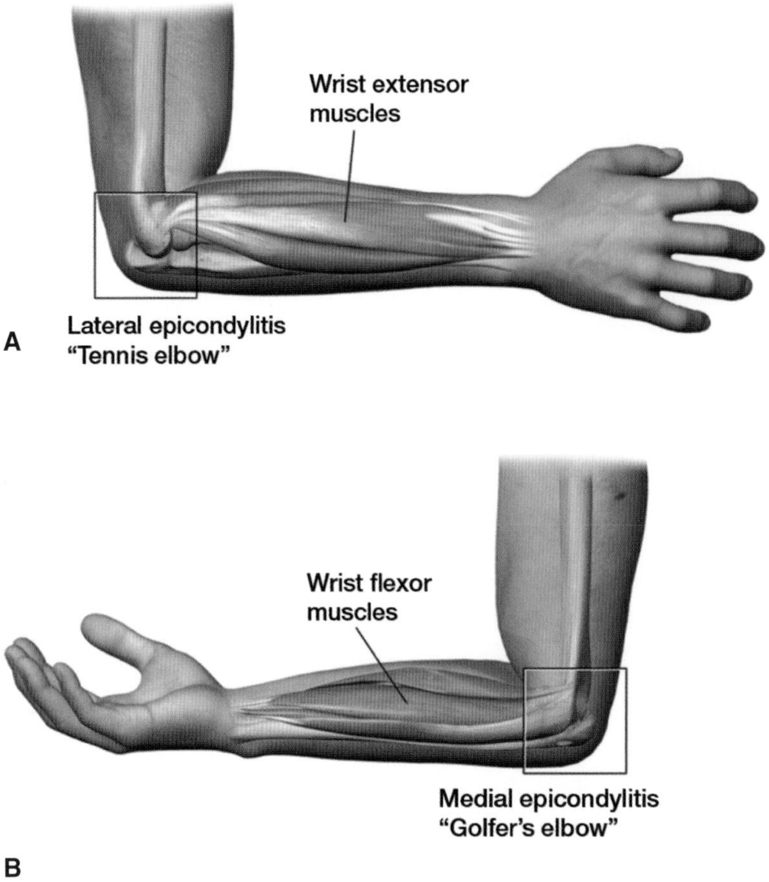


**FIGURE 6-5** Epicondylitis. **A.** Tennis elbow (lateral epicondylitis). **B.** Golfer's elbow (medial epicondylitis).



**Plantar fasciitis** is an inflammation of the plantar fascia (connective tissue in the arch of the foot) that can cause intense pain when walking or running. It may be caused by long periods of weight bearing, sudden changes in activity, or obesity.

Sports injuries often occur to overstressed or poorly conditioned muscles. However, injuries can occur to professional athletes in good physical condition. Two examples are *hamstring injuries* and *shin-splints*. A **hamstring injury** is a strain or tear in one of the hamstring muscles (group of three posterior thigh muscles). This injury is common among sprinters, track hurdlers, baseball players, or football players. **Shin-splints** is tenderness and pain in the muscles in the lower leg following athletic overexertion. It may include a stress fracture (Fx) (small crack in the bone) of the tibia or an inflammation of the periosteum. Shin-splints is actually a collective term describing the pain rather than the condition.

## Paralysis and Paresis

**Paralysis** is the loss of voluntary muscle movement caused by injury or disease. **Paresis** is partial or incomplete paralysis. Below are examples.

- **Hemiparesis:** weakness or paralysis affecting one side of the body
- **Hemiplegia:** total paralysis of one side of the body
- **Paraplegia:** paralysis of both legs and generally the lower trunk
- **Quadriplegia:** paralysis of all four extremities

## DIAGNOSTIC TESTS, TREATMENTS, AND SURGICAL PROCEDURES

Unfortunately for many of the chronic muscle conditions, there is no cure, only treatment of symptoms. For MD, steroids are used to reduce inflammation.

Like MD, there is no cure for MG. Treatment consists of antiacetylcholinesterase medications to keep the neurotransmitter acetylcholine at certain body sites to continue activating muscles. Steroids can reduce muscle inflammation in MG as well. Because there is also an immune component to this disease, immunosuppressant agents (drugs that reduce the body's immune response to itself) can be used to suppress immune reactions.

Amyotrophic lateral sclerosis is a progressive disease of the nervous system that also affects muscles. As nerve cells that control the body's muscles die, the person's ability to control their muscles vanishes. Current treatments cannot reverse this, so treatments are only to slow progression and to make the person more comfortable. As of 2017, the only approved drug to slow progression is Rilutek (riluzole). Other treatments consist of breathing therapy as the muscles needed to breathe start atrophying, occupational and physical therapy for skeletal muscles, and nutritional support.

Treatment of sports injuries commonly consists of rest, ice, compression (bandaging), and elevation, abbreviated "RICE." Intramuscular (IM) injections for pain are sometimes given.

## PRACTICE AND PRACTITIONERS

**Myology** is the branch of science concerned with study of muscles and their accessory structures, including tendons, bursae, and fasciae. The medical specialists who treat disorders of the muscular system are similar to (and in some cases the same as) the specialists who treat disorders of the skeletal system, as discussed in Chapter 5. This includes **orthopedic surgeons**, **kinesiologists**, **occupational therapists**, and **physical therapists**. Many conditions involve joints as well as muscles, and orthopedic physicians diagnose and treat patients with joint disorders.

What is the difference between an abbreviation and an acronym? We speak each letter of an abbreviation, like ALS, and we pronounce an acronym from the sound its letter combination makes. Because RICE spells a common word, it is often pronounced. Most acronyms do not start out as common English words. So, is RICE an acronym? Even though many health care workers treat it as an acronym, it remains an abbreviation and its pronunciation as a word includes the potential for confusing the general population.

**Abbreviation Table** THE MUSCULAR SYSTEM

| ABBREVIATION | MEANING |
|---|---|
| ALS | amyotrophic lateral sclerosis |
| EMG | electromyography |
| Fx | fracture |
| IM | intramuscular |
| MD | muscular dystrophy |
| MG | myasthenia gravis |
| NSAID | nonsteroidal anti-inflammatory drug |
| PT | physical therapy |
| RICE | rest, ice, compression, elevation |
| ROM | range of motion |

**Study Table** THE MUSCULAR SYSTEM

| TERM AND PRONUNCIATION | ANALYSIS | MEANING |
|---|---|---|
| **Structure and Function** | | |
| agonist (AG-on-ist) | from the Greek, *agon* (contest) | muscle that moves a body part when it contracts |
| antagonist (an-TAG-oh-nihst) | a common English word | something (or in common use, someone) opposing or resisting the action of another |
| cardiac muscle (KAHR-dee-ak MUHS-uhl) | *cardi/o* (heart); *-ac* (adjective); from the Latin word *musculus* (muscle) | involuntary, striated heart muscle |
| fascia (FASH-ee-ah) | the Latin word for *band* | fibrous sheath of connective tissue that covers a muscle |
| fascicle (FAS-ih-kul) | from the Latin, *fasciculus (bundle)* | bundle of muscle fibers |
| ligament (LIG-ah-ment) | from the Latin noun *ligamen* (string) | a fibrous connective tissue connecting bones, cartilage, or other tissue structures |
| muscle fiber (MUHS-ul FIGH-bur) | from the Latin, *fibra* (fiber) | the term for a muscle cell |
| nonstriated muscle (non-STRY-ay-ted MUHS-uhl) | non- (adjective); from the Latin verb *striare* (to groove) | muscle that lacks the overlapping myofilaments (muscle proteins) that are found in striated (skeletal) muscles |
| prime mover | two common English words; from the Latin *primus*, meaning first | muscle that has the principal responsibility for a given movement |
| smooth muscle (smooth MUHS-uhl) | common English word; from the Latin word *musculus* (muscle) | involuntary, unstriated muscle of the internal organs and blood vessels |
| skeletal muscle (SKEL-uh-tuhl MUHS-uhl) | *sceleton* (modern Latin for skeleton); -al (adjective); *musculus* (Latin word for muscle) | voluntary, striated muscle connected to the bony framework of the body |
| striated muscle (STRY-ay-ted MUHS-ul) | from the Latin verb *striare* (to groove) | muscle with overlapping myofilaments (muscle proteins); also called skeletal muscle |
| tendon (TEN-dun) | from the Latin verb *tendo* (stretch) | a nonstretching fibrous cord that is part of the muscle complex, such as the Achilles tendon, associated with appendicular muscles |
| tone, tonicity | from the Greek word *tonos* | tension present in resting muscles |

**Study Table** THE MUSCULAR SYSTEM (*continued*)

| TERM AND PRONUNCIATION | ANALYSIS | MEANING |
|---|---|---|
| **Disorders** | | |
| amyotrophic lateral sclerosis (ay-my-oh-TROH-fik) | *a-* (deficient); *my/o* (muscle); lateral (side); *scler/o* (hard); *-osis* (abnormal condition) | a progressive degeneration of the nerve tracts of the spinal cord, causing muscular atrophy; also called Lou Gehrig's disease |
| asthenia (as-THEEN-ee-ah) | *a-* (deficient); *sthenos* (Greek word for strength) | weakness |
| atonia (AY-toh-nee-ah) | *a-* (deficient); *tonia* (tone) | flaccidity; lack of muscle tone; relaxation of muscle |
| atrophy (a-TROH-fee) | *a-* (deficient); *-trophy* (from the Greek word *trophé* meaning "nourishment") | wasting of the muscles |
| carpal tunnel syndrome | carpal (a wrist bone); tunnel (common English word); syndrome (a Greek word meaning "running together") | entrapment of the median nerve in the wrist with chronically swollen and inflamed tendons |
| dysphagia (dis-FEY-juh) | *dys-* (Greek for bad); *-phage* (Greek word for eater) | difficulty swallowing |
| epicondylitis (EP-ih-KON-dih-LYE-tis) | *epi-* (around); *condyl* (rounded end surface of a bone); *-itis* (inflammation) | inflammation of the tissues around the elbow; golfer's or tennis elbow |
| fibromyalgia (FY-broh-MY-al-jee-ah) | *fibr/o* (fiber); *my/o* (muscle); *-algia* (pain) | a chronic disorder characterized by widespread aching and stiffness of muscles and soft tissues, accompanied by fatigue |
| hamstring injury | hamstring muscle | strain or tear of the hamstring muscle group (posterior femoral muscle group) |
| hemiparesis (hem-ee-PAH-ree-sis) | *hemi-* (half); *-paresis* (paralysis) | weakness affecting one side of the body |
| hemiplegia (hem-ee-PLEE-jee-ah) | *hemi-* (half); *-plegia* (paralysis) | total paralysis of one side of the body |
| muscular dystrophy (DIS-tro-fee) | muscular (common English word); *dys-* (difficult); *-trophy* (from the Greek word *trophé* meaning "nourishment") | group of inherited muscle disorders that cause muscle weakness without affecting the nervous system |
| myalgia (mahy-AL-juh) | *my/o* (muscle); -algia (pain) | muscle pain |
| myasthenia gravis (MY-ahs-THEE-nee-ah GRA-viss) | *my/o* (muscle); asthenia (from the Greek word *astheneia* meaning "weakness") | an immunologic disorder characterized by fluctuating weakness, especially of the facial and external eye muscles |

*(continued)*

**Study Table** THE MUSCULAR SYSTEM (*continued*)

| TERM AND PRONUNCIATION | ANALYSIS | MEANING |
|---|---|---|
| myocele (MY-oh-seel) | *my/o* (muscle); *-cele* (hernia) | hernia of a muscle |
| myalgia (my-AL-jee-a) | *my/o* (muscle); (pain); *-algia* (pain) | muscle pain |
| myoma (my-OH-muh) | *my/o* (muscle); *-oma* (tumor) | benign neoplasm of muscle tissue |
| myositis (my-oh-SY-tihs) | *my/o* (s) (muscle); *-itis* (inflammation) | inflammation of muscle |
| myospasm (MY-oh-spaz-uhm) | *my/o* (muscle); *-spasm* (involuntary motion) | involuntary contraction of a muscle |
| paralysis (pah-RAL-ih-sis) | *para-* (not normal); *-lysis* (loosening) | loss of voluntary muscle movements caused by an injury or disease |
| paraplegia (PAR-ah-PLEE-jee-ah) | *para-* (not normal); *-plegia* (paralysis) | paralysis of both legs and the lower trunk |
| paresis (puh-REE-sis) | from the Greek *parienai* (a letting go or slackening) | partial or incomplete paralysis |
| periostitis (PEHR-ee-os-TY-tihs) | *peri-* (around); *oste/o* (bone); *-itis* (inflammation) | inflammation of the periosteum or the covering that surrounds the bone |
| plantar fasciitis (FASH-ee-eye-tis) | plantar (sole of the foot); fasci- (from *fascia,* Latin for band); *-itis* (inflammation) | inflammation of the plantar fascia causing foot and heel pain |
| quadriplegia (kwah-drah-PLEE-jee-ah) | *quadri* (four); *-plegia* (paralysis) | paralysis of all four extremities |
| rotator cuff injury | rotator cuff (four muscles in the shoulder); injury (common English word) | inflammation of the muscles and associated structures in the shoulder (rotator cuff) caused by overuse |
| shin-splints | two common English words used in an uncommon expression | term given to describe pain in the anterior portion of the lower leg during running, walking, and other similar activities |
| tendonitis (ten-doe-NY-tiss); also sometimes spelled tendinitis (TEN-dih-NY-tiss) | *tendon/o* (tendon); *-itis* (inflammation) | inflammation of a tendon |
| **Diagnostic Tests, Treatments, and Surgical Procedures** | | |
| electromyography (ee-LEK-troh-my-OG-rafee) | *electr/o* (electricity); *my/o* (muscle); *-graphy* (process of writing) | abbreviation is EMG; records the strength of muscle contractions by means of electrical stimulation |

**Study Table** THE MUSCULAR SYSTEM (*continued*)

| TERM AND PRONUNCIATION | ANALYSIS | MEANING |
|---|---|---|
| myectomy (my-EKK-tuh-mee) | *my/o* (muscle); *-ectomy* (excision) | excision of part of a muscle |
| physical therapy | common English phrase | treatment to prevent disability and restore function through the use of heat, exercise, and massage to improve circulation, strength, flexibility, and muscle strength |
| skeletal muscle relaxants | *skelet/o* (skeleton); *-al* (adjective suffix); relaxant: that which relaxes | medications used to reduce muscle spasm |
| tendinoplasty (TEN-dih-no-plass-tee) | *tendin/o* (tendon); *-plasty* (surgical repair) | surgical repair of a tendon |
| tenorrhaphy (TEN-oh-raff-ee) | *ten/o* (tendon); *-rrhaphy* (suturing) | suturing of a tendon |
| tenotomy (ten-AW-tuh-mee) | *ten/o* (tendon); *-tomy* (incision) | incision into a tendon |
| **Practice and Practitioners** | | |
| kinesiology (kih-nee-see-AWL-uh-jee) | *kinesi/o* (movement); *-logy* (study of) | study of muscle motion |
| kinesiologist (kih-nee-see-AWL-uh-jist) | *kinesi/o* (movement); *-logist* (one who studies) | a specialist in kinesiology |
| myology (my-AWL-uh-jee) | *my/o* (muscle); *-logy* (study of) | study of muscles |
| occupational therapist (ok-YOU-pey-shun-uhl THER-uh-pist) | *occupationem* (Latin for business); *therapia* (Latin for curing the sick) | practitioner who works to increase independent function through therapy |
| orthopedic (or-thoh-PEE-dik) | *orth/o* (straight); *pedics* (child); note: the word was coined in the 18th century, originating with the study of skeletal disorders in children | pertaining to orthopedics or the study of the musculoskeletal system |
| orthopedic surgeon (or-thoh-PEE-dik SUR-juhn) | *orth/o* (straight); *pedics* (child); surgeon (common English word) | a physician in the field of orthopedics (can be MD or DO) |
| physical therapist (FIZ-i-kul THER-uh-pist) | *physicalis* (Latin for nature); *therapia* (Latin for curing the sick) | practitioner who works to restore correct muscle movement and ability |

## END-OF-CHAPTER EXERCISES

### EXERCISE 6-1 WORD PARTS

**Break each of the following terms into its word parts: prefix, root, or suffix. Give the meaning of each word part and then define the term.**

1. *fibromyalgia*

   root: ____________________

   root: ____________________

   suffix: ____________________

   definition: ____________________

2. *periostitis*

   prefix: ____________________

   root: ____________________

   suffix: ____________________

   definition: ____________________

3. *tendinoplasty*

   root: ____________________

   suffix: ____________________

   definition: ____________________

4. *myology*

   root: ____________________

   suffix: ____________________

   definition: ____________________

5. *electromyography*

   root: ____________________

   root: ____________________

   suffix: ____________________

   definition: ____________________

6. *epicondylitis*

   prefix: ____________________

   root: ____________________

   suffix: ____________________

   definition: ____________________

7. *hemiplegia*

prefix: ____________________

root: ____________________

definition: ____________________

8. *paralysis*

prefix: ____________________

suffix: ____________________

definition: ____________________

## EXERCISE 6-2 WORD BUILDING

**Use the word parts listed to build the terms defined.**

| | | | |
|---|---|---|---|
| -algia | -cele | fasci/o | fibr/o |
| hemi- | -itis | kinesi/o | -logist |
| -logy | muscul/o | my/o | neur/o |
| para- | -paresis | -pathy | -plegia |
| tendin/o | ten/o | -tomy | -trophy |

1. ____________________ incision into a tendon
2. ____________________ physician who diagnoses and treats diseases of the nervous system
3. ____________________ paralysis of both legs and the lower part of the body
4. ____________________ hernia of a muscle
5. ____________________ slight paralysis of one side of the body
6. ____________________ inflammation of the fascia
7. ____________________ pain resulting from movement
8. ____________________ a chronic disorder characterized by widespread aching
9. ____________________ any disease of the muscle
10. ____________________ inflammation of a muscle

## EXERCISE 6-3 MATCHING

**Match the term with its definition.**

| | |
|---|---|
| 1. _________ antagonist | a. fibrous sheath of connective tissue that covers a muscle |
| 2. _________ myoma | b. surgical repair of a tendon |
| 3. _________ tenorrphapy | c. hernia of a muscle |
| 4. _________ tenontoplasty | d. something opposing or resisting the action of another |
| 5. _________ myocele | e. flaccidity; lack of muscle tone; relaxing of muscle |
| 6. _________ atonia | f. suturing of a tendon |
| 7. _________ fascia | g. involuntary contraction of a muscle |
| 8. _________ myospasm | h. a type of muscle structure associated with appendicular muscles |
| 9. _________ atrophy | i. benign neoplasm of muscle tissue |
| 10. _________ tendon | j. a type of muscle tissue connecting bones, cartilage, or other tissue structures |
| 11. _________ prime mover | k. wasting of the muscles |
| 12. _________ ligament | l. muscle that has the principal responsibility for a given movement |



## EXERCISE 6-4 MULTIPLE CHOICE

**Choose the correct answer for the following multiple choice questions.**

1. The three types of muscle tissue are ___________________.
   a. smooth, cardiac, deltoid
   b. cardiac, epicardium, skeletal
   c. cardiac, skeletal, smooth
   d. skeletal, trapezius, deltoid

2. Physicians in which of the following medical specialty(ies) take care of muscular disorders?
   a. neurology
   b. orthopedic
   c. neurology and orthopedics
   d. chiropractic and orthopedics

3. Kinesiology is the study of ___________________.
   a. dance
   b. movement
   c. aerobics
   d. athletics

4. A person who is quadriplegic is paralyzed in ________________ limbs.
   a. one
   b. two
   c. three
   d. four

5. Carpal tunnel syndrome affects the ________________.
   a. wrist
   b. knee
   c. elbow
   d. ankle

6. A muscle antagonist is ________________.
   a. a muscle that resists the action of another
   b. a muscle that has the principal responsibility for a given movement
   c. a type of muscle that connects one muscle to another
   d. none of the above

7. Which muscular disease is usually diagnosed is childhood and affects males?
   a. MG
   b. multiple sclerosis
   c. MD
   d. paraplegia

8. This is a progressive degeneration of the nerve tracts of the spinal cord, causing muscular atrophy, also known as Lou Gehrig's disease:
   a. ALS
   b. asthenia
   c. multiple sclerosis
   d. paraplegia

9. This type of muscle has fibers with noticeable overlapping myofilaments and is involuntary.
   a. cardiac
   b. nonstriated
   c. smooth
   d. skeletal

10. This is an immunologic disorder characterized by fluctuating weakness, especially of the facial and external eye muscle.
    a. MG
    b. fibromyalgia
    c. MD
    d. paraplegia

## EXERCISE 6-5 FILL IN THE BLANK

**Fill in the blank with the correct answer.**

1. ____________________ is the medical term for tennis elbow.
2. The term, which is also the Latin word for string, that names what connects bones to bones to support muscles is ____________________.
3. Pointing the toes downward is called ____________________.
4. ____________________ is the term for weakness.
5. A hernia of a muscle is called ____________________.
6. ____________________ causes intense pain in the heel region and sole of the foot upon walking.
7. A(n) ____________________ records the strength of muscle contractions.
8. The surgical repair of a tendon is called ____________________.
9. ____________________ is the study of muscles.
10. Muscle pain is called ____________________.



## EXERCISE 6-6 ABBREVIATIONS

**Write out the term for the following abbreviations.**

1. ________________________________ MD
2. ________________________________ RICE
3. ________________________________ CTD
4. ________________________________ MG

**Write the abbreviation for the following terms.**

5. ________________ electromyography
6. ________________ amyotrophic lateral sclerosis
7. ________________ intramuscular
8. ________________ fracture
9. ________________ muscular dystrophy

## EXERCISE 6-7 SPELLING

**Select the correct spelling of the medical term.**

1. ___________________ means weakness.
   a. Athenia
   b. Athena
   c. Asthenia
   d. Asthena

2. ___________________ is a chronic disorder characterized by widespread aching and stiffness of muscles and soft tissues, accompanied by fatigue.
   a. Fibromyalgia
   b. Fibromylgia
   c. Fibromyalga
   d. Fibomyalgia

3. The name of this disorder comes from the root word meaning *muscle* and the Greek word meaning *weakness*.
   a. myathenia gravis
   b. myasthenia gravis
   c. myasthenia graviss
   d. myathenia graviss

4. ___________________ means difficulty swallowing.
   a. Disphagia
   b. Disfagia
   c. Dysfagia
   d. Dysphagia

5. ___________________ is also known as Lou Gehrig's disease.
   a. Amotrophic lateral sclerosis
   b. Amyotrophic lateral sklerosis
   c. Amotrophic lateral sclarosis
   d. Amyotrophic lateral sclerosis

6. The muscle movement that closes the angle of a joint is called ___________________.
   a. flextion
   b. flexsion
   c. flexion
   d. flexon

7. Cardiac muscle is considered lightly ___________________, and skeletal muscle is considered heavily ___________________.
   a. stryated
   b. striatted
   c. striated
   d. strieted

8. ___________________ describes paralysis of all four extremities.
   a. Quadraplegia
   b. Quadriplegia
   c. Quadraplesia
   d. Quadriplesia

9. An ___________________ surgeon is a physician who specializes in the musculoskeletal system.
   a. orthopedic
   b. orthapedic
   c. orthopaedik
   d. orthopedik

10. A ___________________ is the connective tissue connecting bones and cartilage.
   a. ligament
   b. ligument
   c. legament
   d. liguhment

## EXERCISE 6-8 CASE STUDY

PHYSICAL THERAPY PROGRESS NOTE

**CHIEF COMPLAINT:** Cervical neck pain with limited movement and right shoulder pain with limited ROM.

**PROGRESS:** The patient states that he is the same as he was the last time he was in for therapy.

**AGGRAVATING FACTORS:** Working.

**PAIN/DISCOMFORT LEVEL:** The patient states that the pain is 5/10.

**TREATMENT:** Treatment today consisted of moist heat and ultrasound of the cervical spine; therapeutic exercise to the neck and shoulder for 45 minutes.

**PATIENT'S PROGRESS:** The patient is doing well with his cervical spine exercises. His neck flexion and neck extension and rotation are relatively improved. His radiating pain is reduced. His right shoulder is very painful. He has pain on flexion and abduction. He has pain on resisted abduction. He has rotator cuff tendonitis, probably caused by impingement.

The patient was put on a four-step treatment approach to decrease pain and increase neck and shoulder movement. He was advised to limit the use of his right arm as much as possible for 2 weeks, use ice and NSAIDs for pain, and keep his arm in a sling. He demonstrated improved ROM following his therapy. He was advised to use the exercise program on a regular basis.

**QUESTIONS**

1. What medical terms are associated with the patient's limited neck movements? Define each one. ______________________________

______________________________

2. What does "tendonitis" mean? ______________________________

______________________________

3. Explain what ROM is. ______________________________

______________________________

4. What does NSAID stand for? ______________________________

______________________________

# 7 The Nervous System

## LEARNING OUTCOMES

***Upon completion of this chapter, you should be able to:***

- Name the major structures and functions of the nervous system.
- Name the parts of a neuron.
- Name the major divisions of the nervous system.
- Pronounce, spell, and define medical terms related to the nervous system.
- Interpret abbreviations associated with the nervous system.

## INTRODUCTION

The nervous system, one of the most complex systems in the body, coordinates the body's involuntary and voluntary actions. It works in conjunction with the endocrine system to maintain **homeostasis**, a term that means "a state of equilibrium." The nervous system also works together with the muscular system to control the body's voluntary and involuntary muscles.

The nervous system has two main divisions: the **central nervous system (CNS)** and the **peripheral nervous system (PNS)**. The CNS consists of the brain and spinal cord. The PNS consists of all the nerves outside the CNS, including the cranial nerves and spinal nerves (see Figure 7-1). The PNS is further divided into the *somatic nervous system* and the *autonomic nervous system*. The autonomic nervous system is then further divided into the *sympathetic nervous system* (fight or flight responses) and the *parasympathetic nervous system* (rest and digest responses), depending on what type of involuntary functions it controls (see Figure 7-2).

## WORD PARTS RELATED TO NERVOUS SYSTEM

The CNS's control center is the brain, so many of the word parts used to describe structures of the nervous system are located in the head. Cephal/o is the word root for head, and encephal/o is the word root for brain. Another word root for brain is cerebr/o, which refers specifically to the cerebrum (the largest part of the brain). Both psych/o and ment/o refer to the mind, the part of the brain responsible for consciousness and higher functions. Table 7-1 lists word parts that make up nervous system terms. Some suffixes that you already learned are also listed.

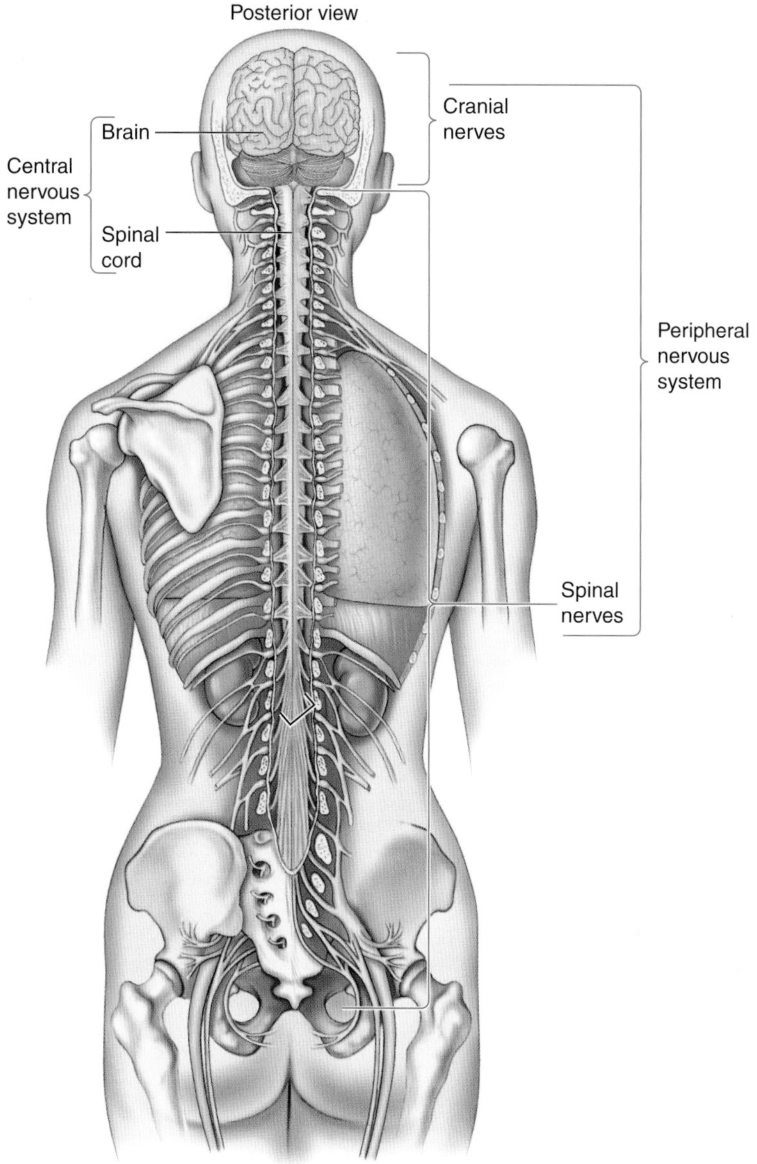


**FIGURE 7-1** A posterior view of the nervous system. The central nervous system consists of the brain and spinal cord, and the peripheral nervous system consists of the cranial nerves and spinal nerves.

## STRUCTURE AND FUNCTION

Nerve tissue, together with its associated connective tissue and blood vessels, makes up both the CNS and the PNS. Nerve tissue is composed of fundamental units called **neurons** (nerve cells), which are separated, supported, and protected by specialized cells called **neuroglia**. Neurons carry electrical messages that coordinate the exchange of information between the body's internal and external environments, and the neuroglia offer protection and support to the nerve tissue. Neurons are grouped together to carry out the highly complex sensing and processing actions required for everything we do.

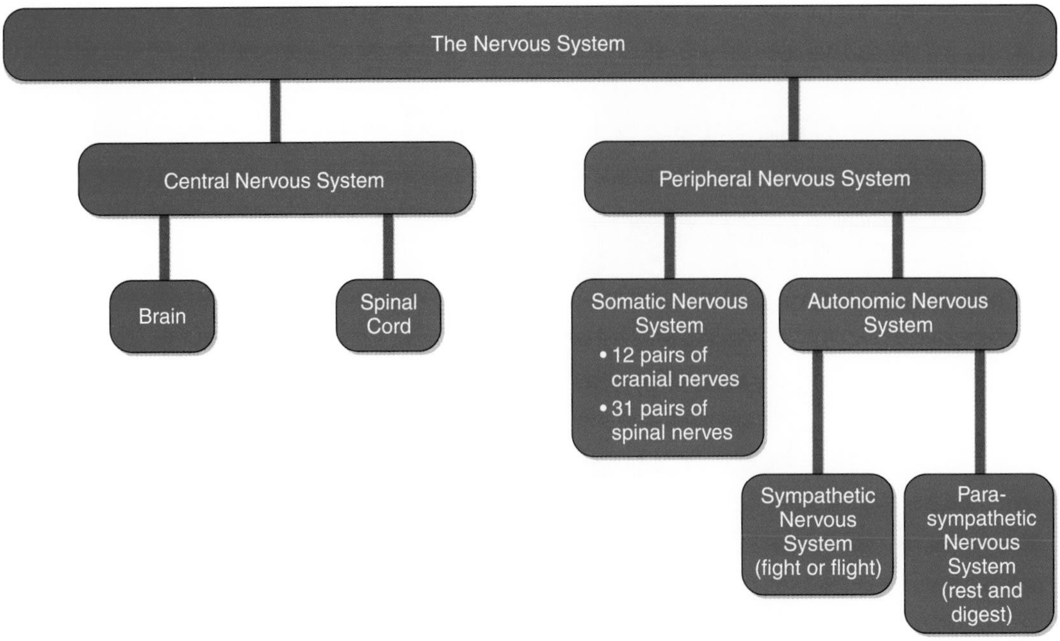


**FIGURE 7-2** The divisions of the nervous system. The chart shows the divisions and subdivisions, but all components work together.

**TABLE 7-1** WORD PARTS RELATED TO THE NERVOUS SYSTEM

| Word Part | Meaning |
|---|---|
| arachn/o | spider |
| cephal/o | head |
| cerebell/o | cerebellum |
| cerebr/o | cerebrum; also, the brain in general |
| cortic/o | outer layer or covering |
| crani/o | cranium, skull |
| encephal/o | brain |
| gangli/o | swelling or knot |
| ganglion/o | swelling or knot |
| gli/o | glue |
| hydr/o | water |
| iatr/o | physician; to treat |
| -mania | morbid attraction to or impulse toward |
| meningi/o | membrane |
| ment/o | referring to the mind |
| -mnesia | memory |
| myel/o | in connection with the nervous system, refers to the spinal cord and medulla oblongata |
| neur/o | nerve, nerve tissue |
| -oid | resembling |

**TABLE 7-1 WORD PARTS RELATED TO THE NERVOUS SYSTEM (*continued*)**

| Word Part | Meaning |
|---|---|
| -paresis | slight paralysis |
| -phasia | speech |
| -phobia | fear |
| -plegia | paralysis |
| psych/o | mind |
| schiz/o | to split |
| spin/o | spine |

## Word Parts Exercise

After studying Table 7-1, write the meaning of each of the word parts.

| WORD PART | MEANING |
|---|---|
| 1. –paresis | 1. ______ |
| 2. cortic/o | 2. ______ |
| 3. ment/o | 3. ______ |
| 4. –plegia | 4. ______ |
| 5. –mnesia | 5. ______ |
| 6. iatr/o | 6. ______ |
| 7. –phobia | 7. ______ |
| 8. encephal/o | 8. ______ |
| 9. cerebr/o | 9. ______ |
| 10. hydr/o | 10. ______ |
| 11. meningi/o | 11. ______ |
| 12. gangli/o | 12. ______ |
| 13. –mania | 13. ______ |
| 14. myel/o | 14. ______ |
| 15. neur/o | 15. ______ |
| 16. arachn/o | 16. ______ |
| 17. schiz/o | 17. ______ |

(*continued*)

## Word Parts Exercise (continued)

| WORD PART | MEANING |
|---|---|
| 18. cephal/o | 18. ________________ |
| 19. psych/o | 19. ________________ |
| 20. –oid | 20. ________________ |
| 21. cerebell/o | 21. ________________ |
| 22. spin/o | 22. ________________ |
| 23. –phasia | 23. ________________ |
| 24. gli/o | 24. ________________ |

The three main parts of a neuron cell are its *cell body*, *dendrites*, and *axon*. The **cell body** contains the nucleus and receives nerve impulses (action potentials) from other cells through the dendrites. The **nucleus** is an organelle found in the central region of the cell body that contains genetic material. The **dendrites**, which project outward from the cell body, act as antennae that receive and transmit messages between the neuron and muscles, skin, other neurons, or glands. The cell body passes these messages to the **axon**, which conducts nerve impulses away from the cell body. Axons are covered by **myelin**, a white fatty material that provides protection and insulation (see Figure 7-3). The connecting points for these message transfers are called **synapses**. Synaptic connections can occur between two nerve cells. The stimulus between the two cells is usually a chemical called a **neurotransmitter**. For example, hormones are typical neurotransmitters.

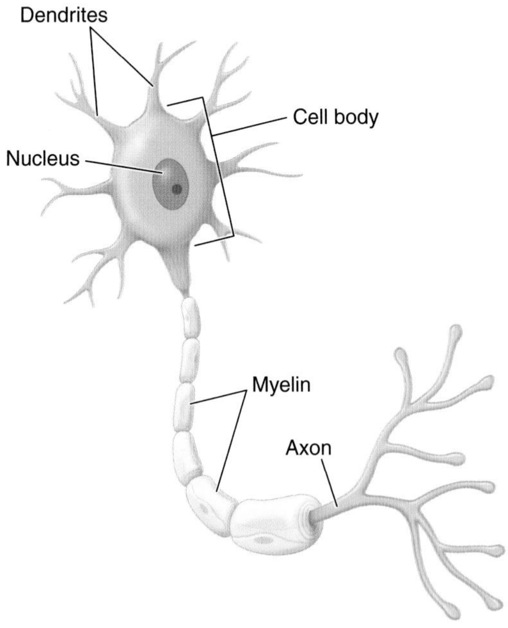


**FIGURE 7-3** Structure of a typical neuron.

Groups of neuron cell bodies within the PNS are called **ganglia** (*ganglion*, singular). Groups of neuron cell bodies within the CNS are called **nuclei** (*nucleus*, singular). Groupings of axons are called **nerves**, wherever they occur in the body.

## Central Nervous System

The CNS is the body's control center. All messages originate and/or terminate either in the brain or in the spinal cord. The brain and spinal cord also interpret the messages and determine the body's responses.

The brain is a large organ that plays a role in many activities, both mental and physical. For example, regions of the brain control bodily functions, such as breathing and temperature regulation, whereas other regions influence walking and other deliberate activities.

The brain is separable into left and right hemispheres each with four lobes: **frontal lobe**, **parietal lobe**, **occipital lobe**, and **temporal lobe** (see Figure 7-4). The names of the lobes relate to their location relative to the skull and the overlying skull bones. For example, *frontal* relates to the front part of the head, *parietal* refers to the sides of the head, *occipital* identifies the back of the head, and *temporal* refers to the temples or area posterior to the eyes on each side of the head.

The major parts of the brain include the following (see Figures 7-4 and 7-5):

- **Cerebrum:** The cerebrum, the largest part of the brain, is where memories and conscious thoughts are stored. It also directs some willed bodily movements. An outer layer of gray matter called the **cerebral cortex** controls higher mental functions.
- **Cerebellum:** The cerebellum, like the larger cerebrum located superiorly to it, also has left and right hemispheres. The cerebellum coordinates voluntary muscles and maintains our balance.
- **Diencephalon:** The diencephalon is the link between the cerebral hemispheres and the brainstem. It contains both the *thalamus* and the *hypothalamus*. The **thalamus** processes sensory information. The **hypothalamus** coordinates the autonomic nervous system and the pituitary gland. It releases hormones, controls body temperature, and is involved with mood.
- **Brainstem:** The brainstem contains connects the brain to the spinal cord. It is made up of the *midbrain*, *pons* (Latin for *bridge*), and *medulla oblongata*. The **midbrain** processes visual and audible sensory information. Visual tracking, such as moving the eyes to read or follow a moving object, is an example of a midbrain function. It also transmits hearing impulses to the brain. The **pons** passes information to the cerebellum and the thalamus to control subconscious activities such as regulating breathing. The **medulla oblongata** sends sensory

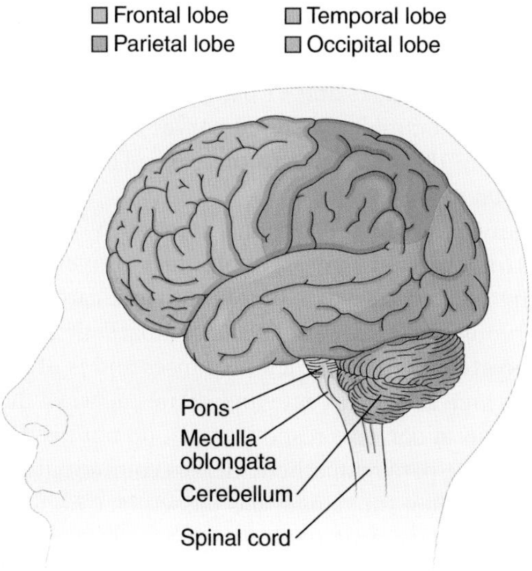


**FIGURE 7-4** Lateral view of the four brain lobes and pons, medulla oblongata, cerebellum, and spinal cord.

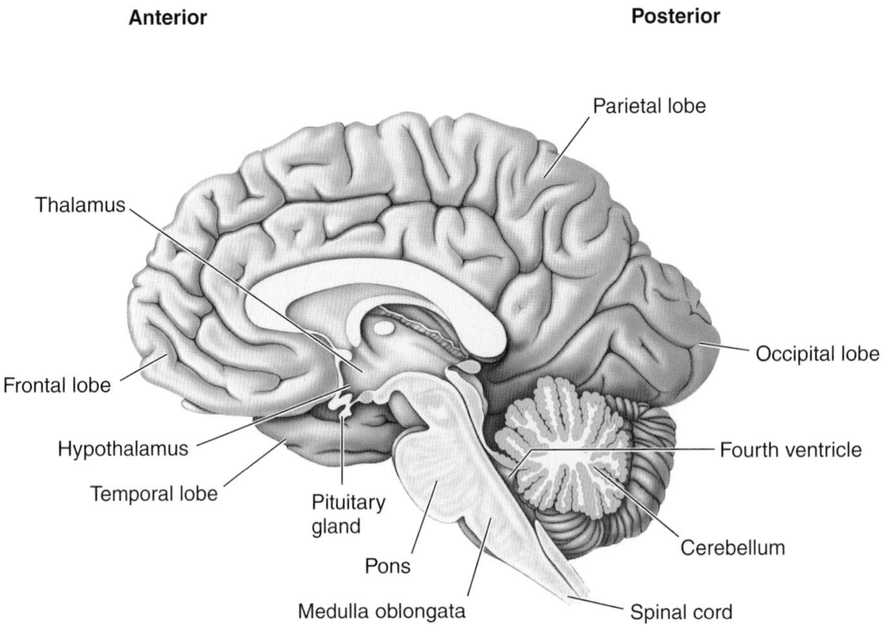


**FIGURE 7-5** A sagittal section of the brain showing important structures.

information to the thalamus to direct the autonomic functions of the heart, lungs, and other body organs. The interconnected cavities within the brain are the **ventricles**. The fourth ventricle is show in Figure 7-5.

The **spinal cord** is the portion of the CNS that is found within the vertebrae that conducts nerve impulses to and from the brain and the body. The brain and spinal cord are surrounded by membranes called **meninges**, which absorb physical shocks that could otherwise damage nerve tissue (see Figure 7-6). The outer layer is the **dura mater**, a dense collection of collagen fibers. The middle layer is the **arachnoid mater**, which is thin, delicate, and weblike. The inner layer, called the **pia mater**, is in direct contact with nerve tissue. Together, the arachnoid and pia mater are two layers of a structure that is called the **leptomeninx**. Cerebrospinal fluid (CSF) is the colorless liquid that circulates in and around the brain and spinal cord that transports nutrients.



## Peripheral Nervous System

The PNS includes 12 pairs of cranial nerves and 31 pairs of spinal nerves that run along the periphery of the body (see Figure 7-1). The cranial and spinal nerves convey directions from the CNS to the PNS and carry information from the PNS back to the CNS. The PNS controls skeletal muscles by means of the cranial and spinal nerves.

Recall that the PNS is divided into the somatic nervous system and the autonomic nervous system. The **somatic nervous system** controls voluntary movement, whereas the **autonomic nervous system** controls involuntary muscles, the smooth and cardiac muscles, and glands. Recall also that the autonomic nervous system is made up of sympathetic and parasympathetic divisions. The **sympathetic nervous system** controls quick responses and is often called the "fight or flight" division because this system increases heart rate and dilates airways during periods of stress. The **parasympathetic nervous system** controls responses that do not need to be fast and is often called the "rest and digest" division. The parasympathetic nerves counterbalance such changes and return the body to a homeostatic state when the danger has passed (see Figure 7-2).

These two divisions of the autonomic nervous system are complementary. The sympathetic nervous system can be thought of as the gas pedal, and the parasympathetic nervous system can be thought of as the brake pedal.

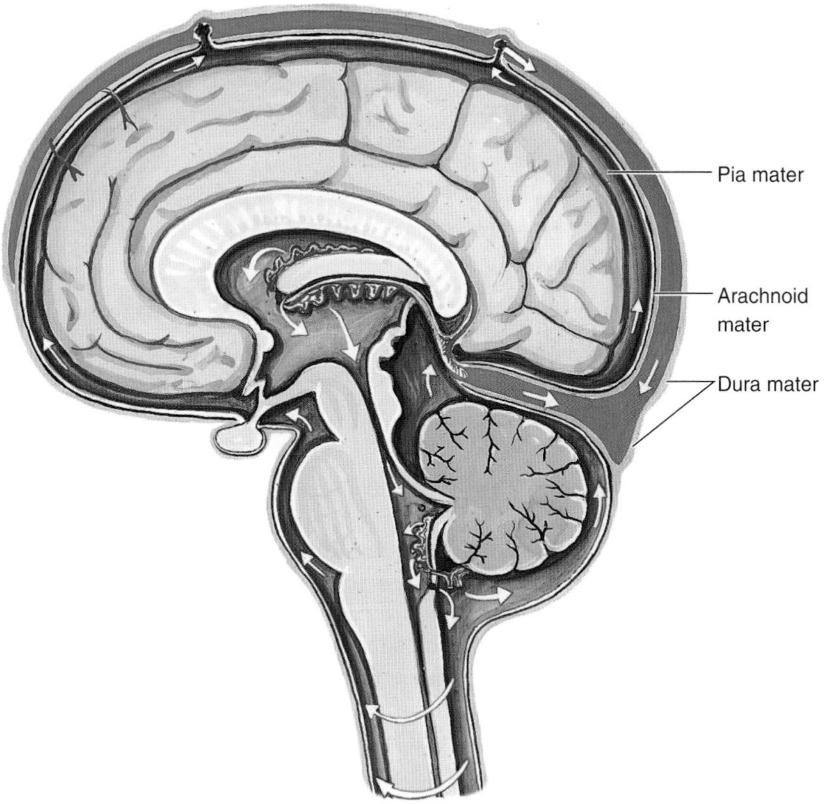


**FIGURE 7-6** The meninges protect the brain and spinal cord. Arrows indicate the flow of cerebrospinal fluid.



## Quick Check

**Fill in the blanks.**

1. The CNS consists of the __________________ and the __________________.
2. The nervous system works in conjunction with the endocrine system to maintain __________________, a term that means "a state of equilibrium."
3. The major parts of the brain include the cerebrum, cerebellum, diencephalon, and __________________.

## DISORDERS RELATED TO THE NERVOUS SYSTEM

Disorders of the nervous system can result from trauma, vascular insults, tumors, systemic degenerative diseases, and seizures. Behavioral disorders are treated as a separate category.

### Trauma

Head injuries can produce skull fractures, hemorrhage, swelling, and direct damage to the brain itself. Brain injury may be relatively mild, involving bruises to brain tissues, or it can be severe,

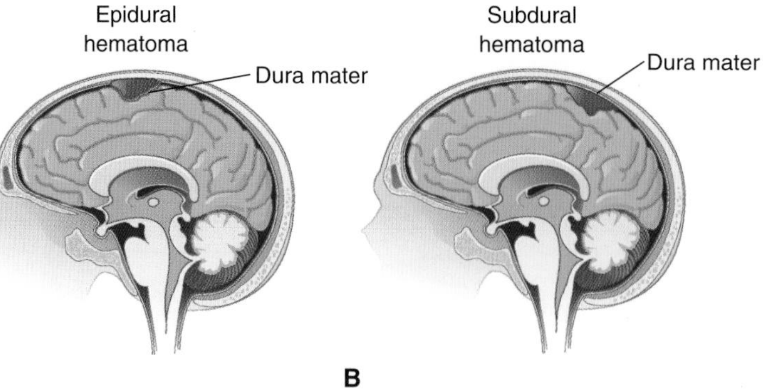


FIGURE 7-7 Hematoma. **A.** Epidural hematoma occurs with a traumatic brain injury when blood accumulates between the dura mater and the skull. **B.** Subdural hematoma occurs between the dura mater and arachnoid mater.

causing tissue destruction and massive swelling. A few common types of brain trauma include the following:

- **Concussion** is an injury to the brain resulting from violent shaking or a hit to the head. A concussion may cause temporary loss of consciousness followed by a short period of amnesia (loss of memory). Dizziness, nausea, and headache are common with a concussion.
- **Epidural hematoma** occurs when blood collects between the dura mater and the skull, causing pressure on the blood vessels and interrupting blood flow to the brain. This condition is caused by a skull fracture or a hit to the head (see Figure 7-7).
- **Subdural hematoma** is a collection of blood trapped in the subdural space, the area beneath the dura mater. It may result from a hit to the front or back of the head (see Figure 7-7).

## Vascular Insults

A vascular insult is an injury to the blood vessels.

- **Cerebrovascular accident (CVA)**: Also known as a stroke, a CVA results from an interruption of oxygen caused by blood vessel blockage or rupture, causing hemorrhage (bleeding) (see Figure 7-8).
- **Transient ischemic attack (TIA)**: A TIA is a temporary interruption in the blood supply to the brain. This is sometimes called a "mini-stroke," but can indicate serious problems and be a forewarning of a stroke.
- **Cerebral aneurysm**: An aneurysm is a localized dilation (widening) of an artery caused by weakness in the vessel wall.



Does not the word "insult" refer to a verbal attack, such as when someone calls someone else a name that causes hurt feelings? Yes, it does, but in the phrase "vascular insult," it means something else. The Latin verb ***insulto*** literally means "to physically jump on." So a vascular insult is a physical event related to that Latin meaning.

## Tumors

Tumors are **lesions** (regions in an organ that are damaged) or neoplasms that may cause localized dysfunction, producing an increase in intracranial pressure (ICP). It is important for the pressure within the cranium to stay within its normal range, as a high ICP usually leads to death if it is not relieved. Tumors may be benign or malignant. Two examples of tumors occurring in the nervous system include *astrocytomas* and *meningiomas*. An **astrocytoma** is a tumor derived from a star-shaped type of neuroglia called an astrocyte. A **meningioma** is a tumor derived from the meninges surrounding the brain and spinal cord.

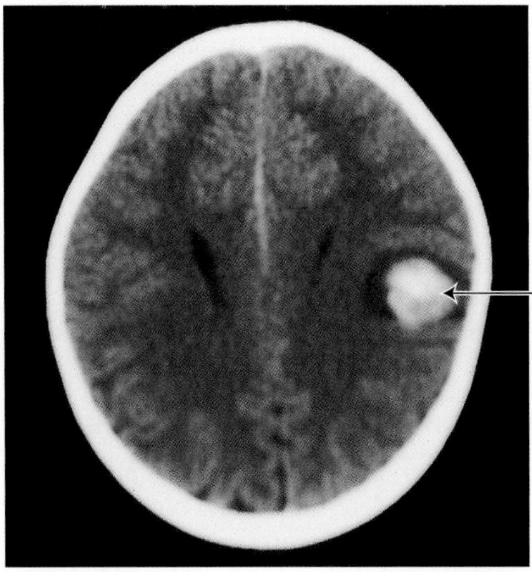


**FIGURE 7-8** Cerebrovascular accident. Computed tomography scan of the brain shows a large hemorrhage in the brain of a 4-year-old boy.

## Systemic Degenerative Diseases

Degenerative diseases develop slowly over time. A progressive deterioration may start out affecting individual body functions and end up involving other body systems. Examples of systemic degenerative diseases include *multiple sclerosis* (MS), *Parkinson's disease* (PD), and *Alzheimer's disease* (AD).

- **MS** is a progressive degenerative disease with symptoms caused by **demyelination**, a patchy loss of the myelin sheath.
- **PD** usually develops after age 60 and occurs with the loss of the neurotransmitter **dopamine** (DA), which inhibits transmission of nerve impulses. When these nerve impulses are no longer inhibited by DA, signs such as tremors and muscle rigidity occur. This can affect posture, balance, speech, and other activities of daily living.
- **AD** is a degenerative, eventually fatal condition involving atrophy of the cerebral cortex, producing a progressive loss of intellectual function.

## Seizures

A **seizure** occurs when there is an abnormal, uncontrolled burst of electrical activity in the brain. Seizures may result from trauma, tumors, fevers, medications, or other causes. Some seizures go unnoticed when the signs are very subtle. Other seizures can cause loss of consciousness or involuntarily body movements.

**Epilepsy** is a chronic disorder characterized by recurrent seizures that result from the excessive discharge of neurons in the brain. Two basic types of epileptic seizures are *grand mal seizures* and *absence seizures*. A **grand mal seizure**, also called a *generalized tonic–clonic seizure*, is severe and characterized by alternating contraction and relaxation of muscles, which produces jerking movements of the face, trunk, and/or extremities. An **absence seizure** (formerly called a *petit mal seizure*) is a milder form of seizure that lasts only a few seconds and does not include convulsive movements. The term *mal* comes from the French language and means "evil."

## Behavioral Disorders

Some behavioral disorders are related to the nervous system. They may be caused by physical changes, substance abuse, medications, or any combination thereof. The categories include anxiety, mood, and psychotic disorders.

- **Anxiety disorders** are characterized by feelings of apprehension or uneasiness, sometimes associated with the anticipation of danger. Common examples include **obsessive–compulsive disorder**

**(OCD)**, which may be signaled by repetitive behaviors; **posttraumatic stress disorder (PTSD)**, which is the development of long-term symptoms following a psychologically traumatic event; and the various **phobias**, which are persistent, irrational fears of specific situations or things.

- **Mood disorders** are a group of mental disorders involving a disturbance of internal emotional states. They include **depression**, which is characterized by loss of interest or pleasure in activities; and **bipolar disorder**, which is characterized by unusual shifts in mood, energy, and activity.
- **Psychotic disorders** are more serious than anxiety or mood disorders because they feature a loss of contact with reality and a deterioration of normal social functioning. An example of a psychosis is **schizophrenia**, which is characterized by abnormal thoughts, hallucinations, delusions, and withdrawal. **Paranoia** is another example characterized by jealousy, delusions of persecution, or perceptions of threat or harm.

## Diagnostic Tests, Treatments, and Surgical Procedures

When evaluating the health of a person's nervous system, medical professionals use various procedures. Sometimes, a patient's mental health is determined by a qualified professional observing and talking with the patient. Other times, diagnostic tests to evaluate the condition of the brain and its function are used. Some examples of diagnostic procedures are listed below.

- **Computed tomography (CT)** is a noninvasive radiologic test that uses a computer to produce cross-sectional images of the soft-tissue structures of the brain and spinal cord. This procedure can reveal problems such as brain tumors and aneurysms.
- **Magnetic resonance imaging (MRI)** uses radio waves and a very strong magnetic field to produce images of the neural soft tissues. It is used to visualize disease-related changes in the brain or spinal cord that conventional X-ray procedures cannot detect. For example, MRI is able to isolate damaged areas of the brain caused by MS.
- **Electroencephalography (EEG)** is the measurement of electrical activity in the brain and the visual trace (electroencephalogram) of that activity. It is used to document increased electrical events of the brain caused by seizures.
- **Lumbar puncture (LP)** requires the insertion of a needle into the subarachnoid space (the area between the arachnoid mater and pia mater) between the third and fourth or fourth and fifth lumbar vertebrae to withdraw CSF for analysis (see Figure 7-9).

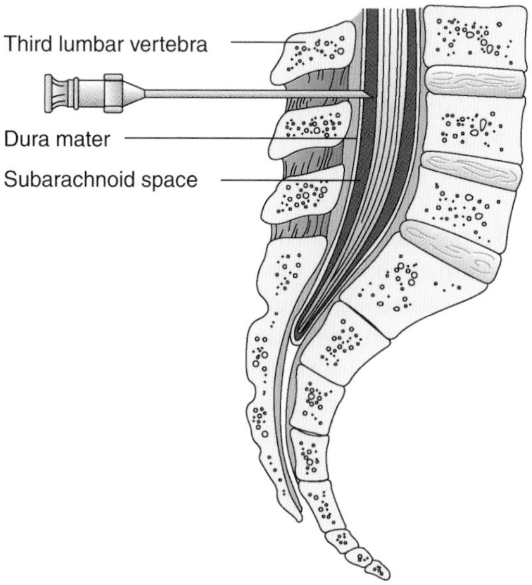


**FIGURE 7-9** Shows the location for a lumbar puncture between L3 and L4.

## PRACTICE AND PRACTITIONERS

The medical specialists who diagnose and treat the nervous system are *neurologists*, *neurosurgeons*, *psychiatrists*, and *psychologists*. **Neurologists** are medical specialists trained in the diagnosis and treatment of neuromuscular disorders. **Neurosurgeons** are physicians specialized in operations on the brain, spinal cord, spinal column, and peripheral nerves. **Psychiatrists** are physicians who treat behavioral and mental health disorders. The health care professional with an advanced academic degree who treats mental and behavioral disorders is a **psychologist**.

What's the difference between a psychiatrist and a psychologist? Using word parts, we can break each word up: psych-olog-ist and psych-iatr-ist. Remember that -logy means "study of" and iatr/o means "physician." The degrees that each profession receives are different: a psychologist has a doctorate degree in the form of a PhD or PsyD, whereas a psychiatrist has an MD or DO and is a medical doctor, meaning they can prescribe medications (unlike a psychologist). This is a key difference and means the two practitioners are not interchangeable; however, they often work together to treat patients.

**Abbreviation Table** THE NERVOUS SYSTEM

| ABBREVIATION | MEANING |
|---|---|
| AD | Alzheimer's disease |
| CNS | central nervous system |
| CSF | cerebrospinal fluid |
| CT | computed tomography |
| CVA | cerebrovascular accident |
| DA | dopamine |
| ECT | electroconvulsive therapy |
| EEG | electroencephalography |
| ICP | intracranial pressure |
| LP | lumbar puncture |
| MRI | magnetic resonance imaging |
| MS | multiple sclerosis |
| OCD | obsessive–compulsive disorder |
| PD | Parkinson's disease |
| PNS | peripheral nervous system |
| PTSD | posttraumatic stress disorder |
| TIA | transient ischemic attack |

**Study Table** THE NERVOUS SYSTEM

| TERM AND PRONUNCIATION | ANALYSIS | MEANING |
|---|---|---|
| **Structure and Function** | | |
| autonomic nervous system (aw-to-NOM-ik NER-vuhs SIS-tuhm) (ANS) | autonomy (self-sufficiency); *-ic* (adjective suffix) | the parts of the PNS that carry messages between the CNS and organs that function autonomously |
| arachnoid mater (ah-RAK-noyd MAY-turh) | from the Greek word *arachne* (spider, cobweb); *-oid* (resembling) | delicate weblike layer of the meninges; middle layer |
| axon (AX-ohn) | *axo-* (axis); *-n* noun ending | the part of a neuron that conducts electrical impulses away from the cell body |
| brainstem (BREYN stem) | common English words | the part of the brain that controls functions, including heart rate, breathing, and body temperature; includes midbrain, pons, and medulla oblongata |
| cell body (sel BOD-ee) | common English words | the main part of a neuron that contains the nucleus |
| central nervous system (SEN-truhl NER-vuhs SIS-tuhm) (CNS) | common English words | the division of the nervous system that includes the brain and spinal cord |
| cerebellum (SERR-uh-bell-uhm) | *cerebr/o* (brain) | the part of the brain that controls the skeletal muscles |
| cerebral cortex (seh-REE-bruhl KOR-tex) | *cerebr/o* (brain); *-al* (adjective suffix) | the gray matter surrounding the cerebrum |
| cerebrospinal fluid (seh-REE-bro-SPY-nuhl) (CSF) | *cerebr/o* (brain); from Latin word *spina*; fluid (common English word) | the fluid in and around the brain and spinal cord |
| cerebrum (seh-REE-bruhm) | *cerebr/o* (brain) | the largest part of the brain; controls conscious thought and stores memories |
| dendrite (DEN-dryte) | from the Greek word *dendrites* (relating to a tree) | process extending from a neuron cell body |
| diencephalon (dy-en-SEFF-uh-lohn) | *di-* (two); *encephal/o* (of or relating to the brain); *-on* (noun suffix) | the part of the brain containing both the thalamus and the hypothalamus |
| dura mater (DOO-ruh MAY-tuhr) | Latin words meaning "hard mother" | the outer meninx, the fibrous membrane protecting the CNS |

**Study Table** THE NERVOUS SYSTEM (*continued*)

| TERM AND PRONUNCIATION | ANALYSIS | MEANING |
|---|---|---|
| frontal lobe (FRUN-tahl lohb) | common English words | the front part of the brain from which voluntary muscle movements and other sensory and motor tasks are directed |
| ganglion (GANG-lee-ohn); plural: ganglia (GANG-lee-uh) | a Greek word meaning "swelling" or "knot" | a group of neuron cell bodies grouped together in the PNS |
| homeostasis (hoh-me-oh-STEY-sis) | *homos* (Greek for "same"); *stasis* (Greek for "existence") | tendency toward equilibrium; remaining normal |
| hypothalamus (HY-po-thal-uh-muhs) | *hypo-* (below, deficient); from the Greek word *thalamus* (a bed, a bedroom) | the hormone and emotion center of the brain that controls autonomic functions |
| leptomeninx (LEPP-toh-ME-ninks) | *lepto-* (light, slender, thin frail); meninx is plural form of *mening/o* (membrane) | collective term for the arachnoid mater and pia mater |
| medulla oblongata (meh-DUH-luh ohb-lohng-GAH-tuh) | a Latin word (marrow); from the Latin *oblongatus* (oblong) | the part of the brainstem that sends sensory information to the thalamus to direct the autonomic functions of the heart, lungs, and other organs |
| meninges (meh-NIHN-jees) | *mening/o* (membrane) | three-layer membrane surrounding the brain and spinal cord |
| mesencephalon (mez-ehn-SEFF-ah-lon) | *mes/o* (middle); *encephal/o* (brain); *-on* (noun suffix) | the middle part of the brain between the diencephalon and the pons; also called the midbrain |
| midbrain (MID-brain) | *mid* = middle | the middle part of the brain between the diencephalon and the pons; also called the mesencephalon |
| myelin (MY-eh-lin) | *myel/o-* (bone marrow; spinal cord) | a fatty white envelope of cells providing protection and electrical insulation to neurons |
| nerve (nurv) | *nervus*, Latin for nerve; common English word | a whitish, cordlike structure composed of one or more bundles of nerve fibers outside the CNS, together with their connective tissues and nourishing blood vessels |

(*continued*)

**Study Table** THE NERVOUS SYSTEM (*continued*)

| TERM AND PRONUNCIATION | ANALYSIS | MEANING |
|---|---|---|
| neuroglia (new-ROG-lee-uh) | *neur/o* (nerve); from the Greek *glia* (glue) | cells within both the CNS and PNS, which, although they are external to neurons, form an essential part of nerve tissue |
| neuron (NUHR-ohn) | *neur/o* (nerve); *-on* (noun suffix) | a nerve cell, including the cell body and its axon |
| neurotransmitter (NOO-roh-TRANS-mitt-ehr) | *neur/o* (nerve); from the Latin *trans* (across); *mittere* (to send) | chemical released by the presynaptic cell (cell before the synapse) that is then picked up by the postsynaptic cell (cell after the synapse) to effect an action |
| nucleus (NEW-klee-uhs); plural: nuclei (NEW-klee-eye) | a Latin word meaning "kernel" | central region of neuron cell body that contains genetic information; a group of neuron cell bodies grouped together in the CNS |
| occipital lobe (AWK-sihp-ih-tuhl lohb) | from Latin word *occiput* (back of the head) | the part of the brain that processes information from the sense of sight and other sensory and motor tasks |
| parasympathetic nervous system (par-uh-sim-puh-THET-ik NER-vuhs SIS-tuhm) | *para-* (beside); *sympatheia* (Greek meaning community of feeling); *-ic* (adjective) | division of the ANS responsible for rest and digest responses |
| parietal lobe (pah-RY-uh-tuhl lohb) | from the Latin adjective *parietalis* (walls); *-al* (adjective suffix) | the part of the brain that processes information from the sense of touch and other sensory and motor tasks |
| peripheral nervous system (puh-RIFF-uh-ruhl NER-vuhs SIS-tuhm) (PNS) | *peri-* (surrounding); from the Greek word *pherein* (to carry); nervous system (common English words) | made up of neurons, neuroglia, and associated tissue, including the cranial and spinal nerves and the sensory and motor nerves that extend throughout the body |
| pia mater (PEE-ah MAY-turh) | Latin words meaning "tender mother" | inner layer of the meninges |
| pons (POHNS) | a Latin word meaning "bridge" | the part of the brainstem that passes information to the cerebellum and the thalamus to regulate subconscious somatic activities |

**Study Table** THE NERVOUS SYSTEM *(continued)*

| TERM AND PRONUNCIATION | ANALYSIS | MEANING | |
|---|---|---|---|
| psychomotor (SY-ko-mo-tuhr) | *psych/o* (of the mind); from the Latin word *motor* (mover) | an adjective used to indicate the relation between psychic activity and muscular movement | |
| somatic nervous system (so-MAT-ik NER-vuhs SIS-tuhm) | *somat/o* (body, bodily); *-ic* (adjective suffix) | the parts of the PNS that carry nerve impulses for conscious activity rather than habitual activity | |
| sympathetic nervous system (sim-puh-THET-ik NER-vuhs SIS-tuhm) | *sympatheia* (Greek meaning community of feeling); *-ic* (adjective) | division of the ANS responsible for fight or flight responses | |
| spinal nerves (SPY-nahl) | from the Latin word *spina* (spine) | the 31 pairs of nerves located along the spinal cord | |
| synapse (SIH-naps) | *syn-* (together); from the Greek word *hapto* (clasp) | the connecting point between nerve cells or between a nerve cell and a receptor or effector cell | |
| temporal lobe (TEM-puh-ruhl lobe) | from the Latin word *temporalis* (time, temple) | the part of the brain that processes information from the senses of hearing, smell, and taste, and other sensory and motor tasks | |
| thalamus (THAL-uh-muhs) | from the Greek word *thalamus* (bed, bedroom) | part of the brain that processes sensory information | |
| ventricles (VEN-trik-uhls) | from the Latin word *ventriculus*, dim. of *venter* (belly) | cavities within the brain | |
| **Disorders** | | | |
| absence seizure (ABB-sens SEE-zhur) | from the Latin word *absentia*, absent | seizure characterized by impaired awareness; milder form of seizure lasting only a few seconds and does not include convulsive movements; formerly known as *petit mal seizures* | French words meaning "small illness" |
| Alzheimer's disease (ALZ-hy-mur) (AD) | named after German physician Alois Alzheimer, who first described it in 1906 | a disease that may begin in late middle life, characterized by progressive mental deterioration that includes loss of memory and visual and spatial orientation | |
| amnesia (am-NEE-zah) | *a-* (without); *-mnesia* (memory) | loss of memory | |

*(continued)*

**Study Table** THE NERVOUS SYSTEM (*continued*)

| TERM AND PRONUNCIATION | ANALYSIS | MEANING |
|---|---|---|
| aneurysm (AN-ur-izm) | from the Greek *ana* (up) and *eurys* (broad) | localized dilation of an artery due to vessel wall weakness |
| anxiety disorder | common English words | a feeling of apprehension or uneasiness that results from anticipation of danger |
| aphasia (uh-FAY-jhah) | *a-* (absence of); from the Greek word *phases* (speech) | loss of speech |
| astrocytoma (A-stroh-sy-TOH-mah) | from the Greek word *astron* (star); *cyt/o* (cell); *-oma* (tumor) | star-shaped tumor that usually develops in the cerebrum; frequently in people younger than 20 years old |
| ataxia (ah-TAK-see-ah) | *a-* (without); from the Greek word *taxis* (order) | lack of muscular coordination |
| bipolar disorder | *bi-* (twice, double); from the Latin word *polus* (the end of an axis) | disorder characterized by manic episodes alternating with depressive episodes |
| cerebral thrombosis (seh-REE-bruhl throm-BO-sihs) | *cerebr/o* (brain); *-al* (adjective suffix); *thromb/o* (of or relating to a blood clot); *-sis* (abnormal condition) | blood clot in the brain |
| cerebrovascular accident (seh-REE-bro-VAS-ku-lahr) (CVA) | *cerebr/o* (brain); *vascul/o* (blood vessel); *-ar* (adjective suffix) | a synonym for *cerebral stroke*, an acute clinical event, related to impairment of cerebral circulation, lasting more than 24 hours |
| cerebrovascular disease (seh-REE-bro-VAS-ku-lahr) | *cerebr/o* (brain); *vascul/o* (blood vessel); *-ar* (adjective suffix) | brain disorder involving a blood vessel |
| concussion (kuhn-KUHSH-uhn) | from the Latin word *concussionem* (a shaking) | brain injury resulting from a hit to the head or violent shaking |
| delirium (duh-LEER-ee-uhm) | from the Latin word *deliro* (to be crazy) | altered state of consciousness |
| delusion (deh-LOO-zhun) | from the Latin word *ludere* (to play) | false belief or wrong judgment despite evidence to the contrary |
| dementia (duh-MEN-shah) | from Latin *de* (apart, away); *mens* (mind) | impaired intellectual function |

**Study Table** THE NERVOUS SYSTEM (*continued*)

| TERM AND PRONUNCIATION | ANALYSIS | MEANING |
|---|---|---|
| demyelination (dee-my-uh-lin-AY-shun) | from the Greek word *myelos* (marrow, inner part of the brain) | loss of myelin |
| depression (dih-PRESH-un) | from the Latin word *depressio* | prolonged period where there is a loss of interest or pleasure in almost all activities |
| dopamine (DOH-puh-meen) (DA) | from the acronym for the amino acid dioxyphenylalanine (DOPA) | neurotransmitter in the CNS and PNS; depletion of dopamine causes PD |
| dysphasia (DISS-fay-jhah) | *dys-* (bad, difficult); from the Greek word *phases* (speaking) | impaired speech |
| encephalitis (en-seff-uh-LY-tiss) | *encephal/o* (of or pertaining to the brain); *-itis* (inflammation) | inflammation of the brain |
| epidural hematoma (EH-pih-dur-ahl hee-mah-TOH-ma) | *epi-* (above); dural (relating to the dura mater); *hemat/o* (blood); *-oma* (tumor) | a collection of blood in the space between the skull and dura mater |
| epilepsy (EPP-ih-lepp-see) | from the Greek *epilepsia* (seizure) | CNS disorder often characterized by seizures |
| glioblastoma (GLY-oh-blass-TOH-mah) | *glio* (glue); from the Greek word *blastos* (germ); *-oma* (tumor) | a cerebral tumor occurring most frequently in adults |
| glioma (gly-OH-muh) | *glio-* (glue); *-oma* (tumor) | tumor of glial tissue |
| grand mal seizure (grahn-mahl SEE-zhur) | French words meaning "big illness" | type of severe seizure with tonic–clonic convulsion; also called tonic–clonic seizure |
| hallucination (hah-LOO-sih-nay-shun) | from the Latin word *alucinor* (to wander in mind) | subjective perception of an object or voice when no such stimulus exists |
| hemiparesis (heh-mee-puh-REE-suhs) | *hemi-* (one-half); *-paresis* (slight paralysis) | partial paralysis of one side of the body |
| hemiplegia (hehm-ee-PLEE-jee-ah) | *hemi-* (one-half); *-plegia* (paralysis) | paralysis of one side of the body |
| Huntington's disease (HUN-ting-tuhnz) | named after American physician George Huntington who described the disorder in 1872 | hereditary disorder of the CNS |

(*continued*)

**Study Table** THE NERVOUS SYSTEM (*continued*)

| TERM AND PRONUNCIATION | ANALYSIS | MEANING |
|---|---|---|
| hydrocephalus (hy-dro-SEFF-uh-lehs) | *hydro-* (water); *cephal/o* (of or pertaining to the head) | excessive CSF in the brain |
| hyperesthesia (hy-per-ess-THEE-zyuh) | *hyper-* (extreme or beyond normal); *esthesi/o* (sensation) | abnormal sensitivity to touch |
| kleptomania (klep-toh-MAY-knee-yah) | from the Greek word *klepto-* (to– steal); from the Latin *-mania* (insanity) | uncontrollable impulse to steal |
| lesion (LEE-zhun) | from the Latin, *laedo* (to injure) | wound or injury; pathologic tissue change |
| meningioma (meh-nihn-jee-OH-muh) | *mening/o* (membrane); *-oma* (tumor) | benign tumor of the meninges |
| meningitis (meh-nihn-JY-tis) | *mening/o* (membrane); *-itis* (inflammation) | inflamed meninges |
| mood disorder | two common English words | a group of mental disorders involving a disturbance of mood not due to any other mental disorder |
| multiple sclerosis (skleh-RO-sihs) (MS) | multiple (from the English word meaning "many"); *scler/o* (hardness); *-osis* (abnormal condition) | disease of the CNS characterized by demyelination and the formation of plaques in the brain and spinal cord |
| myasthenia gravis (MY-ahs-THEE-nee-ah GRA-viss) | *my/o* (muscle); *astheneia* (weakness) | muscle weakness, lack of strength |
| myelitis (my-eh-LY-tiss) | *myel/o* (bone marrow or spine); *-itis* (inflammation) | inflammation of the spinal cord |
| myelomeningocele (MY-loh-mih-NIHN-gee-oh-seel) | *myel/o* (bone marrow or spine); *meningi/o* (membrane); *-cele* (hernia) | protrusion of the membranes of the brain or spinal cord through a defect in the cranium or vertebral column |
| neuralgia (nuh-RALL-jah) | *neur/o* (nerve); *-algia* (pain) | pain in a nerve |
| neuropathy (nuh-ROP-ah-thee) | *neur/o* (nerve); *-pathy* (disease) | a disease involving the cranial, central, or autonomic nervous systems |

**Study Table** THE NERVOUS SYSTEM (*continued*)

| TERM AND PRONUNCIATION | ANALYSIS | MEANING |
|---|---|---|
| obsessive–compulsive disorder (OCD) | common English words | type of anxiety disorder characterized by persistent thoughts and impulses with repetitive responses that interfere with daily activities |
| paralysis (pah-RALL-ih-sihs) | *para-* (abnormal, alongside); *-lysis* (destruction) | loss of one or more muscle functions |
| paranoia (pahr-ah-NOY-ya) | *para-* (abnormal, alongside); from Greek word *noeo* (to think) | a serious mental disorder characterized by unreasonable suspicion or jealousy, along with a tendency to interpret everything others do as hostile |
| paraplegia (pahr-ah-PLEE-jee-ah) | *para-* (abnormal, alongside); *-plegia* (paralysis) | paralysis of the lower extremities and, often, the lower trunk of the body |
| paresthesia (per-ess-THEE-zyuh) | *para-* (abnormal); *esthesi/o* (sensation) | numbness |
| Parkinson's disease (PAR-kin-suhn) (PD) | named for English physician James Parkinson, who described it in 1817 | disease of the nerves in the brain due to an imbalance of dopamine; also called parkinsonism |
| phobia (FOH-bee-ah) | *phob/o* (exaggerated fear); *-ia* (noun suffix) | a fear of something that is not a hazard from a statistical point of view |
| plegia (PLEE-jee-uh) | *-plegia* (paralysis) | paralysis |
| poliomyelitis (pohl-ee-oh-MY-eh-LY-tiss) | *polio-* (denoting gray color); *myel/o* (bone marrow or spine); *-itis* (inflammation) | inflamed gray matter of the spinal cord |
| posttraumatic stress disorder (PTSD) (pohst-truh-MAT-ik stres dis-AWR-der) | *post-* (after); *trauma* (Greek for wound); -ic | development of characteristic long-term symptoms following a psychologically traumatic event that is generally outside the range of usual human experience |
| psychosis (sy-KO-sihs) | *psych/o* (mind); *-sis* (condition of) | a serious disorder involving a marked distortion of, or sharp break from, reality; general term covering severe mental or emotional disorders |

(*continued*)

**Study Table** THE NERVOUS SYSTEM (*continued*)

| TERM AND PRONUNCIATION | ANALYSIS | MEANING |
|---|---|---|
| psychotic disorder (sahy-KOT-ik dis-AWR-der) | *psych/o* (mind); *-ic* (adjective) | a mental and behavioral disorder causing gross distortion or disorganization of a person's mental capacity, affective response, and capacity to recognize reality |
| quadriplegia (kwad-rih-PLEE-jee-ah) | *quadr/i* (four); *-plegia* (paralysis) | paralysis of all four limbs |
| schizophrenia (skits-oh-FREN-ee-ah) | *schiz/o* (denoting split or double sided); from the Greek word *phren* (mind) | a severe mental illness characterized by auditory hallucinations, paranoia, and an inability to distinguish reality from fiction |
| seizure (SEE-zhur) | from the French word *seisir* (to grasp); common English word | sudden disturbance in brain function sometimes producing a convulsion |
| somnambulism (sahm-NAM-bu-lih-sm) | from Latin words *somnus* (sleep) and *ambulo* (walk); *-ism* (a medical condition) | sleep walking |
| subdural hematoma (SUB-dur-ahl hee-mah-TOH-ma) | *sub-* (beneath); *dura* (hard); *-al* (adjective suffix); *hemat/o* (blood); *-oma* (tumor) | a collection of blood trapped in the space beneath the dura mater, between the dura and arachnoid layers of the meninges |
| syncope (SIN-kuh-pee) | from the Greek word *syncope* (a cutting short, a swoon) | fainting |
| transient ischemic attack (TRANS-ee-ent IH-skee-mik) (TIA) | from Greek *isch*, (to restrict), and the suffix *-emia* (blood) | temporary interruption in the blood supply to the brain |
| vertigo (VER-tih-goh) | from the Latin word *verto* (turn) | dizziness |
| **Diagnostic Tests, Treatments, and Surgical Procedures** | | |
| antianxiety agent | *anti-* (against); from the Greek word *angho* (to squeeze, embrace, throttle) | drug used to suppress anxiousness and relax muscles |
| anticonvulsant agent | *anti-* (against); from the Latin *con* (with) and *vulsus* (to tear up) | drug used to decrease seizure activity |

**Study Table** THE NERVOUS SYSTEM (*continued*)

| TERM AND PRONUNCIATION | ANALYSIS | MEANING |
|---|---|---|
| antipsychotic agent | *anti-* (against); *psych/o* (mind); *-tic* (adjective suffix) | drug given to patients to affect behavior and treat psychiatric disorders |
| computed tomography (CT) | *tomos* (Greek "to slice"); *-graph* (instrument for recording) | X-ray imaging using cross-sectional planes of the body |
| craniectomy (KRAY-nee-ek-tuh-mee) | *crani/o* (cranium); *-ectomy* (excision) | excision of part of the skull |
| craniotomy (KRAY-nee-aw-tuh-mee) | *crani/o* (cranium); *-tomy* (cutting operation) | incision into the skull |
| electroconvulsive therapy (ECT) or electroshock therapy (EST) | *electr/o* (electric); from the Latin words *con* (with) and *vulsus* (to tear up) | a controlled convulsion produced by passing an electric current through the brain |
| electroencephalography (ee-LEK-tro-en-sef-ah-LAH-grah-fee) (EEG) | *electr/o* (electric); *encephal/o* (brain); *-graphy* (process of recording) | record of the electrical activity of the brain |
| lobotomy (lo-BAWT-uh-mee) | *lob/o* (lobe); *-tomy* (cutting operation) | incision into a lobe |
| lumbar puncture (LP) | from the Latin word *lumbus* (loin) | insertion of a needle into the subarachnoid space between the third and fourth or fourth and fifth lumbar vertebrae to withdraw fluid for diagnosis |
| magnetic resonance imaging (MRI) | common English words | uses radio waves and a very strong magnetic field to produce images of the soft tissue |
| myelography (my-eh-LOG-rah-fee) | *myel/o* (bone marrow or spine); *-graphy* (process of recording) | radiography of the spinal cord and nerve roots |
| neuroplasty (NURR-oh-plass-tee) | *neur/o* (nerve); *-plasty* (repair) | surgery to repair a nerve |
| sedatives | from the Latin *sedeo* (sit); from the Greek word *hypnotikos* (causing one to sleep) | drugs used to induce calming effect or sleep |

**Study Table** THE NERVOUS SYSTEM (*continued*)

| TERM AND PRONUNCIATION | ANALYSIS | MEANING |
|---|---|---|
| **Practice and Practitioners** | | |
| neurologist (nuhr-AWL-ih-gihst) | *neur/o* (nerve); *-logist* (practitioner) | a medical specialist who treats nervous system disorders |
| neurology (nuhr-AWL-uh-jee) | *neur/o* (nerve); *-logy* (the study of) | medical specialty dealing with the nervous system |
| neurosurgeon (NOO-roh-sur-juhn) | *neur/o* (nerve); from the Greek word *kheirourgos* (working or done by hand) | surgeon who specializes in operations on the nervous system |
| psychiatrist (sy-KY-ah-trist) | *psych/o* (mind); *iatr/o* (of or pertaining to medicine or a physician); *-ist* (one who specializes in) | a medical doctor who specializes in the diagnosis and treatment of psychological disorders |
| psychologist (sy-KOL-oh-jist) | *psych/o* (mind); *-logist* (one who studies a certain field) | a (nonmedical) doctor of psychology who specializes in the diagnosis and treatment of psychological disorders |

# END-OF-CHAPTER EXERCISES

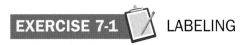

## EXERCISE 7-1 LABELING

**Label the parts of the motor neuron. Select from the terms listed in the table.**

| | | |
|---|---|---|
| axon | dendrites | nucleus |
| cell body | myelin | |

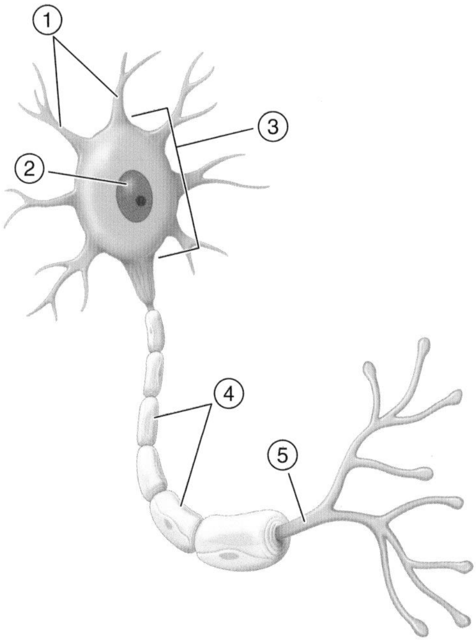


1. ______________________
2. ______________________
3. ______________________
4. ______________________
5. ______________________



## EXERCISE 7-2 WORD PARTS

**Break each of the following terms into its word parts: root, prefix, or suffix. Give the meaning of each word part and then define each term.**

1. *psychosis*

   root: ______________________

   suffix: ______________________

   definition: ______________________

2. *electroencephalography*

 root: ______________________________

 root: ______________________________

 suffix: ______________________________

 definition: ______________________________

3. *astrocytoma*

 root: ______________________________

 root: ______________________________

 suffix: ______________________________

 definition: ______________________________

4. *cerebrovascular*

 root: ______________________________

 root: ______________________________

 suffix: ______________________________

 definition: ______________________________

5. *encephalitis*

 root: ______________________________

 suffix: ______________________________

 definition: ______________________________

6. *epidural*

 prefix: ______________________________

 root: ______________________________

 suffix: ______________________________

 definition: ______________________________

7. *psychiatrist*

 root: ______________________________

 root: ______________________________

 suffix: ______________________________

 definition: ______________________________

8. *meningioma*

 root: ______________________________

 suffix: ______________________________

 definition: ______________________________

## EXERCISE 7-3 WORD BUILDING

Use the word parts listed to build the terms defined.

| | | | |
|---|---|---|---|
| neur/o | -oma | sympathetic | -noia |
| -paresis | para- | -plasty | esthesia |
| gli/a | -itis | -tomy | hemi- |
| di- | -on | lob/o | encephala/o |

1. ________________ inflammation of the brain
2. ________________ tumor of glial tissue
3. ________________ partial paralysis of one side of the body
4. ________________ incision into a lobe
5. ________________ cells that are a part of nerve tissue and are external to neurons
6. ________________ division of the ANS responsible for rest and digestive responses
7. ________________ a mental disorder characterized by unreasonable suspicion or jealousy
8. ________________ surgery to repair a nerve
9. ________________ the part of the brain containing both the thalamus and the hypothalamus
10. ________________ numbness

## EXERCISE 7-4 MATCHING

**Match the term in the first column with its definition in the second column.**

| | | |
|---|---|---|
| 1. ________________ | cerebrum | a. accumulation of fluid on the brain |
| 2. ________________ | cerebral cortex | b. nerve pain |
| 3. ________________ | brainstem | c. contains the mesencephalon (midbrain), pons, and medulla oblongata |
| 4. ________________ | somatic nerves | d. dizziness |
| 5. ________________ | pons | e. hernia of the meninges and the spinal cord |
| 6. ________________ | autonomic nerves | f. outer layer of the cerebrum |
| 7. ________________ | meningomyelocele | g. fainting |
| 8. ________________ | neuralgia | h. smallest part of brain |

9. _______________ convulsion — i. contact point between two nerves

10. _______________ syncope — j. involuntary nerves

11. _______________ vertigo — k. largest part of the brain

12. _______________ hydrocephalus — l. inflammation of a nerve

13. _______________ neuritis — m. seizure

14. _______________ synapse — n. voluntary nerves

## EXERCISE 7-5 MULTIPLE CHOICE

**Choose the correct answer for the following multiple choice questions.**

1. Which term means paralysis on **one side** of the body?
   a. diplegia
   b. paraplegia
   c. monoplegia
   d. hemiplegia

2. Which of the following terms means a disease of the CNS characterized by the formation of plaques in the brain and spinal cord?
   a. amyotrophic lateral sclerosis
   b. PD
   c. MS
   d. poliomyelitis

3. To what does the term *cerebrocranial* refer?
   a. brain and cranium
   b. cerebellum and cranium
   c. cerebrum and brain
   d. cerebrum and cerebellum

4. The axon is a process that extends from a neuron cell body. What is another one?
   a. effector
   b. dendrite
   c. neurotransmitter
   d. ganglia

5. Which of the following means *accumulation of blood under the outermost meningeal layer*?
   a. epidural hematoma
   b. intracerebral hematoma
   c. subdural hematoma
   d. cerebral concussion

6. Which of the following means *hardening of the brain*?
   a. MS
   b. encephalosclerosis
   c. encephalomyelopathy
   d. depilepsy

7. What is cerebral meningitis?
   a. inflammation of the cerebellum
   b. inflammation of the medulla
   c. inflammation of the meninges of the brain
   d. inflammation of the meninges of the spinal cord

8. Which part of the nervous system conducts impulses to skeletal muscle and is under *conscious* control?
   a. autonomic
   b. central
   c. somatic
   d. afferent

9. PD is a disease of the nerves in the brain due to an imbalance of what?
   a. glucose
   b. serotonin
   c. oxygen
   d. DA

10. A craniectomy is an ________________________.
   a. incision into a lobe
   b. incision into the skull
   c. excision of part of the skull
   d. surgery to repair a nerve

11. This is given to reduce seizure activity.
   a. antianxiety agent
   b. anticonvulsant agent
   c. antipsychotic agent
   d. sedative

12. Of the following choices, which is the best place to perform an LP?
   a. between T2 and T3
   b. between T12 and L1
   c. between L5 and S1
   d. between L3 and L4

13. What is another name for an absence seizure?
   a. grand mal seizure
   b. petit mal seizure
   c. somnambulism
   d. syncope

14. A TIA involves primarily the nervous system and which other body system?
   a. respiratory
   b. cardiovascular
   c. muscular
   d. digestive

15. Delirium is ________________.
    a. a false belief or wrong judgment despite evidence to the contrary
    b. a subjective perception of an object or voice when no such stimulus exists
    c. impaired intellectual function
    d. altered state of consciousness

## EXERCISE 7-6 FILL IN THE BLANK

**Fill in the blank with the correct answer.**

1. Abnormal sensitivity to touch is called ________________________.
2. The name for "inflamed" gray matter of the spinal cord is ________________________.
3. Impaired intellectual function is called ________________________.
4. The demyelinization of the spinal cord nerves is called ________________________.
5. The protrusion of the meninges and spinal cord tissue through a spina bifida is called a/an

   ________________________.
6. The term for a blood clot in the brain is ________________________.
7. ________________________ is characterized by a lack of muscular coordination.
8. CNS disorder often characterized by seizures is termed ________________________.
9. ________________________ is synonymous with fainting.
10. Pain in a nerve is ________________________.

## EXERCISE 7-7 ABBREVIATIONS

**Write out the term for the following abbreviations.**

1. ________________________________________ ICP
2. ________________________________________ CSF
3. ________________________________________ LP
4. ________________________________________ EEG
5. ________________________________________ MS
6. ________________________________________ OCD
7. ________________________________________ PD

8. ______________________________ PNS

9. ______________________________ CVA

10. ______________________________ DA

**Write the abbreviation for the following terms.**

11. ____________________ posttraumatic stress disorder

12. ____________________ peripheral nervous system

13. ____________________ cerebrovascular accident

14. ____________________ magnetic resonance imaging

15. ____________________ transient ischemic attack

## EXERCISE 7-8 SPELLING

**Select the correct spelling of the medical term.**

1. ____________________ is the loss, due to brain damage, of the ability to speak or write or to comprehend the written or spoken word.
   a. Aphasia
   b. Afasia
   c. Aphazia
   d. Aphesia

2. ____________________ is a type of psychosis that may manifest itself as paranoia, withdrawal, or psychotic symptoms.
   a. Skitzophrenia
   b. Schizofrenia
   c. Schizophrenia
   d. Skizophrenia

3. ____________________ are the potent chemicals in the synapse between neurons.
   a. Nuerotransmiters
   b. Neurotransmiters
   c. Neurotransmitters
   d. Neuritransmitters

4. ________________________ is a collection of blood in the subdural space.
   a. Subdaral hemitoma
   b. Subdural hemitonia
   c. Subdural henitoma
   d. Subdural hematoma

5. A ________________________ is a protrusion of the membranes of the brain or spinal cord through a defect in the cranium or vertebral column.
   a. myelomeningocele
   b. myelomenengocele
   c. myelomenegocell
   d. meylomeningocele

6. The membranes that surround the brain and spinal cord are called ________________________.
   a. menenges
   b. meninges
   c. meninnges
   d. meningis

7. The plural of nucleus is ________________________.
   a. nuclie
   b. neuclei
   c. nuclius
   d. nuclei

8. TIA stands for transient ________________________ attack.
   a. ichemic
   b. ischemic
   c. ischimic
   d. ischeimic

9. A sudden disturbance in brain function which sometimes produces a convulsion is called a ________________________.
   a. seisure
   b. siezure
   c. seizure
   d. seizur

10. An ________________________ is a localized dilation of an artery due to vessel wall weakness.
   a. aneurysm
   b. aneurism
   c. anurism
   d. anurysm

## EXERCISE 7-9 CASE STUDY

**Read the following excerpt from an emergency room record and answer the questions.**

**CHIEF COMPLAINT:** Mental status changes and aphasia.

**BRIEF HISTORY:** J.D. is an 85-year-old female who presents to the emergency department with difficulty talking. Her daughter states that J.D. has had garbled speech for the past few days, repeatedly says, "How do you do?" and answers the same to any questions asked. This has happened in the past, but the daughter says her mother has always "gotten better." This morning J.D. woke up and has weakness on the right side of her body. There are no other modifying factors or associated signs or symptoms.

**ASSESSMENT:** Probable history of TIA; now CVA with resulting dysphasia and right hemiparesis.

1. What is a TIA? ______________________________
2. What does the acronym CVA represent? ______________________________
3. Break up the medical term *dysphasia* and define its word parts. ______________________________
4. What does the root word *paresis* mean? ______________________________
5. What is the difference between *hemiparesis* and *hemiplegia*? ______________________________
6. Break up the term *hemiplegia* and define the word parts. ______________________________

# The Special Senses of Sight and Hearing

8

**LEARNING OUTCOMES**

***Upon completion of this chapter, you should be able to:***

- Name the structures of the eyes and ears.
- Label diagrams showing major components of the eyes and ears.
- Pronounce, spell, and define medical terms related to the eyes and ears and its disorders
- Interpret abbreviations associated with the eyes and ears.

## INTRODUCTION

We get the English word *sense* from the Latin verb *sentire,* which means "to feel." The phrase *special senses* comes from this word and refers to the five senses related to the organs of sight, hearing, smell, taste, and touch. Sight and hearing are treated in a single chapter because unlike smell, taste, and touch, which rely on chemical responses, sight and hearing include terminology associated with bodily organs that process electromagnetic energy (sight) and mechanical energy (hearing). Sight and hearing will be discussed in two separate sections within this chapter.

## WORD PARTS RELATED TO THE EYE

The word root ocul/o comes from the Latin word *oculus* (eye). The word root *ophthalm/o* comes from the Greek word *ophthalmos*, which also means eye. The Latin word *opticus* means "of sight or seeing" and from this comes words like *optic*. The suffixes -opia and -opsia both mean "vision." Most of the remaining word parts refer to specific structures within the eye. Table 8-1 lists word parts related to the eyes.

### Structure and Function of the Eye

Light waves are part of the electromagnetic spectrum, and our eyes work like a motion picture camera, taking continuous pictures and transmitting them instantaneously to the brain, which converts them to images in motion. Although light energy and brain waves are both part of the electromagnetic spectrum, brain waves have much lower frequencies and, therefore, much longer wavelengths than those of light. Thus, our eyes must also convert detected light frequencies, so that the brain can enable us to "see" objects and their motions.

The eye is the organ of vision that is found within the **orbit**, a bony cavity (socket) formed by seven bones of the skull. Accessory structures of the eyes include the *extraocular muscles*, *eyebrows*, *eyelids*, *eyelashes*, *conjunctiva*, and *lacrimal apparatus*. **Extraocular muscles** are those muscles within the orbit but outside the eyeball that move the eyes. They are not visible from the exterior. **Eyebrows**

## TABLE 8-1 WORD PARTS RELATED TO THE EYE

| Word Part | Meaning |
|---|---|
| blephar/o | eyelid |
| conjunctiv/o | conjunctiva (*conjunctivae*, plural) |
| corne/o | horny |
| dacry/o | tears, lacrimal sac or lacrimal duct |
| dipl/o | two, double |
| irid/o | iris |
| kerat/o | hard, cornea |
| lacrim/o | tear, lacrimal apparatus |
| ocul/o | eye |
| ophthalm/o | eye |
| -opia | vision |
| opt/o | light, eye, vision |
| phac/o | lens |
| presby/o | old age |
| pupil/o | pupil |
| retin/o | retina |
| scler/o | relating to the sclera, hard |
| uve/o | denoting the pigmented middle eye layer |

## Word Parts Exercise

After studying Table 8-1, write the meaning of each of the word parts.

| WORD PART | MEANING |
|---|---|
| 1. retin/o | 1. ________________ |
| 2. kerat/o | 2. ________________ |
| 3. lacrim/o | 3. ________________ |
| 4. opt/o | 4. ________________ |
| 5. ocul/o | 5. ________________ |
| 6. uve/o | 6. ________________ |
| 7. dipl/o | 7. ________________ |
| 8. dacry/o | 8. ________________ |
| 9. irid/o | 9. ________________ |
| 10. ophthalm/o | 10. ________________ |

(*continued*)

**Word Parts Exercise** ***(continued)***

| WORD PART | MEANING |
|---|---|
| 11. phac/o | 11. ______________________________ |
| 12. presby/o | 12. ______________________________ |
| 13. blephar/o | 13. ______________________________ |
| 14. conjunctiv/o | 14. ______________________________ |
| 15. pupil/o | 15. ______________________________ |
| 16. corne/o | 16. ______________________________ |
| 17. scler/o | 17. ______________________________ |

are the crescent-shaped line of hairs on the superior edge of the orbit. The movable upper and lower folds that cover the surface of the eyeballs when they close are called **eyelids** (*palpebrae*), and the stiff hairs projecting from the eyelid margins are the **eyelashes**. The angle formed by the junction of the lateral parts of the upper and lower eyelids is known as the *lateral angle of eye* (*lateral canthus*), and the medial angle formed by their union is the *medial angle* of eye (*medial canthus*) (see Figure 8-1). The **conjunctiva** is the mucous membrane that lines the anterior surface of the eyeball and the underside of the eyelid. This membrane covers and protects the exposed surface of the eyeball (see Figure 8-3).

Several structures associated with tear production and flow make up the **lacrimal apparatus**. Located superior to the outer corner of each eye are the **lacrimal glands**, which secrete tears to cleanse and moisten the eyeball surface. The **lacrimal sac** stores tears. **Lacrimal ducts** are channels that carry tears to the eyes, whereas the **nasolacrimal ducts** carry tears from the lacrimal glands to the nose (see Figure 8-2).

The eyeball is made up of three layers, listed from the outermost to the innermost layer: *fibrous layer*, *vascular layer*, and *inner layer*. The fibrous layer consists of the *sclera* and *cornea*; the vascular layer (also called the *uvea*) is made up of the *choroid*, *ciliary body*, and *iris*; and the inner layer has the *retina* and *optic nerve*. The **sclera**, also known as the white of the eye, helps maintain the shape of eyeball and extends from the cornea to the optic nerve. The **cornea** is the transparent portion that

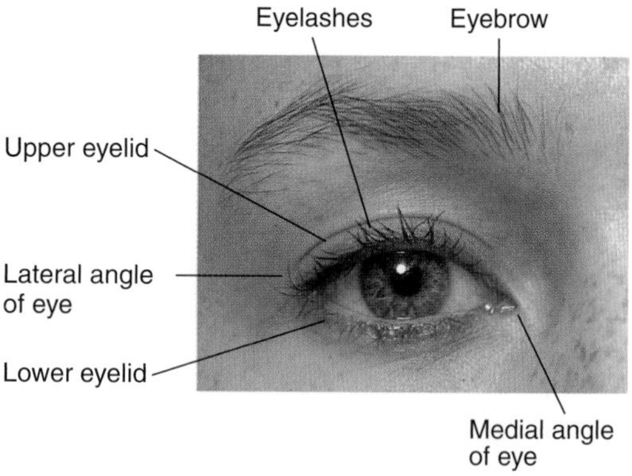


**FIGURE 8-1** Protective structures of the eye.

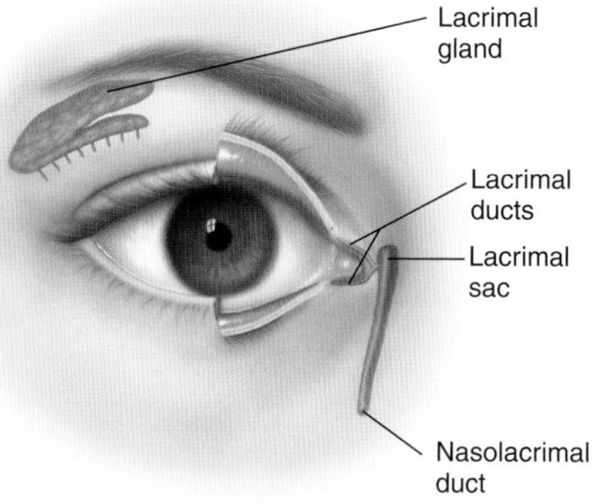


**FIGURE 8-2** Structures of the right lacrimal apparatus.

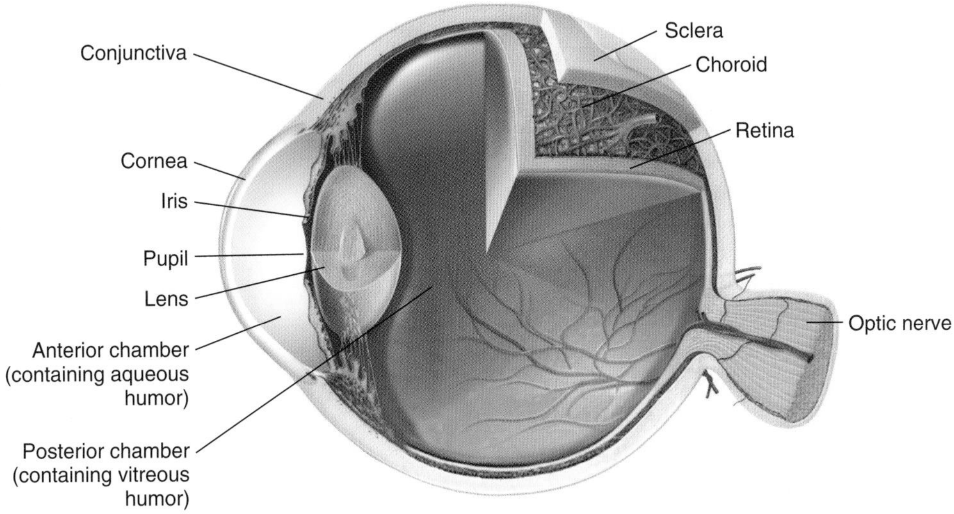


**FIGURE 8-3** Structures of the eyeball.

provides most of the optical power of the eye through its ability to bend light rays to focus on the surface of the retina (see Figure 8-3).

The **choroid** is the opaque layer of the eyeball that contains vessels that supply blood to the eye. The **ciliary body** is a thickened portion between the choroid and iris. Its group of muscles suspends the lens and adjusts it to direct the light entering the eye. The **lens** is a transparent structure posterior to the pupil that bends and focuses light rays on the retina. It is held in place by the ligaments of the ciliary body. The *ciliary muscles* control the shape of the lens to allow for far and near vision. The **iris** is the pigmented muscular ring that surrounds and controls the size of the **pupil**, the opening in the middle of the iris through which light enters the eye (see Figure 8-3).

The innermost layer of the eye that contains visual receptors (rod and cones) is the **retina**. The first cranial nerve, called the **optic nerve**, carries nerve impulses from the retina to the brain to give us the sense of sight. It exits the eyeball through the optic foramen (opening) in the orbit (see Figure 8-3).

The interior spaces (chambers) of the eyeball contain fluid. The *anterior chamber* is the space between the cornea and the lens, and it is filled with a watery fluid called the **aqueous humor**. The *posterior chamber* is the large open space between the lens and retina that contains a semi-gelatinous liquid, the **vitreous humor** (see Figure 8-3).

## Quick Check #1

**Fill in the blanks.**

1. The three layers of the eyeball are the ______________________ layer, the ______________________ layer, and the ______________________ layer.

2. The ______________________ contains vessels for supplying blood to the eye.

3. The opening in the middle of the iris is the ______________________.

**Photoreceptors** are the specialized visual receptor cells in the retina. There are two types of photoreceptors: rods and cones. **Rods** are black and white receptors that respond to dim light, and **cones** are color receptors that provide color vision and sharp vision (visual acuity). These photosensitive cells receive the light waves that come in through the cornea and convert them into nerve impulses. These nerve impulses are carried to the brain through the optic nerve. An oval area of the retina is called the **macula** and at its center is a pit called the **fovea centralis**, which is saturated with cones and thus permits the best possible color vision. The **optic disc** is the location where nerve fibers from the retina converge to form the optic nerve. Because it has no photoreceptors, it is referred to as the *blind spot* (see Figure 8-4).

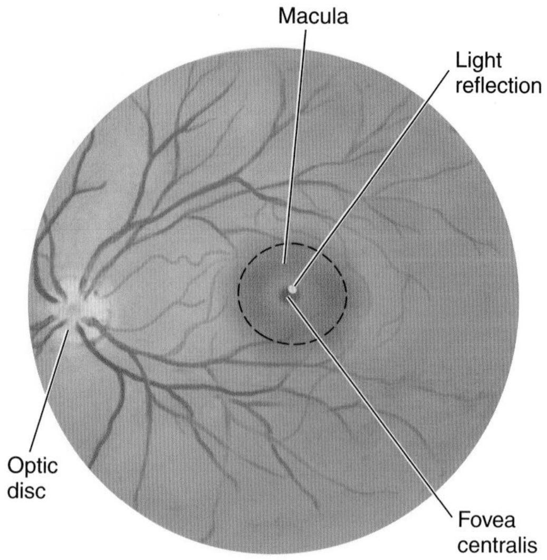


**FIGURE 8-4** Structures of the internal right eye.

**Refraction**, the bending of light rays, is the ability of the eye to change the direction of light in order to focus it on the retina. Light rays are refracted by the cornea and lens to focus an image on the retina. We are able to see because of **accommodation**, the automatic adjustment of focusing the eye by flattening or thickening the lens (see Figure 8-5).

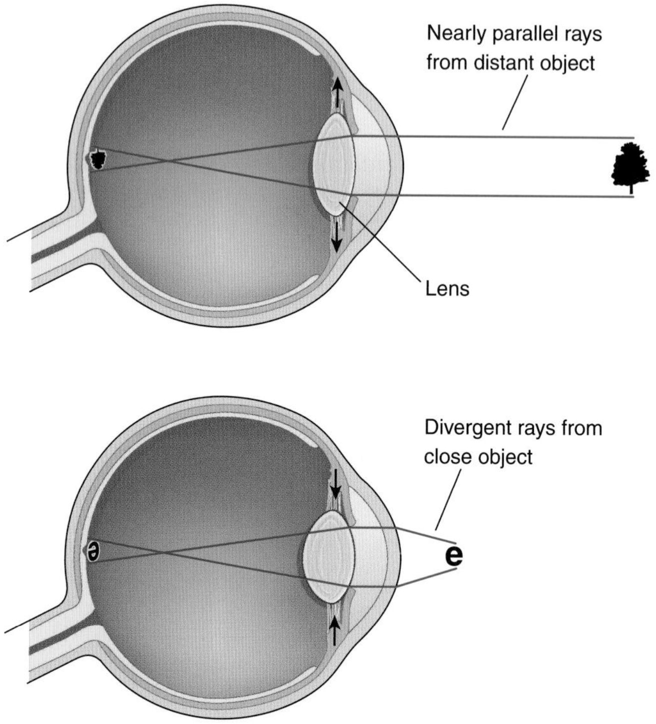


**FIGURE 8-5** Accommodation. The ciliary muscles control the shape of the lens to allow for far and near vision. The top figure has an elongated lens allowing the eye to focus on distant objects. The bottom figure has a shortened lens, allowing the eye to focus on close objects.

## Disorders Related to the Eye

Refractive errors, infections, and disorders of the eyelids are common. Refractive errors can be corrected with glasses, contact lenses, or operations that include the reshaping of the cornea. Other eye conditions can be treated with medications or surgery.

### *Refractive Errors*

**Hyperopia** is the medical term for *farsightedness*, a condition in which the image falls behind the retina. With hyperopia, people cannot see things clearly if they are close to the eyes but can see distant objects. **Myopia** is the medial term for *nearsightedness*, a condition in which the image falls in front of the retina. People with myopia cannot see things clearly unless they are close to the eyes (see Figure 8-6). **Presbyopia** is farsightedness caused by aging. Another refractive error is called **astigmatism**, which means the light coming into the eye does not focus on a single point; this condition is caused by an irregularity of the curve of the cornea or lens that distorts light entering the eye. Corrective lenses can usually compensate for any refractive error.

### *Infections*

**Conjunctivitis**, commonly known as *pinkeye*, is an inflammation of the conjunctiva. The inflammation causes small blood vessels in the conjunctiva to become more prominent, giving the sclera a pink or red color. **Keratitis** is an inflammation of the cornea that occurs when the cornea has been scratched or otherwise damaged. An inflamed lacrimal sac is called **dacryocystitis**.

### *Disorders of the Eyelids*

**Blepharoptosis** is drooping of the upper eyelid. **Ectropion** is a condition in which the eyelid is turned outward away from the eyeball. **Entropion** is a condition that causes the eyelid to roll inward against the eyeball. A **hordeolum**, commonly called a **sty**, is an infection of the oil gland of an eyelash.

### *Other Disorders of the Eye*

**Xerophthalmia**, also known as dry eyes, occurs when the surface of the eye becomes dry, often from wearing contact lenses or from a diminished flow of tears.

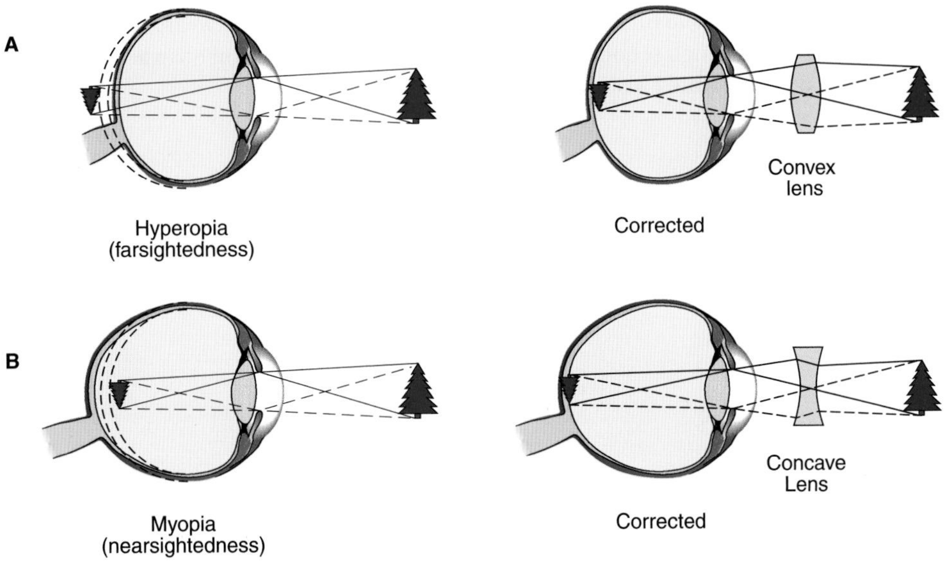


FIGURE 8-6 Refractive errors. **A.** Hyperopia or farsightedness. The image falls behind the retina, making it difficult to see up close. The corrective lens places the image properly on the retina. **B.** Myopia or nearsightedness. The image falls in front of the retina, making it difficult to see far. The corrective lens places the image properly on the retina.

**Glaucoma** is a disease characterized by an increase in intraocular pressure (IOP) that causes damage to the optic nerve. If left untreated, it can result in permanent blindness. Symptoms frequently go unnoticed by the patient until the optic nerve has been damaged.

A cloudiness or opacity of the lens is called a **cataract** (see Figure 8-7). Disease, injury, chemicals, or exposure to various physical elements may cause cataracts. Surgery to replace the clouded lens with an artificial intraocular lens is a common treatment for cataracts.

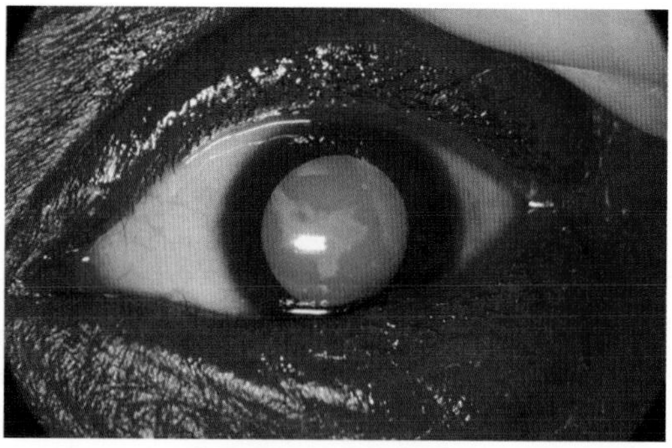

**FIGURE 8-7** Cataract.

## Diagnostic Tests, Treatments, and Surgical Procedures of the Eye

An **ophthalmoscope** is the instrument by which practitioners can examine the interior of the eye by looking through the pupil.

A popular procedure to correct vision problems, such as myopia, hyperopia, and astigmatism, is **laser-assisted in situ keratomileusis (LASIK)**. This procedure uses a laser to create a corneal flap and reshape the cornea. Treatment for a detached retina or retinal tear may include scleral buckling. A **scleral buckle** is a permanent silicone band that attaches to the scleral peripheral behind the eye, pulling the retina together (see Figure 8-8).

## Practice and Practitioners of the Eye

An **ophthalmologist** provides eye care ranging from examining eyes and prescribing corrective lenses to performing surgery. Such a wide range of activities and responsibilities requires ophthalmologists to have completed an undergraduate college degree, a doctorate in medicine, a 1-year internship, and 3 or more additional years of specialized clinical training in the field of **ophthalmology** (medical specialty concerned with the eye). **Optometry** is the profession concerned with examination of the eyes and related structures. An **optometrist** is a doctor of optometry (O.D.) who examines eyes and prescribes corrective lenses. In the United States, optometrists have completed a preprofessional undergraduate education plus 4 years of professional education at an accredited college of optometry. The technicians who fill eyeglass prescriptions and dispense eyewear are called **opticians**. This occupation requires a high school diploma and successful completion of an accredited optician program, which consists about 1 year of study.

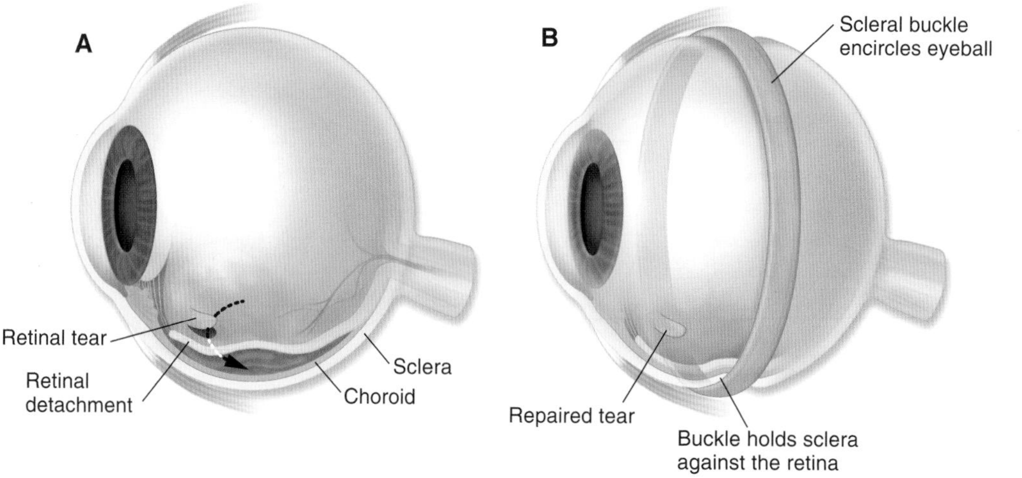


**FIGURE 8-8** Scleral buckle. **A.** Detached retina. The arrow shows the movement of fluid. **B.** Repair of retinal tear by attached a band (buckle) around the sclera to keep the retina from pulling away.

## WORD PARTS RELATED TO THE EAR

The three root words that mean ear are aur/o, auricul/o, and ot/o. These refer to the structure of the ear, but more commonly you will see words related to the function of the ear. Acous/o, acus/o, and accost/o all mean hearing, from the Greek *akoustikos* (pertaining to hearing). The Latin word for "pertaining to hearing" is *auditorius*, which gives us the word part audi/o and makes up words like *auditory* and *audible*. Table 8-2 list word parts related to the ear.

### Structure and Function of the Ear

The ear is an organ of hearing and equilibrium (balance). The ear is divided into three sections: the external ear, middle ear, and internal ear. The **external ear** consists of the auricle (outer ear), external acoustic meatus (passageway), and tympanic membrane (eardrum). It directs sound waves into the ear. Numerous ceruminous glands line the external acoustic meatus and secrete **cerumen**, better known as *earwax*. Cerumen protects the ear by preventing dust, insects, and some bacteria from

**TABLE 8-2 WORD PARTS RELATED TO THE EAR**

| Word Part | Meaning |
|---|---|
| acous/o, acus/o, acoust/o | hearing |
| audi/o | sound |
| aur/o | ear |
| auricul/o | ear |
| myring/o | tympanic membrane (eardrum) |
| ot/o | ear |
| staped/o | stapes (smallest ear bone) |
| tympan/o | eardrum |

**Word Parts Exercise**

After studying Table 8-2, write the meaning of each of the word parts.

| WORD PART | MEANING |
|---|---|
| 1. audi/o | 1. ______ |
| 2. ot/o | 2. ______ |
| 3. acous/o, acus/o, acoust/o | 3. ______ |
| 4. myring/o | 4. ______ |
| 5. tympan/o | 5. ______ |
| 6. aur/o | 6. ______ |
| 7. staped/o | 7. ______ |
| 8. auricul/o | 8. ______ |

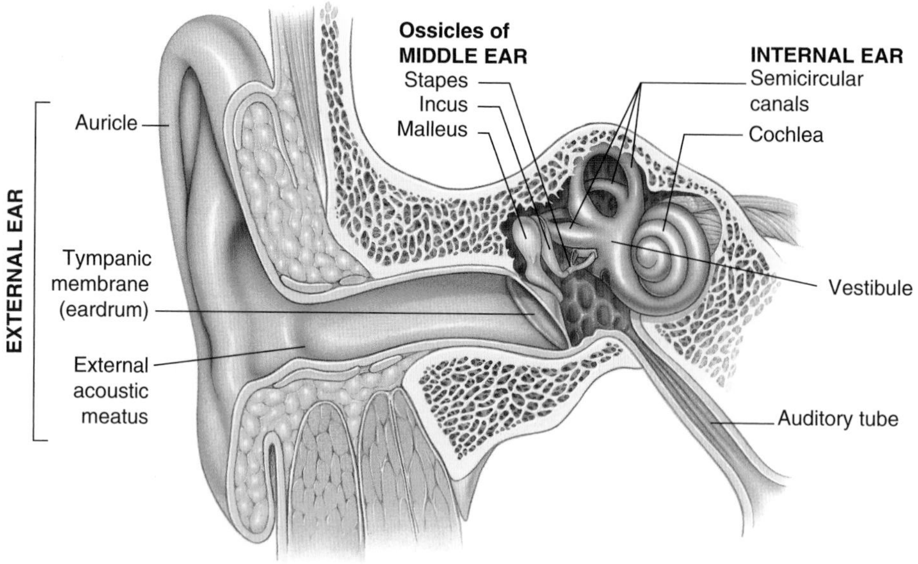


**FIGURE 8-9** Structures of the external, middle, and internal ear.

entering the middle ear. The **middle ear** consists of the tympanic cavity with its auditory ossicles (bones), associated muscles, and the auditory tube. The **internal ear** contains the vestibule, which includes the bony labyrinth of semicircular canals and the cochlea (see Figure 8-9).

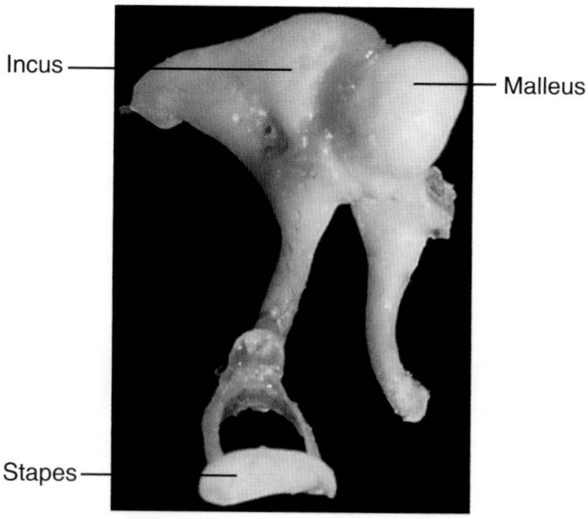


**FIGURE 8-10** The auditory ossicles.

Sound waves entering the ear vibrate the **tympanic membrane** (eardrum). Just beyond the tympanic membrane is the middle ear. A tiny *tympanic cavity* in the skull houses the **auditory ossicles**, three small bones called the **malleus**, **incus**, and **stapes** (see Figure 8-10). These are also sometimes referred to as the hammer, anvil, and stirrup because of their shapes. Sound waves affect these tiny bones and cause them to transmit sound vibrations to the internal ear. Also found inside the middle ear is the **auditory tube**, which reaches from the tympanic cavity to the nasopharynx to help equalize pressure in the ear with outside atmospheric pressure (see Figure 8-9).

The internal ear has a **bony labyrinth** (maze) that contains the sensory receptors for hearing and balance. Major structures of the bony labyrinth include the **semicircular canals** (organ of balance) and **cochlea** (organ of hearing). Receptors in the cochlea change sound waves into nerve impulses that the brain can process.

## Disorders Related to the Ear

Ear disorders can occur in any part of the ear. **Impacted cerumen**, an accumulation of earwax in the external acoustic meatus, may cause hearing loss. An earache, termed **otalgia** or **otodynia**, may be caused by trauma or infection. **Otitis** is any inflammation of the ear but can be divided into otitis externa (inflammation of the outer ear), otitis media (OM) (inflammation of the middle ear), or otitis interna (inflammation of the inner ear), with otitis media being the most common type.

Hearing loss may range from a partial loss of hearing that includes only a certain range of frequencies to leaving a person completely **deaf** (unable to hear). **Conductive hearing loss** occurs when sound waves are not conducted through the external ear to the ossicles of the middle ear. **Sensorineural hearing loss** occurs when there is damage to the cochlea of the internal ear or to the nerve pathways to the brain. **Presbycusis** is a progressive hearing loss that occurs with aging. **Anacusis** is total deafness.

### Quick Check #2

**Fill in the blanks.**

1. What are the medical terms for the ossicles, sometimes referred to as the hammer, anvil, and stirrup? ______________________

2. Identify the types of hearing loss. ______________________

3. Identify the structure in the labyrinth that changes sound waves into nerve impulses. ______________________

Other inflammatory ear conditions are **myringitis**, inflammation of the tympanic membrane; **mastoiditis**, inflammation of the mastoid air cells, which are intercommunicating cavities in the mastoid process of the temporal bone; and **labyrinthitis**, an inflammation of the labyrinth.

Two other disorders of the ear include **otosclerosis** (hardening of the stapes, resulting in sound being unable to travel from the outer ear to the internal ear) and **Ménière's syndrome**, a chronic disease of the internal ear characterized by vertigo, tinnitus, and periodic hearing loss. **Vertigo** is dizziness and/or a loss of balance. **Tinnitus** is a ringing, buzzing, or roaring sound in the ears.

## Diagnostic Tests, Treatments, and Surgical Procedures of the Ear

Some disorders of the ear are treated by surgical intervention. Some of these procedures include the following:

- **Otoplasty:** surgical repair of the auricle of the ear
- **Mastoidectomy:** surgical removal of the mastoid process of the temporal bone
- **Myringectomy** or **tympanectomy:** surgical removal of all or part of the tympanic membrane
- **Myringotomy:** surgical incision of the eardrum to create an opening for placement of drainage tubes
- **Tympanoplasty:** surgical correction of a damaged tympanic membrane
- **Stapedectomy:** surgical removal of the stapes
- **Labyrinthotomy:** a surgical incision into the labyrinth

## Practice and Practitioners of the Ear

**Audiology** is the specialty dealing with hearing and hearing disorders. An **audiologist** is the specialist who measures hearing and treats hearing impairments. An **otoscope** is an instrument with light and lenses used to visually examine the external ear and eardrum. **Otology** is the study of the ear and its related structures. An **otologist** is the specialist who diagnoses and treats diseases of the ear and its related structures. An **otorhinolaryngologist** is a physician who specializes in the diagnosis and treatment of diseases that involve not only the ear but also nose and throat.

## ABBREVIATIONS

The following table lists common abbreviations relating to the eyes and ears. The Latin words *dexter* and *sinister* mean, respectively, "right" and "left." These two Latin words give us many English words, such as ambidextrous (able to use either hand equally well), dextrous (good with one's hands), and sinister (odd or spooky—probably because 83% of the population is right-handed). The first letter of each of these two words, namely, D and S, have also found their way into abbreviations for the eyes and ears. AD means right ear because *A* refers to audi/o "the ear," and *D* refers to *dexter* "the right side." Likewise, AS refers to the left ear. The root ocul/o refers to the eye, and thus OD is the right eye, and OS is the left eye. The abbreviation OU means both eyes and is derived from the Latin term *oculus uterque*, meaning "both eyes."

Are abbreviations good or bad? The good thing about abbreviations is that they save time. The bad thing about them is that time saved seldom equals accuracy lost. Looking up the abbreviation AU will get you many answers, one of which is "both ears" and another of which is "aortic stenosis." Heart surgery is not going to help someone who is suffering hearing loss in both ears. By the way, neither of those meanings has a connection with Australia, which is also among the many meanings given for the AU abbreviation.

**Abbreviation Table** SIGHT AND HEARING

| ABBREVIATION | MEANING |
|---|---|
| AD | right ear |
| AS | left ear |
| AU | both ears |
| EOM | extraocular movement |
| IOP | intraocular pressure |
| LASIK | laser-assisted in situ keratomileusis |
| OD | right eye |
| O.D. | doctor of optometry |
| OM | otitis media |
| OS | left eye |
| OU | both eyes |

**Study Table** SIGHT AND HEARING

| TERM AND PRONUNCIATION | ANALYSIS | MEANING |
|---|---|---|
| **Structure and Function: Eye** | | |
| accommodation (ah-KOM-moh-DAY-shun) | common English word | the process that allows the shape of the lens to change for near and far vision |
| aqueous humor (A-kwee-us HUE-mor) | from the Latin word *aqua* (water) + humor, from the Latin word *umor* (body fluid) | watery substance filling the space between the lens and the cornea |
| canthus (KAN-thus) | from the Greek word *kanthus* (corner of the eye) | angle where the upper and lower eyelids meet |
| choroid (KOH-royd) | derived from the Greek words *chorion* (skin, leather; a spot or plot of ground) and *eidos* (form, likeness, appearance, resemblance) | opaque middle layer of the eyeball |
| ciliary body (SIL-ee-her-ee) | from the Latin word *ciliaris* (pertaining to eyelashes) + body | set of muscles and suspensory ligaments that adjust the shape of lens |
| cones | from the Greek word *konos* (cone) | color receptors on the retina that have high visual acuity |
| conjunctiva (kon-JUNK-tih-vuh); plural: conjunctivae (kon-JUNK-tih-vay) | from the Latin words *con* (with) and *jungere* (to join) | the mucous membrane covering the anterior of the eyeball and inner eyelid |
| cornea (KOR-nee-uh) | from the Latin word *cornus* (horn) | transparent shield of tissue forming the outer wall of the eyeball |
| dacryocyst (DACK-ree-oh-sist) | from the Greek words *dakryon* (tear) and *kytis* (bag) | dilated upper portion of nasolacrimal duct; tear sac, lacrimal sac |
| extraocular muscles (EX-trah-AWK-yu-lahr MUS-ulz) | *extra-* (outside); *ocul/o* (eye); *-ar* (adjective suffix) | muscles within the orbit but outside the eyeball |
| eyebrows (EYE-browz) | common English word | arched line of hairs on the superior edge of the orbit |
| eyelashes | common English word | stiff hairs projecting from the margins of the eyelids |
| eyelids | common English word | movable folds that cover the front of the eyes when they close; also called *palpebrae* |
| fovea centralis (FOH-avee-ah sen-TRAH-lis) | *fovea*, a Latin word meaning "small pit" + *centralis*, a Latin word meaning "central" | a depression in the middle of the retina that is the area of sharpest vision |

*(continued)*

**Study Table** SIGHT AND HEARING (*continued*)

| TERM AND PRONUNCIATION | ANALYSIS | MEANING |
|---|---|---|
| iris (EYE-rihs); plural: irides (IHR-ih-deez) | a Greek word meaning "lily," "iris of the eye," originally "messenger of the gods," personified as the rainbow | the anterior part of the vascular tunic; it is the colored part of the eye |
| lacrimal apparatus (LAK-rih-mul app-ah-RAT-uhs) | from the Latin words *lacrima* (tear) + *ad* (toward) and *parare* (to make ready) | collectively: the lacrimal gland, lacrimal lake, lacrimal canaliculi (small canals), and lacrimal sac, along with the nasolacrimal duct |
| lacrimal ducts (LAK-rih-mul DUKTZ) | from the Latin words *lacrima* (tear) | channels that carry tears to the eyes |
| lacrimal glands (LAK-rih-mul GLANDZ) | from the Latin words *lacrima* (tear) | glands that secrete tears |
| lacrimal fluid (LAK-rih-mahl FLOO-id) | from the Latin words *lacrima* (tear) and *fluidus* (fluid) | a watery, physiologic saline; *tears* |
| lacrimal sac (LAK-rih-mul SAK) | from the Latin words *lacrima* (tear) | dilated upper part of the nasolacrimal duct |
| lateral angle of eye | common English words | angle formed by the union of the lateral parts of the upper eyelid and lower eyelid; also called *lateral canthus* |
| lens (lenz) | common English word | the refractive structure of the eye, lying between the iris and the vitreous humor |
| medial angle of eye | common English words | angle formed by the union of the upper eyelid and lower eyelid; also called *medial canthus* |
| nasolacrimal ducts | naso- (nose); from the Latin word *lacrima* (tear) | ducts that carry tears from the lacrimal glands to the nose |
| ocular (OK-yoo-lahr) | *ocul/o* (eye); *-ar* (adjective suffix) | adjective referring to the eye |
| optic disc (OP-tik DISK) | *opt/o* (light, eye, vision); *-ic* (adjective suffix) | oval area in eye without light receptors; *blind spot* |
| optic nerve (OP-tik nuhrv) | *opt/o* (light, eye, vision); *-ic* (adjective suffix) + nerve | the cranial nerve responsible for vision |
| orbit (OR-biht) | from the Latin word *orbita* (wheel track, course, orbit) | bony depression in the skull that houses the eyeball |
| palpebra (pal-PEE-brah) | a Latin word meaning "eyelid" | eyelid |

**Study Table** SIGHT AND HEARING (*continued*)

| TERM AND PRONUNCIATION | ANALYSIS | MEANING |
|---|---|---|
| photoreceptors (FOH-toh-ree-SEPP-tohrs) | from the Greek word *phos* (light) and the Latin word *recipere* (to receive) | retinal cones and rods |
| pupil (PYOO-pihl) | from the Latin word *pupilla* (little girl-doll) so called from the tiny image one sees of oneself reflected in the eye of another | the dark part in the center of the iris through which light enters the eye |
| retina (RETT-ih-nah) | from Medieval Latin *retina* probably from the Latin word *rete* (net) | light-sensitive membrane forming the innermost layer of the eyeball |
| rods | a common English word | black and white receptors on the retina that respond to dim light |
| sclera (SKLER-ah); plural: sclerae (SKLER-ay) | from the Greek word *skleros* (hard) | the outer surface of the eye; part of the fibrous tunic; white part of eye |
| uvea (YOO-vee-ah) | from the Latin word *uva* (grape) | vascular layer of the eye |
| vitreous body (VIH-tree-uhs BOD-ee) | from the Latin word *vitreus* (of glass, glassy) + body | a transparent jellylike substance filling the interior of the eyeball |
| vitreous humor (VIH-tree-uhs HYU-mohr) | from the Latin word *umor* (body fluid) | the fluid component of the vitreous body |
| **Disorders: Eye** | | |
| amblyopia (am-blee-OH-pee-ah) | from the Greek word *ambly* (dim); *-opia* (eye, vision) | condition that occurs when visual acuity is not the same in both eyes; also called *lazy eye* |
| astigmatism (ah-STIG-mah-tizm) | *a-* (without) + from the Greek word *stigmatos* gen. of *stigma* (a mark, spot, puncture) | fuzzy vision caused by the irregular shape of one or both eyeballs |
| blepharitis (bleff-ah-RY-tiss) | *blephar/o* (eyelid); *-itis* (inflammation) | inflammation of the eyelid |
| blepharoconjunctivitis (BLEFF-ah-roh-kon-junk-tih-VY-tiss) | *blephar/o* (eyelid); *conjunctiv/o* (mucous membrane covering the anterior surface of the eyeball and inner eyelid); *-itis* (inflammation) | inflammation of the palpebral conjunctiva, the inner lining of the eyelids |
| blepharoplegia (BLEFF-ah-roh-pleej-ee-uh) | *blephar/o* (eyelid); *-plegia* (paralysis) | paralysis of an eyelid |

(*continued*)

**Study Table** SIGHT AND HEARING (*continued*)

| TERM AND PRONUNCIATION | ANALYSIS | MEANING |
|---|---|---|
| blepharoptosis (BLEFF-ahr-opp-TOH-sis) | *blephar/o* (eyelid); *-ptosis* (falling, downward placement, prolapse) | drooping eyelid |
| blepharospasm (BLEFF-ahr-oh-SPAZ-um) | *blephar/o* (eyelid); from the Greek *spasmos* (spasm, convulsion) | involuntary contraction of the eyelid |
| cataract (KAT-ah-rakt) | from the Latin word *cataracta* (waterfall) | complete or partial opacity of the ocular lens |
| conjunctivitis (kon-junk-tih-VY-tiss) | *conjunctiv/o* (mucous membrane covering the anterior surface of the eyeball); *-itis* (inflammation) | inflammation of the conjunctiva; pinkeye |
| dacryocele (DAKK-ree-oh-seel) | *dacry/o* (tears); *-cele* (hernia) | enlargement of the lacrimal sac with fluid |
| dacryocystitis (DAKK-ree-oh-SIST-it is) | *dacryocyst/o* (tear sac); *-itis* (inflammation) | inflammation of the tear sac |
| dacryolith (DAKK-ree-oh-lith) | *dacry/o* (tears); *-lith* (stone) | a "stone" in the lacrimal apparatus |
| dacryorrhea (DAK-ree-uh-REE-yuh) | *dacry/o* (tears); *-rrhea* (discharge) | excessive discharge of tears |
| diplopia (dih-PLOH-pee-uh) | *diplo-* (from the Greek *diploos* meaning "double"); *-opia* (eye, vision) | condition in which a single object is perceived as two objects; double vision |
| ectropion | *ex-* (out); *trope* (Greek "that which turns") | eversion (turning out) of the eyelid |
| entropion | *en-* (in); *trope* (Greek "that which turns") | inversion (turning in) of the eyelid |
| glaucoma (glaw-KOH-mah) | from the Greek word *glaucoma* (cataract, opacity of the lens) (note: cataracts and glaucoma not distinguished until around 1705) | disease of the eye characterized by increased intraocular pressure and atrophy of the optic nerve |
| hordeolum (hor-DEE-oh-lum) | from the Latin word *hordeum* (barley) | an infection of a gland in the eye; also called *sty* |
| hyperopia (hy-pur-OH-pee-ya) or presbyopia (pres-be-OH-pee-ah) | *hyper-* (above normal); *-opia* (eye, vision) | Farsightedness |
| iridomalacia (IHR-ih-doh-muh-LAY-shee-uh) | *irid/o* (iris); *-malacia* (softening) | softening of the iris |
| iritis (eye-RY-tiss) | *ir/o* (iris); *-itis* (inflammation) | inflammation of the iris |

**Study Table** SIGHT AND HEARING (*continued*)

| TERM AND PRONUNCIATION | ANALYSIS | MEANING |
|---|---|---|
| keratitis (ker-ah-TYE-tis) | *kerat/o* (hard, cornea); *-itis* (inflammation) | inflammation of the cornea |
| lacrimal (LAK-rih-muhl) | *lacrim/o* (tear, lacrimal apparatus); *-al* (adjective suffix) | referring to or related to tears or the tear ducts and glands |
| lacrimation (LAK-rih-MAY-shun) | *lacrim/o* (tear, lacrimal apparatus); *-ation* (noun suffix) | secretion of tears, especially in excess |
| myopia (my-OHP-ee-ah) | from the Greek word *myops* (nearsighted) | Nearsightedness |
| oculodynia (AWK-yu-loh-DIN-ee-ah) | *ocul/o* (eye); *-dynia* (pain) | pain in the eyeball; also called *ophthalmalgia* |
| oculopathy (AWK-yu-loh-path-ee) | *ocul/o* (eye); *-pathy* (disease) | any disease of the eyes; also called *ophthalmopathy* |
| ophthalmolith (off-THAL-moh-lith) | *ophthalm/o* (eye); *-lith* (stone) | a stone in the lacrimal apparatus; also called *dacryolith* |
| ophthalmomalacia (off-THAL-moh-muh-LAY-shee-uh) | *ophthalm/o* (eye); *-malacia* (softening) | softening of the eyeball |
| ophthalmopathy (off-THAL-moh-path-ee) | *ophthalm/o* (eye); *-pathy* (disease) | any disease of the eyes; also called *oculopathy* |
| presbyopia (prez-bee-OH-pee-ah) | from the Greek word *presbys* (old man); *-opia* (eye, vision) | farsightedness resulting from loss of elasticity of the lens due to aging |
| retinitis (rett-ih-NY-tiss) | *retin/o* (retina); *-itis* (inflammation) | inflammation of the retina |
| retinopathy (rett-ihn-AWP-uh-thee) | *retin/o* (retina); *-pathy* (disease) | disease of the retina |
| scleroiritis (skler-oh-EYE-RY-tiss) | *sclera/o* (sclera); *ir/o* (iris); *-itis* (inflammation) | inflammation of the sclera and iris |
| strabismus (stra-BIZ-muhs) | from the Greek word *strabismos*, from *strabos* (squinting, squint-eyed) | lack of parallelism in the visual axes; also called *crossed eyes* |
| xerophthalmia (zee-roh-OFF-thal-mee-ah) | from the Greek word *xeros* (dry); *ophthalm/o* (eye); *-ia* (condition) | dry eyes |
| **Diagnostic Tests, Treatments, and Surgical Procedures: Eye** | | |
| blepharectomy (bleff-ah-REK-tuh-mee) | *blephar/o* (eyelid); *-ectomy* (excision) | surgical removal of part or all of an eyelid |
| blepharoplasty (BLEFF-ah-roh-plass-tee) | *blephar/o* (eyelid); *-plasty* (surgical repair) | surgery to correct a defective eyelid |
| blepharotomy (BLEFF-uh-rot-uh-mee) | *blephar/o* (eyelid); *-tomy* (incision into) | surgical incision of an eyelid |

(*continued*)

**Study Table** SIGHT AND HEARING (*continued*)

| TERM AND PRONUNCIATION | ANALYSIS | MEANING |
|---|---|---|
| conjunctivoplasty (kon-JUNK-tih-voh-plass-tee) | *conjunctiv/o* (conjunctiva); *-plasty* (surgical repair) | surgery on the conjunctiva |
| dacryocystectomy (dakk-ree-oh-sist-EKK-toh-mee) | *dacryocyst/o* (tear sac); *-ectomy* (excision) | surgical removal of the lacrimal sac |
| dacryocystotomy (dakk-ree-oh-sist-AW-toh-mee) | *dacryocyst/o* (tear sac); *-tomy* (incision into) | incision into the lacrimal sac |
| lacrimotomy (lakk-rih-MAW-toh-mee) (uncommon) | *lacrim/o* (tear, lacrimal apparatus); *-tomy* (incision into) | incision into the lacrimal sac or lacrimal duct |
| ophthalmoscope (OFF-THAL-moh-skope) | *ophthalm/o* (eye); *-scope* (instrument for viewing) | device for examining the interior of the eyeball by looking through the pupil |
| ophthalmoscopy (OFF-thal-MAW-skuh-pee) | *ophthalm/o* (eye); *-scopy* (use of instrument for viewing) | examination of the eye with an ophthalmoscope |
| phacolysis (fah-KAWL-ih-sis) | *phac/o* (lens); *-lysis* (destruction) | operative removal of the lens in pieces |
| refraction (re-FRAK-shun) | from late Latin *refractio*, from *refringere* (to break up) | deflection of a ray of light into the eye for accommodation or correction of vision as it passes from one medium to another of different densities |
| retinectomy (ret-ihn-EK-tuh-mee) | *retin/o* (retina); *-ectomy* (excision) | surgical removal of part of the retina |
| retinopexy (RETT-ihn-oh-pexx-ee) | *retin/o* (retina); *-pexy* (surgical fixation) | surgical fixation of a detached retina |
| retinotomy (rett-ihn-AW-tuh-mee) | *retin/o* (retina); *-tomy* (incision into) | incision through the retina |
| scleral buckle (SKLEER-ul BUCK-ul) | *scler/o* (hard) | an operation to place a silicone band on the scleral periphery to tighten the retina |
| **Practice and Practitioners: Eye** | | |
| ophthalmologist (off-thul-MAWL-uh-jist) | *ophthalm/o* (eye); *-logist* (one who studies a specific field) | physician whose specialty is the diagnosis and treatment of eye disorders |
| ophthalmology (off-thul-MAWL-uh-jee) | *ophthalm/o* (eye); *-logy* (study of) | medical specialty dealing with the eye |
| optician (opp-TISH-ihn) | *opt/o* (light, eye, vision) | person who fills prescriptions for ophthalmic lenses, dispenses glasses, and makes and fits contact lenses |
| optometrist (opp-TOM-uh-trist) | *opt/o* (light, eye, vision); *-metrist* (one who measures) | one trained in examining the eyes and prescribing corrective lenses |

**Study Table** SIGHT AND HEARING (*continued*)

| TERM AND PRONUNCIATION | ANALYSIS | MEANING |
|---|---|---|
| optometry (opp-TOM-uh-tree) | *opt/o* (light, eye, vision); *-metry* (measurement) | science of examining eyes for impaired vision and other disorders |
| **Structure and Function: Ear** | | |
| auditory tube (AW-dih-uh-tor-ee TOOB) | from the Latin word *auditorius* (pertaining to hearing) | Canal that connects the middle ear to the pharynx (throat); also called *pharyngotympanic tube* and *eustachian tube* |
| auricle (AW-rik-uhl) | *auri-* (ear) | external portion of the ear that directs sound waves; also called *pinna* |
| cerumen (she-ROO-men) | from the Latin word *cera* (wax) | waxy substance produced by glands of the external acoustic meatus |
| external acoustic meatus (EKS-tur-nul uh-KOOS-tick mee-AY-tus) | from the Latin, *externus* (outside) + from the Greek, *akoustikos* (pertaining to sound) + from the Latin, *meatus* (passage) | Passage leading inward from the auricle to the tympanic membrane (eardrum); also called *external auditory canal* |
| eustachian tube (yu-STAY-shun) | named after Bartolomeo Eustachi (died 1574), who discovered the passages from the ears to the throat | canal that connects the middle ear to the pharynx (throat); also called the *auditory tube* and *pharyngotympanic tube* |
| incus (INK-uhs) | a Latin word meaning “anvil” | one of the auditory ossicles (the anvil) |
| labyrinth (LAB-uh-rinth) | from the Greek word *labyrinthos* (maze, large building with intricate passages) | canals of the inner ear |
| malleus (MAL-ee-uhs) | a Latin word meaning “hammer” | one of the auditory ossicles (the hammer) |
| ossicles (OSS-ih-kulz) | from the Latin word *ossiculum* (a small bone) | three small bones in the middle ear: the malleus (hammer), the incus (anvil), and the stapes (stirrup) |
| pinna (PIN-ah) | a Latin word meaning “feather,” “wing,” “fin,” “lobe” | external portion of the ear that directs sound waves; also called *auricle* |
| stapes (STAY-peez) | a Modern Latin word meaning “stirrup” | one of the auditory ossicles (the stirrup) |
| tympanic cavity (tim-PAN-ik) | *tympan/o* (eardrum); *-ic* (adjective suffix) + cavity | air chamber between the external acoustic meatus and the internal ear that contains the ossicles |

(*continued*)

**Study Table** SIGHT AND HEARING (*continued*)

| TERM AND PRONUNCIATION | ANALYSIS | MEANING |
|---|---|---|
| tympanic membrane (tim-PAN-ik MEM-brayn) | *tympan/o* (eardrum); *-ic* (adjective suffix) | eardrum |
| **Disorders: Ear** | | |
| anacusis (ann-ah-KU-sis) | *a-* (without); cusis, from the Greek word *akousis* (hearing) | total deafness |
| conductive hearing loss (kon-DUK-tihv) | common English words | hearing loss caused by interference with sound transmission in the external acoustic meatus, middle ear, or ossicles |
| deaf (def) | common English word | unable to hear |
| labyrinthitis (lab-ih-rin-THIGH-tis) | *labyrinth/o* (internal ear); *-itis* (inflammation) | inflammation of the labyrinth |
| mastoiditis (mas-toy-DYE-tis) | mastoid (mastoid process); *-itis* (inflammation) | inflammation of any part of the mastoid air cells of the mastoid process of the temporal bone |
| Ménière's (men-YEHRS) syndrome | named for Prosper Ménière, the French physician who first described the illness in 1861 | chronic disease of the internal ear characterized by vertigo, tinnitus, and periodic hearing loss |
| myringitis (mir-in-JIGH-tis) | *myring/o* (tympanic membrane); *-itis* (inflammation) | inflammation of the tympanic membrane |
| otalgia (oh-TAHL-jee-ah) | *ot/o* (ear); *-algia* (pain) | pain in the ear |
| otitis (oh-TY-tihs) | *ot/o* (ear); *-itis* (inflammation) | inflammation of the ear (otitis externa = the outer ear; otitis media = the middle ear; otitis interna = the inner ear) |
| otodynia (oh-toh-DIN-ee-uh) | *ot/o* (ear); *-dynia* (pain) | earache |
| otopathy (oh-TOP-ahth-ee) | *ot/o* (ear); *-pathy* (disease) | any disease of the ear |
| otoplasty (oh-toh-PLAS-tee) | *ot/o* (ear); *-plasty* (surgical repair) | surgical repair of the auricle of the ear |
| otorrhea (oh-toh-REE-uh) | *ot/o* (ear); *-rrhea* (discharge) | fluid discharge from the ear |
| otosclerosis (OH-toh-skler-OH-sihs) | *ot/o* (ear); *scler/o* (hardening); *-osis* (abnormal condition) | formation of spongy bone in the internal ear producing hearing loss |
| presbycusis (PREZ-be-KOO-sihs) | *presby-* (old); cusis, from the Greek word *akousis* (hearing) | hearing loss that occurs with aging |
| sensorineural hearing loss (SENTZ-oh-rih-NOO-rahl) | *sensor-* (sensory); *neur/o* (nervous system); *-al* (adjective suffix) | hearing loss caused by a neural condition |

**Study Table** SIGHT AND HEARING (*continued*)

| TERM AND PRONUNCIATION | ANALYSIS | MEANING |
|---|---|---|
| tinnitus (TIN-nih-tuhs) | from the Latin word *tinnire* (to ring) | sensation of noises (such as ringing) in the ears |
| vertigo (VUR-tih-go) | a Latin word meaning "dizziness" | sensation of spinning or whirling; dizziness; can be caused by infection or other disorder in the inner ear |
| **Diagnostic Tests, Treatments, and Surgical Procedures: Ear** | | |
| audiogram (AW-dee-oh-gram) | *audi/o* (sound, hearing); *-gram* (record or picture) | a graphic record produced by the results of hearing tests with an audiometer |
| audiometer (aw-dee-AWM-ih-tehr) | *audi/o* (sound, hearing); *-meter* (measurement) | electrical device for measuring hearing |
| audiometry (aw-dee-AWM-ih-tree) | *audi/o* (sound, hearing); *-metry* (process of measuring) | measuring hearing with an audiometer |
| cochlear implant (KOK-lee-ahr IM-plant) | from the Latin word *cochlea* (snail shell); *-ar* (adjective suffix) + implant | surgically implanted hearing aid in the cochlea |
| labyrinthotomy (lab-ih-rin-THAH-toh-mee) | *labyrinth/o* (internal ear); *-tomy* (incision into) | a surgical incision into the labyrinth |
| mastoidectomy (mas-toy-DECK-toh-mee) | mastoid (mastoid process) + *-ectomy* (excision) | surgical removal of the mastoid process |
| myringectomy (mir-ini-JECK-toh-mee) | *myring/o* (tympanic membrane); *-ectomy* (excision) | surgical removal of all or part of the tympanic membrane; also called *tympanectomy* |
| myringoplasty (mih-RIN-go-PLASS-tee) | *myring/o* (tympanic membrane); *-plasty* (surgical repair) | surgical repair of the tympanic membrane (eardrum) |
| myringotomy (mih-rin-GOT-uh-mee) | *myring/o* (tympanic membrane); *-tomy* (incision into) | incision or surgical puncture of the eardrum; also called *tympanotomy* |
| otoplasty (OH-toh-plass-tee) | *ot/o* (ear); *-plasty* (surgical repair) | surgical repair of the auricle of the ear |
| otoscope (OH-toh-skope) | *ot/o* (ear); *-scope* (instrument for viewing) | device for looking into the ear |
| otoscopy (oh-TOSS-kuh-pee) | *ot/o* (ear); *-scopy* (use of an instrument for viewing) | looking into the ear with an otoscope |
| Rinne test (rihn-eh) | named after Heinrich A. Rinne, German otologist (1819–1868) | hearing test using a tuning fork; checks for differences in bone conduction and air conduction |
| stapedectomy (stay-peh-DECK-toh-mee) | *staped/o* (stapes); *-ectomy* (excision) | surgical removal of the stapes |

(*continued*)

**Study Table** SIGHT AND HEARING *(continued)*

| TERM AND PRONUNCIATION | ANALYSIS | MEANING |
|---|---|---|
| tuning fork (TOO-ning) | common English words | an instrument that vibrates when struck and is used to test hearing and vibratory sensations |
| tympanectomy (TIM-puh-NEK-tuh-mee) | *tympan/o* (eardrum); *-tomy* (incision into) | surgical removal of the eardrum; also called *myringectomy* |
| tympanocentesis (TIM-puh-noh-senn-TEE-sihs) | *tympan/o* (eardrum); *-centesis* (surgical puncture for aspiration) | puncture of the tympanic membrane with a needle to aspirate middle ear fluid |
| tympanoplasty (TIM-puh-no-plass-tee) | *tympan/o* (eardrum); *-plasty* (surgical repair) | surgery performed on the eardrum |
| tympanotomy (TIM-puh-NOT-oh-mee); | *tympan/o* (eardrum); *-tomy* (incision) | incision or surgical puncture of the eardrum; also called *myringotomy* |
| Weber test (VAY-behr) | named after Wilhelm Edward Weber, German physicist (1804–1891) | hearing test using a tuning fork; distinguishes between conductive and sensorineural hearing loss |
| **Practice and Practitioners: Ear** | | |
| audiologist (awd-ee-AWL-oh-jist) | *audi/o* (sound, hearing); *-logist* (one who studies a certain field) | specialist who measures hearing efficiency and treats hearing impairment |
| audiology (awd-ee-AWL-oh-jee) | *audi/o* (sound, hearing); *-logy* (the study of a certain field) | specialty dealing with hearing and hearing disorders |
| otologist (oh-TOL-oh-jist) | *ot/o* (ear); *-logist* (one who studies a certain field) | specialist in otology, the branch of medical science concerned with the study, diagnosis, and treatment of diseases of the ear and its related structures |
| otology (oh-TOL-oh-jee) | *ot/o* (ear); *-logy* (the study of a certain field) | branch of medical science concerned with the study, diagnosis, and treatment of diseases of the ear and its related structures |
| otorhinolaryngologist (oh-TOH-REYE-no-lair-in-GOL-oh-jist) | *ot/o* (ear); *rhin/o* (nose); *g/o* (throat); *-logist* (one who studies a certain field) | physician who specializes in the diagnosis and treatment of ear, nose, and throat disorders |

## END-OF-CHAPTER EXERCISES

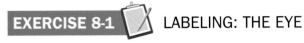

### EXERCISE 8-1 LABELING: THE EYE

**Using the following list, choose the correct terms to label the diagram correctly.**

| | | |
|---|---|---|
| anterior chamber (containing aqueous humor) | choroid | conjunctiva |
| cornea | fovea centralis | iris |
| lens | optic nerve | posterior chamber (containing vitreous humor) |
| pupil | retina | sclera |

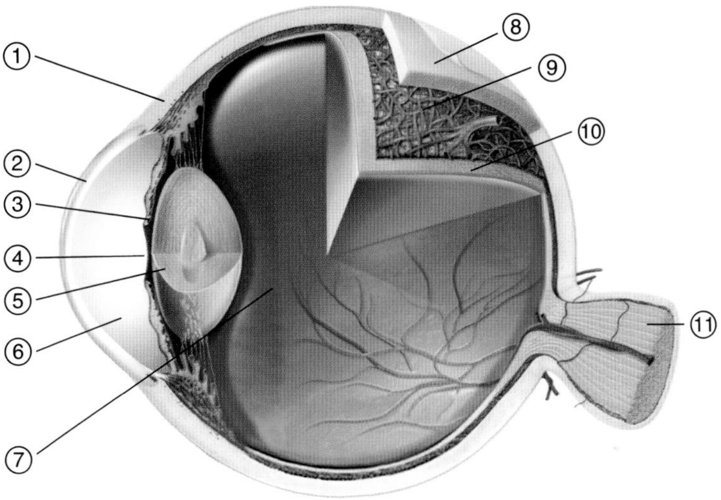


1. ______________________
2. ______________________
3. ______________________
4. ______________________
5. ______________________
6. ______________________
7. ______________________
8. ______________________
9. ______________________
10. ______________________
11. ______________________

## EXERCISE 8-2 WORD PARTS

**Break each of the following terms into its word parts: prefix, root, or suffix. Give the meaning of each word part and then define the term.**

1. *extraocular*

   prefix: ____________________

   root: ____________________

   suffix: ____________________

   definition: ____________________

2. *xerophthalmia*

   root: ____________________

   root: ____________________

   suffix: ____________________

   definition: ____________________

3. *scleroiritis*

   root: ____________________

   root: ____________________

   suffix: ____________________

   definition: ____________________

4. *blepharoconjunctivitis*

   root: ____________________

   root: ____________________

   suffix: ____________________

   definition: ____________________

5. *audiometry*

   root: ____________________

   suffix: ____________________

   definition: ____________________

6. *otosclerosis*

   root: ____________________

   root: ____________________

   suffix: ____________________

   definition: ____________________

7. *mastoidectomy*

root: ______________________

suffix: ______________________

definition: ______________________

8. *otorhinolaryngologist*

root: ______________________

root: ______________________

root: ______________________

suffix: ______________________

definition: ______________________

## EXERCISE 8-3 WORD BUILDING

**Use the word parts listed to build the terms defined.**

| | | | | |
|---|---|---|---|---|
| -lith | -centesis | irid/o | -rrhea | -malacia |
| tympano | myringo | -pexy | -tomy | -lysis |
| phac/o | ot/o | -dynia | retin/o | -itis |
| cyst/o | dacryo | | | |

1. ______________________ a "stone" in the lacrimal apparatus
2. ______________________ operative removal of the lens in pieces
3. ______________________ surgical removal of the lacrimal sac
4. ______________________ surgical fixation of a detached retina
5. ______________________ softening of the iris
6. ______________________ puncture of the tympanic membrane with a needle to aspirate middle ear fluid
7. ______________________ earache
8. ______________________ incision or surgical puncture of the eardrum
9. ______________________ fluid discharge from the ear
10. ______________________ inflammation of the ear

## EXERCISE 8-4 MATCHING: THE EYE

**Match the term with its definition.**

1. __________ ophthalmology
2. __________ vitreous humor
3. __________ pupil
4. __________ iris
5. __________ sclera
6. __________ cornea
7. __________ conjunctiva
8. __________ ophthalmoscope
9. __________ retina
10. __________ lacrimal

a. transparent shield of tissue covering the iris
b. adjective associated with tears
c. sensitive inner nerve layer of the eye that contains the rods and cones
d. the "colored" part of the eye
e. the dark part in the very center of the eye
f. mucous membrane that covers the anterior surface of the eyeball and lines the underside of each eyelid
g. gelatinous liquid between the lens and retina
h. part of the outermost layer of the eye, which is white in color
i. a device for examining the interior of the eyeball by looking through the pupil
j. name of the medical specialty dealing with the eye

## EXERCISE 8-5 MATCHING: THE EAR

**Match the term with its definition.**

1. __________ audiologist
2. __________ cerumen
3. __________ otoscope
4. __________ tympanoplasty
5. __________ labyrinth
6. __________ auditory ossicles
7. __________ otitis media
8. __________ tympanic membrane
9. __________ auditory tube
10. __________ cochlea

a. the eardrum
b. maze-like portion of the inner ear
c. specialist treating abnormal hearing
d. device for looking into the ear
e. inflammation of the middle ear
f. part of the bony labyrinth (internal ear)
g. wax-like secretion in the external auditory canal
h. passageway that connects the middle ear to the nasopharynx
i. surgical repair on the tympanic membrane
j. three small bones in the middle ear: the malleus, incus, and stapes

## EXERCISE 8-6 MULTIPLE CHOICE

**Choose the correct answer for the following multiple choice questions.**

1. The medical specialist who treats ear disorders is called a(n) ____________________.
   a. ophthalmologist
   b. otologist
   c. audiologist
   d. optometrist

2. A term for eardrum is ____________________.
   a. tympanic membrane
   b. malleus
   c. oval window
   d. none of the above

3. The function(s) of the ear include ____________________.
   a. equilibrium
   b. hearing
   c. sound vibrations
   d. both A and B

4. The ability of the eye to adjust to variations in distance is ____________________.
   a. eversion
   b. strabismus
   c. accommodation
   d. presbycusis

5. An inflammation of the tear sac is called ____________________.
   a. dacryocystitis
   b. scleroiritis
   c. blepharitis
   d. keratitis

6. The layer of the eye that contains the rods and cones is the ____________________.
   a. sclera
   b. choroid
   c. uvea
   d. retina

7. Hearing loss that is due to nerve damage is ____________________.
   a. conductive hearing loss
   b. sensorineural hearing loss
   c. tympanitis
   d. tinnitus

8. The cornea is the transparent part of the eye and is an extension of the ____________________.
   a. choroid
   b. iris
   c. sclera
   d. both a and c

9. The ciliary body is ____________________.
    a. a group of muscles that suspends the lens
    b. the curved portion of the eye that refracts light
    c. the area between the lens and retina
    d. the protective layer of the eye

10. Farsightedness is called ____________________.
    a. myopia
    b. hyperopia
    c. presbyopia
    d. both b and c

## EXERCISE 8-7 FILL IN THE BLANK

**Fill in the blank with the correct answer.**

1. A cloudiness or opacity of the lens is called a ____________________.
2. Difficulty hearing due to the aging process is termed ____________________.
3. The medical term for double vision is ____________________.
4. Another name for dizziness due to an internal ear disturbance is ____________________.
5. ____________________ is a ringing or buzzing of the ears.
6. The external ear component is called the pinna or ____________________.
7. Another name for a sty is ____________________.
8. ____________________ means pain in the ear or an earache.
9. An irregularity of the curve of the cornea that distorts the light entering the eye is called ____________________.
10. An inflammation of the cornea is called ____________________.
11. The ____________________ contains the sensory receptors for hearing.
12. The internal ear contains the ____________________ canals and cochlea.
13. The passageway that goes from the middle ear to the nasopharynx is the ____________________.
14. ____________________ is the medical term for a drooping eyelid.
15. A ____________________ hearing loss is one in which the external or middle ear cannot conduct the sound vibrations to the internal ear.

## EXERCISE 8-8 ABBREVIATIONS

**Write out the term for the following abbreviations.**

1. ______________________________ AD
2. ______________________________ OM
3. ______________________________ OD
4. ______________________________ AS
5. ______________________________ OU
6. ______________________________ OS
7. ______________________________ LASIK

**Write the abbreviation for the following terms.**

8. ____________ both ears
9. ____________ extraocular movement
10. ____________ right ear
11. ____________ intraocular pressure
12. ____________ left eye
13. ____________ doctor of optometry

## EXERCISE 8-9 SPELLING

**Select the correct spelling of the medical term.**

1. ________________ is the medical condition known as double vision.
   a. Diplopia
   b. Diploplia
   c. Dioplia
   d. Diplopea

2. The mucous membrane covering the anterior of the eyeball and the inner eyelid is the ________________.
   a. conjuctivah
   b. conjunktiva
   c. conjunctiva
   d. conjuncteva

3. The adjective ____________________ is used to describe tears.
   a. lacrimul
   b. lacrimal
   c. lacrimle
   d. lacramal

4. An eye disease characterized by an increase in intraocular pressure is ____________________.
   a. glacoma
   b. glaucoma
   c. gluacoma
   d. glocoma

5. An ____________________ is a health care professional who examines eyes and prescribes corrective lenses.
   a. optomatrist
   b. optomotrist
   c. optomitrist
   d. optometrist

6. The purpose of the ____________________ is to funnel sound waves into the auditory canal.
   a. aricle
   b. oricle
   c. auricel
   d. auricle

7. A synonym for otodynia is ____________________.
   a. otalgia
   b. otoalgia
   c. otalga
   d. otoalga

8. The three auditory ossicles are the incus, the stapes, and the ____________________.
   a. maleus
   b. malleus
   c. mallius
   d. malleous

9. A ____________________ is a puncture of the tympanic membrane with a needle to aspirate middle ear fluid.
   a. timpanacentesis
   b. timpanocentesis
   c. tympanocentesis
   d. tympanocentisis

10. An ____________________ is a specialist who measures hearing efficiency and treats hearing impairments.
    a. audiologist
    b. adiologist
    c. audilogist
    d. auddiologist

## EXERCISE 8-10 CASE STUDY

**Read the following report and define the italicized medical terms.**

**PREOPERATIVE DIAGNOSIS:** Chronic (1) *otitis media*

**OPERATIVE PROCEDURE:** Bilateral (2) *myringotomy* and placement of tubes

**INDICATIONS:** Recurrent ear infections with persistent fluid buildup despite prolonged medical treatment

**PROCEDURE:** The patient was brought to the operating suite and placed under general mask anesthesia. The ear canals were cleaned of dry (3) *cerumen* and crust. Myringotomies were done bilaterally. Cultures were taken of the fluid present in the middle ear spaces. Ear tubes were placed in the myringotomy sites bilaterally. Antibiotic drops and cotton balls were placed in (4) the *external acoustic meatus*.

The patient tolerated the procedure well and was taken to the recovery room.

1. ______________________________

2. ______________________________

3. ______________________________

4. ______________________________

# The Endocrine System

9

## LEARNING OUTCOMES

***Upon completion of this chapter, you should be able to:***

- Name the major endocrine glands and the hormones each gland secretes.
- Pronounce, spell, and define medical terms related to the endocrine system and its disorders.
- Interpret abbreviations associated with the endocrine system.

## INTRODUCTION

The **endocrine system** consists of ductless *glands* and organs that secrete *hormones* directly into the bloodstream. **Glands** are cell groupings that function as a secretory organ. In the case of the endocrine system, the secretion is called a **hormone**. Hormones are transported in the bloodstream to stimulate specific cells or tissues. Working together with the nervous system, the endocrine system helps to maintain **homeostasis** (chemical balance) throughout the body. The nervous system also contributes to this process by either stimulating or delaying hormone release according to feedback mechanisms.

## WORD PARTS RELATED TO THE ENDOCRINE SYSTEM

Endocrine comes from *endo-* (within) and the Greek *krinein* (to separate) and refers to secreting internally. This can be contrasted to **exocrine glands**, which secrete hormones through ducts instead of directly into the bloodstream, as endocrine glands do. An example of an exocrine gland is a sweat gland, which secretes onto the skin surface. *Aden/o* is the root for gland and comes from the Greek word for gland, *aden*. Be careful not to confuse aden/o with adren/o. Adren/o refers specifically to the adrenal glands, found by the kidneys and comes from the Latin ad- (near) and ren/o (kidney). Table 9-1 lists word parts that make up endocrine system terms.

**TABLE 9-1** WORD PARTS RELATED TO THE ENDOCRINE SYSTEM

| Word Part | Meaning |
|---|---|
| acr/o | extremities |
| aden/o | gland |
| adren/o | adrenal glands |
| adrenal/o | adrenal glands |
| calc/i | calcium |
| crin/o | to separate or secrete |

**TABLE 9-1 WORD PARTS RELATED TO THE ENDOCRINE SYSTEM**

| Word Part | Meaning |
|---|---|
| endocrin/o | secreting internally |
| gluc/o | sugar, glucose, glycogen |
| glyc/o | sugar, glucose, glycogen |
| hypophys/o | pituitary gland |
| -ine | suffix used in the formation of names of chemical substances |
| -megaly | enlargement |
| -oma | tumor |
| pancreat/o | pancreas |
| parathyr/o | parathyroid gland |
| parathyroid/o | parathyroid gland |
| thyr/o | thyroid gland |
| thyroid/o | thyroid gland |
| -tropin | suffix meaning nourishment or stimulation |

## Word Parts Exercise

After studying Table 9-1, write the meaning of each of the word parts.

| WORD PART | MEANING |
|---|---|
| 1. endocrin/o | 1. ____________ |
| 2. hypophys/o | 2. ____________ |
| 3. adren/o, adrenal/o | 3. ____________ |
| 4. -ine | 4. ____________ |
| 5. -tropin | 5. ____________ |
| 6. -oma | 6. ____________ |
| 7. pancreat/o | 7. ____________ |
| 8. acr/o | 8. ____________ |
| 9. aden/o | 9. ____________ |
| 10. thyr/o, thyroid/o | 10. ____________ |
| 11. -megaly | 11. ____________ |
| 12. gluc/o, glyc/o | 12. ____________ |
| 13. crin/o | 13. ____________ |
| 14. parathyr/o, parathyroid/o | 14. ____________ |
| 15. calc/i | 15. ____________ |

## STRUCTURE AND FUNCTION

Several glands make up the endocrine system. These include the **pineal**, **pituitary** (anterior lobe, intermediate, and posterior lobes), **thyroid**, **parathyroid** (two paired glands, superior and inferior), **thymus**, **adrenal** (cortex and medulla), **pancreas** (pancreatic islets), **testes** (in males), and **ovaries** (in females) (see Figure 9-1). The hormones and primary functions of each of these glands are noted in **Table 9-2**.

What do the words *endocrine* and *hormone* actually mean? Endocrine glands are so-called because they secrete hormones directly into the bodily fluids that surround them and eventually find their way into the bloodstream. In other words, endocrine gland secretions do not travel through ducts. Glands that direct their secretions through ducts are called exocrine glands. The word *hormone* comes from Greek and means "to urge on or set in motion." So, a hormone is a chemical "messenger" transported through blood to other parts of the body. When the hormone reaches its target destination, the "message" has been delivered and can be acted upon.

### Pituitary Gland

Located in the brain, the **pituitary gland**, or *hypophysis*, is suspended from the base of the hypothalamus. (The *hypothalamus* coordinates the autonomic nervous system and the activities of the pituitary gland.) The pituitary gland controls the activities of other endocrine glands by releasing

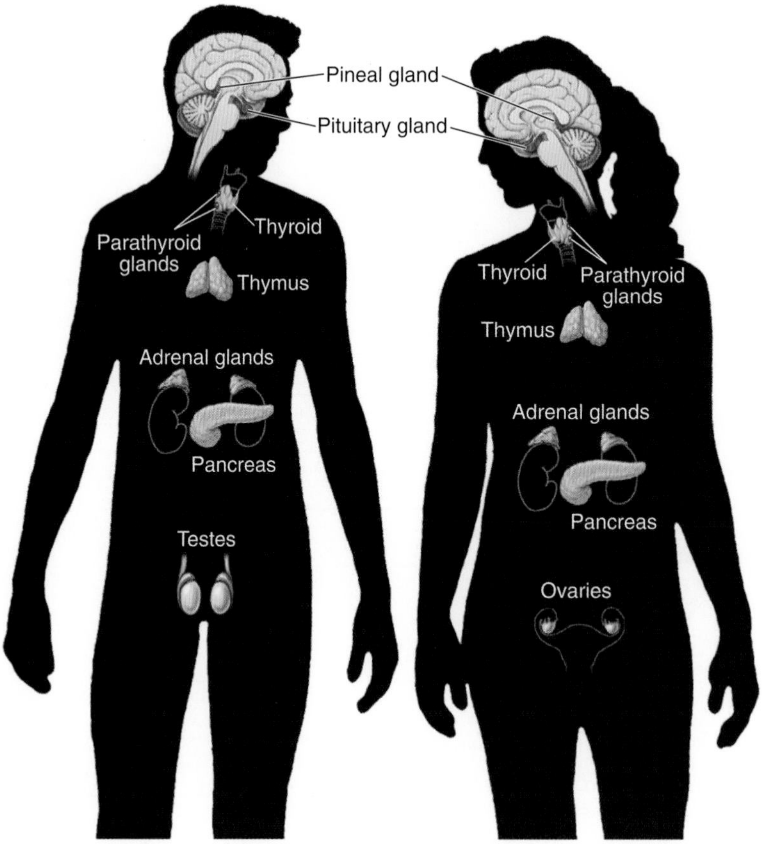


**FIGURE 9-1** The endocrine system.

**TABLE 9-2** SUMMARY OF THE ENDOCRINE GLANDS, HORMONES, AND HORMONE FUNCTIONS

| Gland | Hormone | Hormone Function |
|---|---|---|
| pineal gland | melatonin | affects sleep–wake cycles and reproduction |
| pituitary gland | | regulates activities of other glands; referred to as the "master gland" |
| anterior lobe | growth hormone (GH) | growth and development of bones, muscles, and other organs |
| | thyroid-stimulating hormone (TSH) | growth and development of thyroid gland |
| | adrenocorticotropic hormone (ACTH) | growth and development of adrenal cortex |
| | follicle-stimulating hormone (FSH) | stimulates production of sperm in males and growth of ovarian follicles in females |
| | luteinizing hormone (LH) | stimulates the production of testosterone in males and secretion of estrogen and progesterone in females |
| | prolactin hormone (PRL) | stimulates milk secretion in the mammary glands |
| intermediate lobe | melanocyte-stimulating hormone (MSH) | regulates skin pigmentation |
| posterior lobe | antidiuretic hormone (ADH) | stimulates the reabsorption of water by the kidneys |
| | oxytocin | stimulates the uterus to contract during labor and delivery |
| thyroid gland | thyroxine ($T_4$); also called tetraiodothyronine ($T_4$) | influences growth and development, both physical and mental |
| | triiodothyronine ($T_3$) | maintenance and regulation of metabolism |
| | calcitonin (CT) | decreases the blood level of calcium |
| parathyroid gland | parathyroid hormone (PTH) | increases the blood level of calcium |
| thymus | thymosin | aids T-cell development; T cells play a role in immunity |
| adrenal gland | | consists of outer region (cortex) and inner region (medulla) |
| cortex | cortisol | regulates carbohydrates, proteins, fat metabolism; anti-inflammatory effect; helps the body cope during stress |
| | aldosterone | regulates water and electrolyte balance |
| | androgen (sex hormone) | develops male secondary sex characteristics |
| medulla | epinephrine (adrenaline) | acts as a vasoconstrictor, cardiac stimulant (increases heart rate and cardiac output), and antispasmodic; releases glucose into the bloodstream (giving the body a spurt of energy) |
| | norepinephrine (noradrenaline) | acts as a vasoconstrictor; elevates blood pressure and heart rate |
| pancreas (islets of Langerhans) | insulin | transports glucose into the cells; decreases blood glucose levels |
| | glucagon | promotes release of glucose by liver; increases blood glucose levels |
| ovaries | estrogen | promotes growth, development, and maintenance of female sex organs |

(*continued*)

**TABLE 9-2 SUMMARY OF THE ENDOCRINE GLANDS, HORMONES, AND HORMONE FUNCTIONS (*continued*)**

| Gland | Hormone | Hormone Function |
|---|---|---|
| ovaries | progesterone | prepares uterus for pregnancy; promotes development of mammary glands |
| testes | testosterone | promotes growth, development, and maintenance of male sex organs |

special hormones that regulate glandular functions. The pituitary gland is divided into an **anterior lobe**, or *adenohypophysis*, and a **posterior lobe**, or *neurohypophysis*.

The anterior lobe secretes several hormones essential for the development of sex glands, muscles, bones, thyroid gland, and other organs. The posterior lobe secretes two hormones that are produced in the hypothalamus, **antidiuretic hormone (ADH)** and **oxytocin (OXT)**. ADH helps the body regulate fluid balance by reducing urination. OXT enhances labor contractions during childbirth and promotes milk release during lactation (milk secretion). During ejaculation in males, a spurt of OXT stimulates reproductive tract contractions to aid sperm release. In both sexes, it also appears to play a role in social bonding.

## Thyroid Gland and Parathyroid Gland

The **thyroid gland** is a butterfly-shaped gland lying in front and to the sides of the upper part of the trachea (windpipe) and lower part of the larynx (voicebox) (see Figure 9-2). It secretes hormones needed for cell growth, metabolism, and calcium regulation. Thyroid hormones include *triiodothyronine* ($T_3$), *thyroxine* ($T_4$), and *calcitonin* (CT). **Triiodothyronine ($T_3$)** and **thyroxine ($T_4$)** play roles in many body functions including growth and development, metabolic rate, body temperature, and heart rate. **CT** helps control calcium levels in the blood by decreasing the blood level of calcium.

There are four **parathyroid glands** consisting of a superior and inferior pair, which are located on the posterior surface of the thyroid gland (see Figure 9-3). The hormone **parathyroid hormone (PTH)**, also called *parathyrin* or *parathormone*, helps maintain correct calcium levels in the blood by increasing the blood level of calcium.

## Adrenal Glands

The **adrenal glands**, or *suprarenal glands*, consist of two triangular-shaped glands, each located on the superior border the kidneys. Each adrenal gland is divided into an outer part called the **adrenal cortex** and an inner part called the **adrenal medulla** (see Figure 9-4). The adrenal cortex secretes the steroid hormones, **cortisol**, which helps the body cope with stress, and **aldosterone**, which helps with sodium regulation. It also produces **androgens**, which contribute to the development of male sex characteristics.

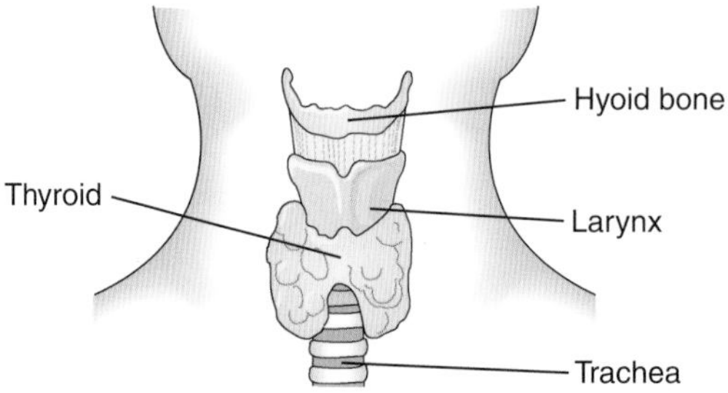


**FIGURE 9-2** The thyroid gland and adjacent structures.

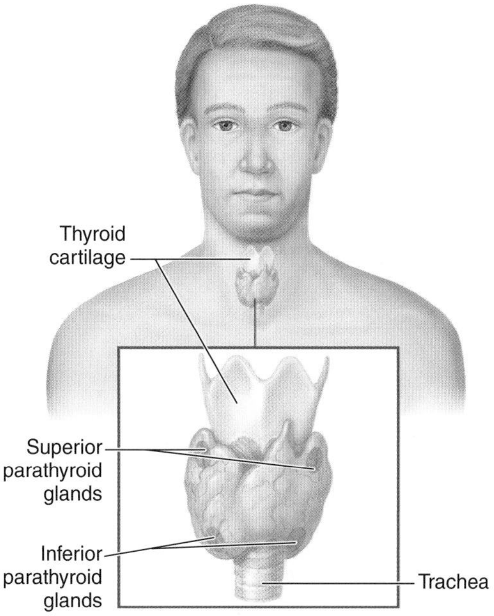


**FIGURE 9-3** The parathyroid glands consist of four glands, a superior and inferior pair. They are found on the posterior surface of the thyroid gland but are highlighted in this anterior view.

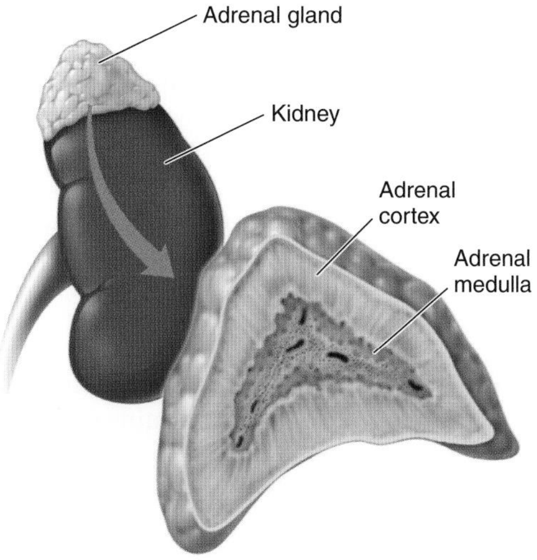


**FIGURE 9-4** The adrenal glands are positioned above each kidney and have an outer adrenal cortex and an inner adrenal medulla.

The adrenal medulla secretes **epinephrine** (*adrenaline*), which stimulates the sympathetic nervous system. It also secretes **norepinephrine** (*noradrenaline*), a hormone structurally similar to epinephrine that also stimulates the sympathetic nervous system.

## Pancreas

The pancreas is a feather-shaped organ located posterior to the stomach. It contains clusters of specialized cells called the **pancreatic islet** (*islets of Langerhans*), which produce *insulin* and *glucagon*. These chemicals control blood glucose (sugar) levels and glucose metabolism throughout the body. **Insulin**, produced by the β cells of the pancreas, decreases blood glucose. **Glucagon**, produced by the α cells of the pancreas, increases blood glucose.

## Gonads

Reproductive organs that produce sex cells are called **gonads**. The female gonads are the **ovaries**, and the male gonads are the **testes**. The ovaries secrete estrogen and progesterone. **Estrogen** affects the development of female organs, regulates the menstrual cycle, and plays a role in pregnancy. **Progesterone** stimulates the uterus in preparation for and maintenance of pregnancy. The testes secrete **testosterone**, a hormone that affects development of sexual organs in males and secondary sexual characteristics. We discuss the reproductive system and these hormones in Chapter 15.

### Quick Check

**Fill in the blanks.**

1. Another name for the pituitary gland is the __________________________.
2. Another name for the adrenal gland is the __________________________ because it is located on the superior border of the kidney.
3. __________________________ glands secrete hormones directly into the bloodstream.

# DISORDERS RELATED TO THE ENDOCRINE SYSTEM

Disorders of the endocrine system are almost always the result of an excess or a deficit in hormone production. In other words, either too much or too little of a hormone causes a problem. If there is too much, surgery or radiation may be needed. If there is too little, replacement therapy is the usual treatment.

## Disorders of the Pituitary Gland

One cause of pituitary disorders can be an **adenoma**, a benign tumor that causes excessive hormone secretion. This condition may also destroy pituitary cells and cause too little hormone secretion.

**Diabetes insipidus** is a disorder in which the posterior lobe of the pituitary gland no longer releases sufficient amounts of ADH or because the response to ADH is impaired. This results in **polydipsia** (excessive thirst) and **polyuria** (excessive urination).

**Gigantism**, or *giantism*, is a disorder caused by excessive secretion of growth hormone (GH) before puberty, resulting in abnormally long bones (see Figure 9-5). When excessive GH secretion occurs in adulthood, this results in **acromegaly**, which is characterized by abnormally thick bones in the extremities, especially the hands and feet.

## Disorders of the Thyroid Gland

As with other endocrine disorders, an excess or deficiency of thyroid hormone production results in homeostatic imbalance. **Hypothyroidism**, deficient hormone production by the thyroid gland, is characterized by decreased metabolic rate, weight gain, and tiredness. Excessive thyroid hormone production leads to **hyperthyroidism**, characterized by increased metabolic rate, weight loss, and rapid heartbeat. A form of hyperthyroidism is **Graves disease**, which is an autoimmune disorder (condition in which the body's antibodies are directed against itself) resulting in **goiter** (neck swelling) and **exophthalmos** (eye protrusion) (see Figure 9-6).

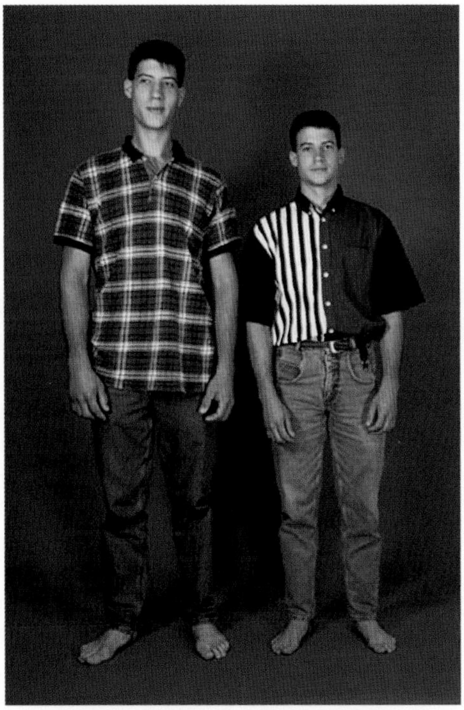

**FIGURE 9-5** A 22-year old man with gigantism is shown next to his identical twin, who does not have the condition.

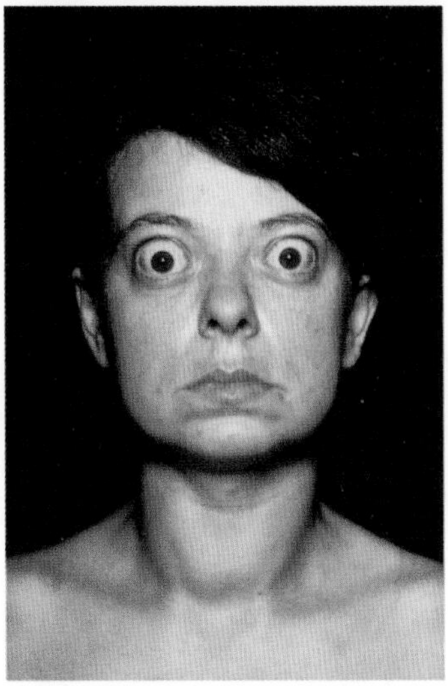

**FIGURE 9-6** A young woman exhibiting the signs of Graves disease, including goiter and exophthalmos.

What causes thyroid enlargement? Enlargement of the thyroid gland (goiter) is caused by a deficiency of iodine in the diet. Iodine is necessary to make thyroid hormones. Recall that these hormones have the word part *iodo* in their names. Although this condition is no longer common in the United States, it still affects people in less developed parts of the world. The reason for its rarity in the United States is that in 1924, members of the Michigan State Medical Society championed the fight against goiter by convincing salt producers to include small amounts of iodine in their product. The discovery that goiter was a result of too little iodine in the diet had previously been noted by French physician J. B. Boussingault nearly a century earlier.

## Disorders of the Adrenal Gland

Inflammatory conditions and viral infections involving the adrenal glands can cause a decrease in hormone production. Benign tumors are often the cause of increased hormone production from the adrenal glands.

**Addison disease** is a progressive disorder caused by an insufficient amount of cortisol and aldosterone production in the adrenal gland or a failure of the pituitary gland to produce a stimulating hormone targeting the adrenal gland. It is characterized by skin darkening, weakness, and loss of appetite (see Figure 9-7).

**Cushing's syndrome** is caused by an excessive amount of cortisol production by the adrenal glands. It is characterized by fat pads in the chest and abdomen and a "moon face" appearance.

The naming of disorders for persons who first identified them is a well-established practice. Recently, using the possessive form of the founder's name in the names of the disorders has been questioned, and one may, therefore, see and hear both *Addison's disease* and *Addison disease*. The problem is one of tradition versus logic. Those who eschew tradition in favor of logic say that Addison's disease is not something that 19th century British physician Thomas Addison contracted but rather a disorder he identified. Likewise, Harvey Cushing identified and did not contract Cushing's syndrome. In this book, the traditional naming was used because when you search these terms on the Internet, the apostrophe appears more often. Medical dictionaries, however, often do not include the apostrophe.

There is an exception: Graves disease, although a traditional spelling, is not a true possessive. The rule for forming possessives specifies that this should be Graves' disease. Robert Graves was an Irish physician who described exophthalmic goiter in 1835. In this one case, therefore, tradition defies not only logic but also the rules of grammar and punctuation.

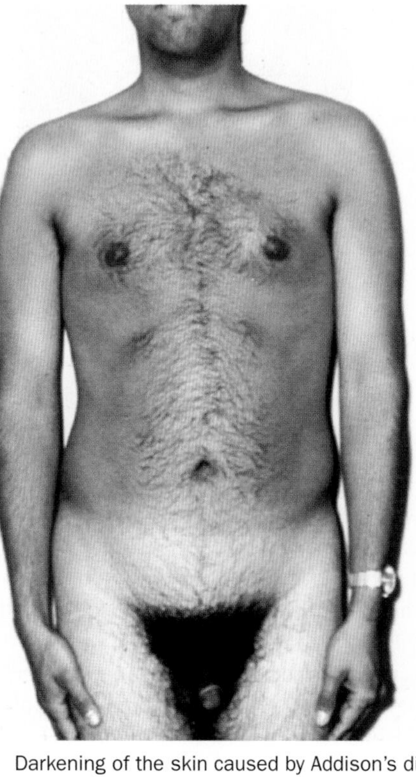

**FIGURE 9-7** Darkening of the skin caused by Addison's disease.

### Disorders of the Pancreas

**Diabetes mellitus (DM)** is a disorder caused by insulin deficiency and/or insulin resistance. This results in poor carbohydrate metabolism and high blood glucose level. There are two main types: **Type 1 DM** is a metabolic disorder caused by insufficient production of insulin and usually develops in childhood. Symptoms in the early stages include **glycosuria** (excess glucose in the urine) and **hyperglycemia** (excess glucose in the blood). **Type 2 DM** is caused by either a lack of insulin or the body's inability to use insulin efficiently. It usually develops in middle-aged or older adults.

## DIAGNOSTIC TESTS, TREATMENTS, AND SURGICAL PROCEDURES

Hormone replacement therapy is often used to correct endocrine disorders, where the problem is a low hormone level. Examples of disorders treatable by hormone replacement are hypothyroidism and DM. In hypothyroidism, patients are given a medication called levothyroxine to replace low thyroxine levels. In diabetes, patients are given medications to treat high glucose levels. Most commonly, Type I patients are given insulin. In Type II, diet and exercise may be enough to control glucose levels. If they do need medications, these patients are more likely to receive oral medications to help decrease blood glucose. In Addison's disease, where the hormone lacking is cortisol, **corticosteroids** may also be administered for their immunosuppressant and anti-inflammatory properties.

## PRACTICE AND PRACTITIONERS

**Endocrinology** is the medical practice of treating endocrine and hormonal disorders. The practitioner, an **endocrinologist**, specializes in caring for patients with endocrine diseases and hormonal dysfunctions that may involve sexual development, body growth, or other bodily functions.

**Abbreviation Table** THE ENDOCRINE SYSTEM

| ABBREVIATION | MEANING |
|---|---|
| ACTH | adrenocorticotropic hormone |
| ADH | antidiuretic hormone |
| CT | calcitonin |
| DM | diabetes mellitus |
| FBS | fasting blood sugar |
| FSH | follicle-stimulating hormone |
| GH | growth hormone |
| GTT | glucose tolerance test |
| $HbA_{1c}$ | hemoglobin A1c (glycosylated hemoglobin) |
| LH | luteinizing hormone |
| MSH | melanocyte-stimulating hormone |
| PRL | prolactin |
| PTH | parathyroid hormone |
| TSH | thyroid-stimulating hormone |
| $T_3$ | triiodothyronine |
| $T_4$ | thyroxine, tetraiodothyronine |

**Study Table THE ENDOCRINE SYSTEM**

| TERM AND PRONUNCIATION | ANALYSIS | MEANING |
|---|---|---|
| **Structure and Function** | | |
| adenogenous (ad-eh-NAW-jeh-nuhs) | *aden/o* (gland); *-genous* (originating) | originating in a gland |
| adenohypophysis (AD-eh-noh-hy-POFF-ih-sihs) | *aden/o* (gland); *hypophys/o* (pituitary gland) | the anterior lobe of the pituitary gland |
| adrenal cortex (ah-DREE-nahl kor-teks) | *adren/o* (adrenal glands); *cortex* (a Latin word meaning "bark"); | the outer region of the adrenal gland |
| adrenal glands (ah-DREE-nahl glands) | *adren/o* (adrenal glands) | triangular-shaped glands located above each kidney that secretes hormones that aid in metabolism, electrolyte balance, and stress reactions; each has an outer cortex and an inner medulla; *suprarenal glands* |
| adrenal medulla (ah-DREE-nahl med-OOL-uh) | *adren/o* (adrenal glands); *medulla* (a Latin word meaning "marrow, innermost part") | the inner region of the adrenal gland |
| adrenaline (ah-DREN-ah-lihn) | *adren/o* (adrenal glands); *-ine* (a suffix used to form names of chemical substances) | chemical secreted by the adrenal medulla that increases blood circulation, breathing rate, and carbohydrate metabolism; *epinephrine* |
| adrenocorticotropic hormone (ah-DREE-oh-KOR-tih-ko-TROH-pik HOR-mohn) (ACTH) | *cortic/o* (from *cortex* [bark]); from the Greek word *trophe* (nourishment); *-in* (a suffix used to form names of biochemical substances) | pituitary secretion that stimulates the adrenal glands |
| androgen (AN-droh-jen) | *andro-* (masculine); *-gen* (suffix meaning "source of") | male hormone secreted by the adrenal cortex |
| aldosterone (al-DOSS-teh-rone) | ald (ehyd) + ster(ol) + *-one* (chemical suffix) | one of the corticosteroids, hormones produced by the adrenal glands |
| antidiuretic hormone (AN-tee-dy-uh-RET-ik HOHR-mohn) (ADH) | *anti-* (against); from the Greek *dia* (through); *-uresis* (urination); from the Greek word *hormon* (to set in motion) | hormone secreted by the posterior pituitary gland to prevent the kidneys from expelling too much water |
| calcitonin (kal-sih-TOH-nihn) (CT) | *calci-* (calcium); from the Greek *tonos* (to stretch); *-in* (suffix used to form names of biochemical substances) | hormone secreted by the thyroid that lowers blood calcium level |
| corticosteroids (KOR-tih-ko-STEHR-oyds) | *cortic/o* (from Latin word *cortex* [bark]); from Steros (solid); *-oid* (resemblance to) | steroids produced by the cortices of the adrenal glands; *cortisol* |

**Study Table** THE ENDOCRINE SYSTEM (*continued*)

| TERM AND PRONUNCIATION | ANALYSIS | MEANING |
|---|---|---|
| cortisol (KOR-tih-suhl) | from the Latin word *corticus* (cortex) | main glucocorticoid produced in the adrenal cortex; inhibits inflammation and immune response |
| endocrine (EN-doh-krin) | *endo-* (within, inner); from the Greek word *krino* (to separate) | adjective describing a gland that delivers its secretions directly into bloodstream |
| epinephrine (EP-ih-NEFF-rihn) | *epi-* (upon); *nephr/o* (kidney); *-ine* (suffix used to form the names of chemical substances) | chemical secreted by the adrenal medulla that increases blood circulation, breathing rate, and carbohydrate metabolism; *adrenaline* |
| estrogen (EHS-troh-jen) | from the Greek word *oistrus* (estrus); *-gen* (producing) | hormone secreted by the female ovaries |
| exocrine gland (EX-oh-krihn GLAND) | *exo-* (outside of); from the Greek word *krino* (to separate) | gland that delivers its secretions through a duct onto the skin or other epithelial surface |
| follicle stimulating hormone (FOL-i-kuhl STIM-yuh-leyt-ing HOR-mohn) (FSH) | from the Latin words *folliculus* (little bag) and *stimulatus* (rouse to action); from the Greek word *hormon* (to set in motion) | hormone promoting gonadal growth |
| glands (GLANDZ) | From the Latin, *glans* (acorn) | organized group of cells that function as a secretory or excretory organ |
| glucagon (GLOO-ka-guhn) | *gluc/o* (glucose); from the Greek word *ago* (to lead) | hormone secreted by the pancreas that increases blood glucose level |
| homeostasis (hoh-mee-uh-STEY-sis) | from two Greek words *homos* (same) and *stasis* (existence) | tendency toward equilibrium; remaining normal |
| hormone (HOHR-mohn) | from the Greek word *hormon* (to set in motion) | chemical messenger that is secreted by an endocrine gland directly into the bloodstream |
| hydrocortisone (hy-droh-KOR-tih-sone) | *hydro-* (water); *cortic/o* (from the Greek word *cortex* meaning "bark"); *-one* (chemical suffix) | an adrenal gland hormone secretion |
| hypophysis (hy-POFF-ih-sihs) | *hypophys/o* (pituitary gland) | major endocrine gland in the brain that controls growth, development, and functioning of other endocrine glands; *pituitary gland* |

(*continued*)

**Study Table** THE ENDOCRINE SYSTEM (*continued*)

| TERM AND PRONUNCIATION | ANALYSIS | MEANING |
|---|---|---|
| hypothalamus (high-poh-THAL-uh-mus) | *hypo-* (below); from the Greek word, *thalamus* (bed, bedroom) | part of the brain located near the pituitary gland that secretes releasing hormones that control the release of other hormones by the pituitary gland |
| insulin (IN-soo-lihn) | from the Latin word *insula* (island) | hormone produced in the pancreas that decreases blood glucose level |
| islets of Langerhans (EYE-lets LAN-gehr-hans) | after German pathologist Paul Langerhans, who described it in 1869; islets are the regions of the pancreas that contain its hormone-producing cells | clusters of specialized cells in the pancreas that secrete insulin (β cells) and glucagon (α cells) |
| luteinizing hormone (LOO-tee-uh-nahyz-ing HOHR-mohn) (LH) | from the Latin word *luteus* (yellow); from the Greek word *hormon* (to set in motion) | hormone that stimulates the final ripening of follicles, oocyte release, and conversion of the ruptured follicle into the corpus luteum |
| melanocyte-stimulating hormone (MEL-an-oh-syte STIM-yuh-leyt-ing HOHR-mohn) (MSH) | *melan/o* (black); *-cyte* (cell); from the Latin word *stimulatus* (rouse to action); from the Greek word *hormon* (to set in motion) | hormone secreted from the anterior lobe of the pituitary gland that is involved with pigmentation changes |
| melatonin (mel-ah-TONE-ihn) | melanophore + Greek *tonos* (to stretch); *-in* (suffix used to form names of biochemical substances) | hormone secreted by the pineal gland that is involved with sleep–wake cycles and reproduction |
| neurohypophysis (NUHR-oh-hy-POFF-ih-sihs) | *neur/o* (nerve); *hypophys/o* (pituitary gland) | posterior lobe of the pituitary gland that stores and releases OXT and ADH, which are produced in the hypothalamus |
| noradrenaline (nor-ah-DREN-ah-lihn) | *nor-* (chemical prefix); *adrenal/o* (adrenal glands); *-ine* (a suffix used to denote chemical substances) | chemical secreted by the adrenal medulla that aids the body during stress and increases blood pressure; *norepinephrine* |
| norepinephrine (NOR-ehp-ih-NEFF-rihn) | *nor-* (chemical prefix); *epi-* (upon); from the Greek word *nephros* (kidney); *-ine* (a suffix used to denote chemical substances) | chemical secreted by the adrenal medulla that aids the body during stress and increases blood pressure; *noradrenaline* |
| ovaries (OH-vayr-ees) | from the Latin word *ovum* (egg) | female gonads; two oval-shaped glands that are located in the pelvic cavity and secrete the hormones estrogen and progesterone |

**Study Table** THE ENDOCRINE SYSTEM (*continued*)

| TERM AND PRONUNCIATION | ANALYSIS | MEANING |
|---|---|---|
| oxytocin (ox-ih-TOH-sihn) (OXT) | from the Greek word *oxytokos* (swift birth); *-in* (suffix used to form names of biochemical substances) | hormone secreted by the posterior pituitary gland that stimulates uterine contractions and milk ejection from mammary glands |
| pancreas (PAN-kree-uhs) | from the Greek word *pancreas* (sweet bread) | feather-shaped organ that lies posterior to the stomach that contains islets of Langerhans (α cells and β cells that secrete glucagon and insulin respectively) |
| parathyroid gland (pahr-ah-THY-royd gland) | *para-* (prefix denoting involvement of two like parts; also denoting adjacent, alongside, near); *thyr/o* (thyroid gland) | secretes PTH |
| parathyroid hormone (pahr-ah-THY-royd HOHR-mohn), parathormone (pahr-ah-THOR-mohn) (PTH) | *para-* (prefix denoting involvement of two like parts; also denoting adjacent, alongside, near); *thyr/o* (thyroid gland); from the Greek word *hormon* (to set in motion) | a hormone secreted by the parathyroid gland that regulates calcium and phosphorus levels in the blood and bones |
| pineal gland (PIHN-ee-ahl gland) | from the Latin word *pinus* (pine); *-al* (adjective ending) | small, cone-shaped gland that secretes melatonin, which affects sleep–wake cycles and reproduction |
| pituitary gland (pih-TOO-ih-tahr-ee gland) | from the Latin word *pituita* (phlegm) | major endocrine gland in the brain that controls growth, development, and functioning of other endocrine glands; *hypophysis* |
| progesterone (proh-JES-ter-ohn) | from the Latin *pro* (for); from the Latin *gestare* (to carry about); *-one* (chemical suffix) | female hormone secreted by the ovary that stimulates uterus in preparation for and maintenance of pregnancy |
| prolactin (pro-LAK-tihn) (PRL) | from the Latin *pro* (for); from the Latin *lacteus* (milky) | a secretion of the anterior lobe of the pituitary gland that stimulates milk production |
| suprarenal glands (SOO-prah-REEN-ahl glands) | *supra-* (above); *ren-* (kidney); *-al* (pertaining to) | triangular-shaped glands located above each kidney that secretes hormones that aid in metabolism, electrolyte balance, and stress reactions; each has an outer cortex and an inner medulla; *adrenal glands* |

(*continued*)

**Study Table** THE ENDOCRINE SYSTEM *(continued)*

| TERM AND PRONUNCIATION | ANALYSIS | MEANING |
|---|---|---|
| testes (TES-tees) | from the plural form of the Latin *testis* (testicle) | male gonads; two oval organs that lie in the scrotum that secrete testosterone |
| testosterone (teh-STAH-steh-rone) | from the Latin *testis* (testicle); ster(ol); *-one* (chemical suffix) | male hormone secreted by the testes that affects development of sexual organs in males and secondary sexual characteristics |
| thymus (thigh-MUS) | from the Greek word *thymos* (a warty excrescence) | gland located in the neck whose function is immunologic |
| thyroid gland (THIGH-royd gland) | *thyr/o* (thyroid gland) | bilobed gland located in the neck that secretes thyroid hormone that is needed for cell growth and metabolism |
| thyroid-stimulating hormone (THIGH-royd STIM-yoo-late-ing HOR-mohn) (TSH) | *thyr/o* (thyroid gland) | hormone produced in the anterior lobe of the pituitary that stimulates the growth and function of the thyroid gland; *thyrotropin* |
| thyrotropin (thigh-ROT-roh-pihn) | *thyr/o* (thyroid gland); from the Greek *trophe* (nourishment); *-in* (suffix used to form names of biochemical substances) | hormone produced in the anterior lobe of the pituitary that stimulates the growth and function of the thyroid gland; *thyroid-stimulating hormone* |
| thyroxine (thy-ROK-sihn) ($T_4$) | *thyr/o* (thyroid gland); *-ine* (suffix used to form names of biochemical substances) | a secretion of the thyroid gland |
| triiodothyronine (try-EYE-oh-doh-THY-roh-neen) ($T_3$) | *tri-* (three); *iodo* (iodine); *thyr/o* (thyroid gland); *-ine* (a suffix used to form names of chemical substances) | another secretion of the thyroid gland that is often synthesized from thyroxine ($T_4$) by bodily organs |
| **Disorders** | | |
| acromegaly (AK-roh-mehg-alee) | from the Greek *akron* (extremity); *-megaly* (enlargement) | enlargement of the extremities (mostly hands and feet) caused by excessive secretion of Addison's GH *after* puberty |
| Addison's disease (AD-uh-suhns dih-ZEEZ) | after the British physician, Thomas Addison, who first described the condition in 1855 | disorder in which the adrenal glands to not produce sufficient cortisol; characterized by skin darkening, weakness, and loss of appetite |
| adenitis (ad-eh-NY-tihs) | *aden/o* (gland); *-itis* (inflammation) | inflammation of a gland |

**Study Table** THE ENDOCRINE SYSTEM (*continued*)

| TERM AND PRONUNCIATION | ANALYSIS | MEANING |
|---|---|---|
| adenohypophysitis (AD-eh-noh-hy-poff-ih-SY-tihs) | *aden/o* (gland); *hypophys/o* (pituitary gland); *-itis* (inflammation) | inflammation of the anterior pituitary, often related to pregnancy |
| adenoma (ad-en-OH-muh) | *benignus* (Latin for *aden/o* (gland) *–oma* (tumor) | benign (nonmalignant) neoplasm in which the tumor cells form glands or gland-like structures |
| adrenalitis (ah-dree-nah-LY-tiss) | *adrenal/o* (adrenal glands); *-itis* (inflammation) | inflammation of an adrenal gland |
| adrenalopathy (ah-dree-nah-LOP-ah-thee); | *adrenal/o* (adrenal glands); *-pathy* (disease) | any disease of the adrenal glands; *adrenopathy* |
| adrenomegaly (ah-dree-noh-MEG-ah-lee) | *adren/o* (adrenal gland); *-megaly* (enlargement) | enlargement of the adrenal glands |
| adrenopathy (ah-dree-NOP-ah-thee) | *adrenal-* (adrenal glands); *-pathy* (disease) | any disease of the adrenal glands; *adrenalopathy* |
| Cushing's syndrome (KOOSH-ingz SIN-druhm) | named after Harvey Cushing, American physician, who described the disorder in 1932 | a hormonal disorder caused by too much cortisol; characterized by fat pads in the chest and abdomen and a "moon face" appearance |
| diabetes insipidus (DY-ah-BEET-ehs ihn-SIP-ih-duhs) | *diabetes*, a Greek word meaning "a compass," "a siphon"; *insipidus* (lacking flavor or zest) | condition brought about by the posterior pituitary's failure to produce enough ADH |
| diabetes mellitus (DY-ah-BEET-ehs meh-LY-tuhs) (DM) | *diabetes*, a Greek word meaning "a compass, a siphon"; *mellitus*, a Latin word meaning "sweetened with honey" or "honey-sweet" | condition brought about by insufficient production of insulin in the pancreas or the failure of the body's cells to absorb glucose |
| exophthalmos (ek-sof-THAL-mos) | *ex* (out) + *ophthalmos* (eye) | protruding or bulging eyes from their sockets |
| gigantism (JEYE-gan-tizm) | *giant* (common English word); *-ism* (condition) | abnormal overgrowth of the body due to excessive secretion of the GH *before* puberty; *giantism* |
| glycosuria (GLY-koh-SYUR-ee-ah) | *glyc/o/s* (sugar); *-uria* (urine) | sugar (glucose) in the urine |
| goiter (GOY-tuhr) | from the Latin word *gutter* (throat) | chronic enlargement of the thyroid gland |
| Graves disease (grahvz dih-ZEEZ) | named after Robert James Graves (1796–1853), an Irish physician who first described exophthalmic goiter in 1835 | a common form of hyperthyroidism resulting from overproduction of thyroxine caused by a false immune system response |

*(continued)*

**Study Table** THE ENDOCRINE SYSTEM *(continued)*

| TERM AND PRONUNCIATION | ANALYSIS | MEANING |
|---|---|---|
| Hashimoto's thyroiditis (Hah-shee-moh-tohz thahy-roi-DAHY-tis) | Hashimoto (Japanese surgeon, 1881–1934); *thyr/o* (thyroid gland); *-itis* (inflammation) | an autoimmune disorder that attacks the thyroid gland causing hypothyroidism |
| hyperglycemia (hy-puhr-gly-SEEM-ee-ah) | *hyper-* (above normal); *glyc/o* (sugar); *-ia* (condition) | excessive sugar (glucose) in the blood |
| hyperpituitarism (HY-puhr-pih-TOO-iht-ahr-izm) | *hyper-* (above normal); from the Latin word *pituita* (phlegm) | excessive hormone secretion by the pituitary gland |
| hyperthyroidism (HY-puhr-THY-royd-izm) | *hyper-* (above normal); *thyr/o* (thyroid); *-ism* (condition) | excessive production of thyroid hormone by the thyroid gland; overactive thyroid |
| hypophysitis (hy-poh-fih-SY-tihs) | *hypophys/o* (pituitary gland); *-itis* (inflammation) | inflammation of the pituitary gland |
| hypopituitarism (hy-poh-pih-TOO-ih-tahr-izm) | *hypo-* (below normal); from the Latin word *pituita* (phlegm); *-ism* (condition) | condition of diminished hormone secretion from the anterior pituitary gland |
| hypothyroidism (hahy-puh-THAHY-roi-diz-uhm) | *hypo-* (below normal); thyroid refers to the thyroid gland; *-ism* (state of) | decrease in thyroid hormone production |
| pituitarism (pih-TOO-iht-ahr-izm) | from the Latin word *pituita* (phlegm); *-ism* (condition) | pituitary dysfunction |
| polydipsia (pol-ee-DIP-see-uh | *poly-* (much) + the Greek word *dipsa* (thirst) | excessive thirst that is usually indicative of diabetes |
| polyuria (pol-ee-YOO-ree-uh) | *poly-* (much) + the Greek word *ouron* (urine) | excessive urination |
| thyroaplasia (THY-roh-a-PLAY-zee-ah) | *thyr/o* (thyroid gland); aplasia from the Greek *a plassein* (not to form) | congenital condition characterized by low thyroid output |
| thyroiditis (thy-roy-DY-tihs) | *thyr/o* (thyroid gland); *-itis* (inflammation) | inflammation of the thyroid gland |
| thyromegaly (thy-roh-MEG-ah lee) | *thyr/o* (thyroid gland); *-megaly* (enlargement) | enlargement of the thyroid gland |
| toxic goiter (TOK-sik GOI-ter) | from two Latin words *toxicus* (poisoned); *gutter* (throat) | a goiter that forms excessive secretions causing signs and symptoms of hyperthyroidism |
| Type 1 diabetes mellitus (DY-ah-BEET-ehs meh-LY-tuhs) | *diabetes*, a Greek word meaning "a compass, a siphon"; *mellitus*, a Latin word meaning "sweetened with honey" or "honey-sweet" | condition brought about by insufficient production of insulin in the pancreas and generally appearing in childhood |

**Study Table** THE ENDOCRINE SYSTEM (*continued*)

| TERM AND PRONUNCIATION | ANALYSIS | MEANING |
|---|---|---|
| Type 2 diabetes mellitus (DY-ah-BEET-ehs meh-LY-tuhs) | *diabetes*, a Greek word meaning "a compass, a siphon"; *mellitus*, a Latin word meaning "sweetened with honey" or "honey-sweet" | condition brought about by insufficient production of insulin in the pancreas or the failure of the body's cells to absorb glucose |
| **Diagnostic Tests, Treatments, and Surgical Procedures** | | |
| adenectomy (ad-eh-NEK-toh-mee) | *aden/o* (gland); *-ectomy* (excision) | excision of a gland |
| adenotomy (ad-eh-NOT-oh-mee) | *aden/o* (gland); *-tomy* (cutting operation) | incision of a gland |
| adrenalectomy (ah-dree-nah-LEK-toh-mee) | *adrenal/o* (adrenal glands); *-ectomy* (excision) | surgical removal of one adrenal gland or both adrenal glands |
| fasting blood sugar (FSB) | *fasting* (to not eat) | test for diabetes; after drinking glucose, the patient fasts and then their blood is tested for glucose; *glucose tolerance test* (GTT) |
| glycosylated hemoglobin (glye-KOS-ih-late-ed HE-muh-gloh-bin) ($HbA_{1c}$) | *glyco-* (glucose, sugar); *hem-* (blood) | blood test that indicates the amount of glucose in the blood over the previous few (no more than 3) months; used to indicate how well DM is being controlled |
| hypoglycemic (HY-poh-gly-SEE-mik) | *hypo-* (below normal); *glyc/o* (sugar); *-ic* (pertaining to) | drug used to lower blood glucose |
| hypophysectomy (HY-poh-fih-SEK-toh-mee) | *hypophys/o* (pituitary gland); *-ectomy* (excision) | surgical removal of the hypophysis (pituitary gland) |
| parathyroidectomy (PAHR-ahthy-royd-EK-toh-mee) | *parathyr/o* (parathyroid gland); *-ectomy* (excision) | surgical excision of the parathyroid gland |
| thyroidectomy (THY-royd-EK-toh-mee) | *thyr/o* (thyroid gland); *-ectomy* (excision) | removal of the thyroid gland |
| thyroparathyroidectomy (THY-roh-pehr-ah-THY-roy-DEK-toh-mee) | *thyr/o* (thyroid gland); *parathyr/o* (parathyroid gland); *-ectomy* (excision) | removal of the thyroid and parathyroid glands |
| thyrotomy (thy-ROT-oh-mee) | *thyr/o* (thyroid gland); *-tomy* (cutting operation) | surgery performed on the thyroid gland |
| **Practice and Practitioners** | | |
| endocrinologist (en-do-krih-NOL-oh-jist) | *endocrin/o* (endocrine); *-logist* (one who specializes) | medical specialist in endocrinology |
| endocrinology(en-do-krih-NOL-oh-jee) | *endocrin/o* (endocrine); *-logy* (study of) | medical specialty of the endocrine system |

## END-OF-CHAPTER EXERCISES

### EXERCISE 9-1 LABELING

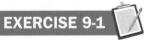

**Using the following list, choose the correct terms to label the diagram correctly.**

| | | |
|---|---|---|
| adrenal glands | parathyroid glands | testes |
| ovaries | pineal gland | thymus |
| pancreas | pituitary gland | thyroid |

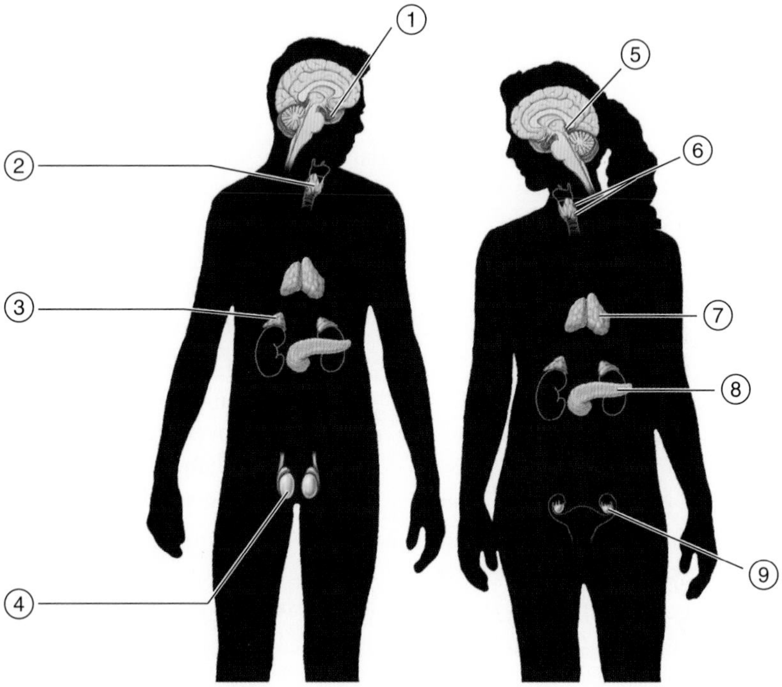


1. ______________ 4. ______________ 7. ______________
2. ______________ 5. ______________ 8. ______________
3. ______________ 6. ______________ 9. ______________

### EXERCISE 9-2 WORD PARTS

**Break each of the following terms into its word parts: prefix, root, or suffix. Give the meaning of each word part and then define the term.**

1. adenogenous

   root: ______________________________

   suffix: ______________________________

   definition: ______________________________

2. epinephrine

   prefix: ____________________

   root: ____________________

   suffix: ____________________

   definition: ____________________

3. suprarenal

   prefix: ____________________

   root: ____________________

   suffix: ____________________

   definition: ____________________

4. adrenomegaly

   root: ____________________

   suffix: ____________________

   definition: ____________________

5. hyperglycemia

   prefix: ____________________

   root: ____________________

   suffix: ____________________

   definition: ____________________

6. adenotomy

   root: ____________________

   suffix: ____________________

   definition: ____________________

7. thyroparathyroidectomy

   root: ____________________

   root: ____________________

   suffix: ____________________

   definition: ____________________

8. endocrinology

   root: ____________________

   suffix: ____________________

   definition: ____________________

## EXERCISE 9-3 WORD BUILDING

Use *adren/o* **to build the medical words meaning:**

1. enlargement of the adrenal gland ____________________
2. surgical removal of an adrenal gland ____________________
3. disease of the adrenal glands ____________________

Use *thyr/o or thyroid/o* **to build the medical words meaning:**

4. condition of minimal functioning of the thyroid gland ____________________
5. inflammation of the thyroid gland ____________________
6. incision of the thyroid gland ____________________
7. enlargement of the thyroid gland ____________________

Use *pancreat/o* **to build the medical words meaning:**

8. tumor of the pancreas ____________________
9. inflammation of the pancreas ____________________
10. originating in the pancreas ____________________

## EXERCISE 9-4 MATCHING

**Match the term with its definition.**

| | | |
|---|---|---|
| 1. ______________ | adrenalopathy | a. synonym for epinephrine |
| 2. ______________ | hyperpituitarism | b. thyroid-stimulating hormone, secreted by the anterior lobe of the pituitary gland |
| 3. ______________ | adenogenous | c. enlargement of the thyroid gland |
| 4. ______________ | antidiuretic hormone | d. disease of the adrenal glands |
| 5. ______________ | adrenaline | e. synonym for pituitary gland |
| 6. ______________ | master gland, hypophysis | f. hormone secreted by the thyroid to decrease blood calcium level |
| 7. ______________ | calcitonin | g. originating in a gland |
| 8. ______________ | goiter | h. removal of the thyroid and parathyroid glands |
| 9. ______________ | parathyroid gland | i. hormone released by the posterior lobe of the pituitary gland |
| 10. ______________ | thyrotropin | j. secretes PTH (parathyroid hormone) |
| 11. ______________ | thyromegaly | k. excessive pituitary secretion |
| 12. ______________ | adenohypophysitis | l. inflammation of the anterior pituitary gland |
| 13. ______________ | thyroparathyroidectomy | m. chronic enlargement of the thyroid |

## EXERCISE 9-5 MULTIPLE CHOICE

**Choose the correct answer for the following multiple choice questions.**

1. The master gland is known as the ____________________.
   a. pituitary gland
   b. thymus gland
   c. thyroid gland
   d. pineal gland

2. The ovaries produce which two hormones?
   a. insulin and glucagon
   b. estrogen and progesterone
   c. testosterone and thymosin
   d. $T_3$ and $T_4$

3. Endocrine means ____________________.
   a. to cringe from within
   b. to secrete within
   c. to cry inside
   d. disease of the gland

4. Over-secretion of GH in an adult produces a condition called ___________________.
   a. hyperthyroidism
   b. adenitis
   c. acromegaly
   d. tetany

5. ___________________ is an enlargement of the thyroid gland.
   a. Hypothyroidism
   b. Goiter
   c. Thyroidectomy
   d. Addison's disease

6. A chemical secreted from an endocrine gland is called a/an ___________________.
   a. hormone
   b. lymph
   c. neurotransmitter
   d. insulin

7. Hypersecretion of GH may cause ___________________.
   a. insulin
   b. diabetes
   c. hypothyroidism
   d. gigantism

8. ___________________ is associated with excessive hormone secretion from the adrenal cortex.
   a. Cushing's syndrome
   b. Exophthalmos
   c. Goiter
   d. Gigantism

9. The two-lobed gland in the neck is called the ___________________.
   a. Adam's apple
   b. thymus
   c. pituitary gland
   d. thyroid gland

## EXERCISE 9-6 FILL IN THE BLANK

**Fill in the blank with the correct answer.**

1. Another term for enlargement of the thyroid gland besides goiter is ___________________.

2. Insufficient insulin production or insulin resistance results in the condition called

   ___________________.

3. An abnormally high level of glucose in the blood is termed ___________________.

4. Excessive urination is called ___________________.

5. The term ____________________ means sugar (glucose) in the urine.

6. The hormone ____________________ increases blood glucose level.

7. The enlargement of extremities caused by the overproduction of GH in adults is ____________________.

8. ____________________ is the tendency toward equilibrium.



## EXERCISE 9-7 ABBREVIATIONS

**Write out the term for the following abbreviations.**

1. ____________________________________ GTT
2. ____________________________________ PTH
3. ____________________________________ $T_4$
4. ____________________________________ FBS
5. ____________________________________ ADH
6. ____________________________________ $HbA_{1c}$
7. ____________________________________ GH
8. ____________________________________ PTH

**Write the abbreviation for the following terms.**

9. ______________ adrenocorticotropic hormone
10. ______________ follicle-stimulating hormone
11. ______________ diabetes mellitus
12. ______________ calcitonin
13. ______________ melanocyte-stimulating hormone
14. ______________ triiodothyronine
15. ______________ prolactin
16. ______________ thyroid-stimulating hormone
17. ______________ luteinizing hormone

## EXERCISE 9-8 SPELLING

**Select the correct spelling of the medical term.**

1. An ____________________ is a physician who specializes in caring for patients with endocrine diseases and hormonal dysfunctions.
   a. enocreenologist
   b. endokrineologist
   c. endocrineologist
   d. endocrinologist

2. A medication that can be taken orally to lower the circulating level of blood glucose is called a ____________________.
   a. hypogysemic
   b. hyperglycemic
   c. hypoglycemic
   d. hyperglysemik

3. ____________________ is one of the hormones produced in the pancreas that regulates blood sugar.
   a. Insullin
   b. Insulin
   c. Insalin
   d. Insulen

4. One of the main disorders of the pancreas is called ____________________.
   a. diabetes mellitus
   b. diabetis mellitus
   c. diabetis melletes
   d. diabetes mellitus

5. The ____________________ is located posterior to the stomach.
   a. pancreas
   b. pancrease
   c. pankreas
   d. pankrease

6. In addition to insulin, the pancreas also produces ____________________, which increases blood sugar.
   a. glukagon
   b. glucagun
   c. glucagon
   d. glucagone

7. The ____________________ gland controls the activities of the other endocrine glands.
   a. pituatary
   b. pitooatary
   c. patuitary
   d. pituitary

8. A ____________________ is a chronic enlargement of the thyroid gland.
   a. goyter
   b. goiter
   c. goitar
   d. goytar

9. Enlargement of the extremities, especially the hands and feet, that is caused by excessive GH after puberty is called ____________________.
   a. acromeguly
   b. acromegaly
   c. acrohmegaly
   d. akromegaly

10. The male sex hormone secreted by the adrenal cortex is ____________________.
   a. andragen
   b. androhgen
   c. androjen
   d. androgen

## EXERCISE 9-9 CASE STUDY

ENDOCRINOLOGY OFFICE CONSULTATION

After reading the case study, answer the following questions.

**OFFICE NOTE:** This 59-year-old woman has previously been in good health. On a routine physical examination, she was noted to have a thyroid nodule on the right lobe of the thyroid gland. She complained of hoarseness, dysphasia, local tenderness, and a slight enlargement on the right side of her neck. She also stated that she feels anxious and cannot sleep throughout the night.

On physical examination, the right side of the neck was visibly enlarged, and a nodule was felt; it was noted that the patient's eyes were bulging outward. A blood test to check her thyroid hormone levels indicated a high value of TSH. No other modifying factors or associated signs or symptoms were present.

1. What does dysphasia mean? ____________________

____________________

2. What is a medical term for an "enlargement of the thyroid gland"? ____________________

____________________

3. What does TSH stand for? ____________________

____________________

10

# The Cardiovascular System

## LEARNING OUTCOMES

***Upon completion of this chapter, you should be able to:***

- Understand blood flow through the heart and through the body.
- Name the elements that form blood.
- Pronounce, spell, and define medical terms related to the cardiovascular system and its disorders.
- Interpret abbreviations associated with the muscular system.

## INTRODUCTION

The **cardiovascular system** is made up of the heart and blood vessels, which transport blood. The blood vessels include all the **arteries** (carrying blood *away* from the heart), **veins** (carrying blood *toward* the heart), and **capillaries** (vessels between the arteries and veins). Together they form a transportation system that delivers oxygen and nutrients to the body's cells, returns carbon dioxide and wastes to be eliminated, and helps regulate body temperature. The heart pumps the blood within the blood vessels to all parts of the body. When we discuss the cardiovascular system, we can divide it into the *pulmonary circuit* and the *systemic circuit*. The **pulmonary circuit** is the passage of blood from the heart's right ventricle, through the lung's pulmonary arteries, and then back through the pulmonary veins to the heart's left atrium. The **systemic circuit** is the circulation of blood the through the arteries, capillaries, and veins of the general system (see Figure 10-1).

## WORD PARTS RELATED TO THE CARDIOVASCULAR SYSTEM

The term *cardiovascular* introduces two word parts: cardi/o, which comes from the Greek *kardia* (heart), and vas/o, which comes from the Latin *vas* (vessel). The third component to this system besides the heart and vessels is blood. The root words hem/o and hemat/o both mean blood, as does the suffix –emia. Table 10-1 lists word parts related to the cardiovascular system terms.

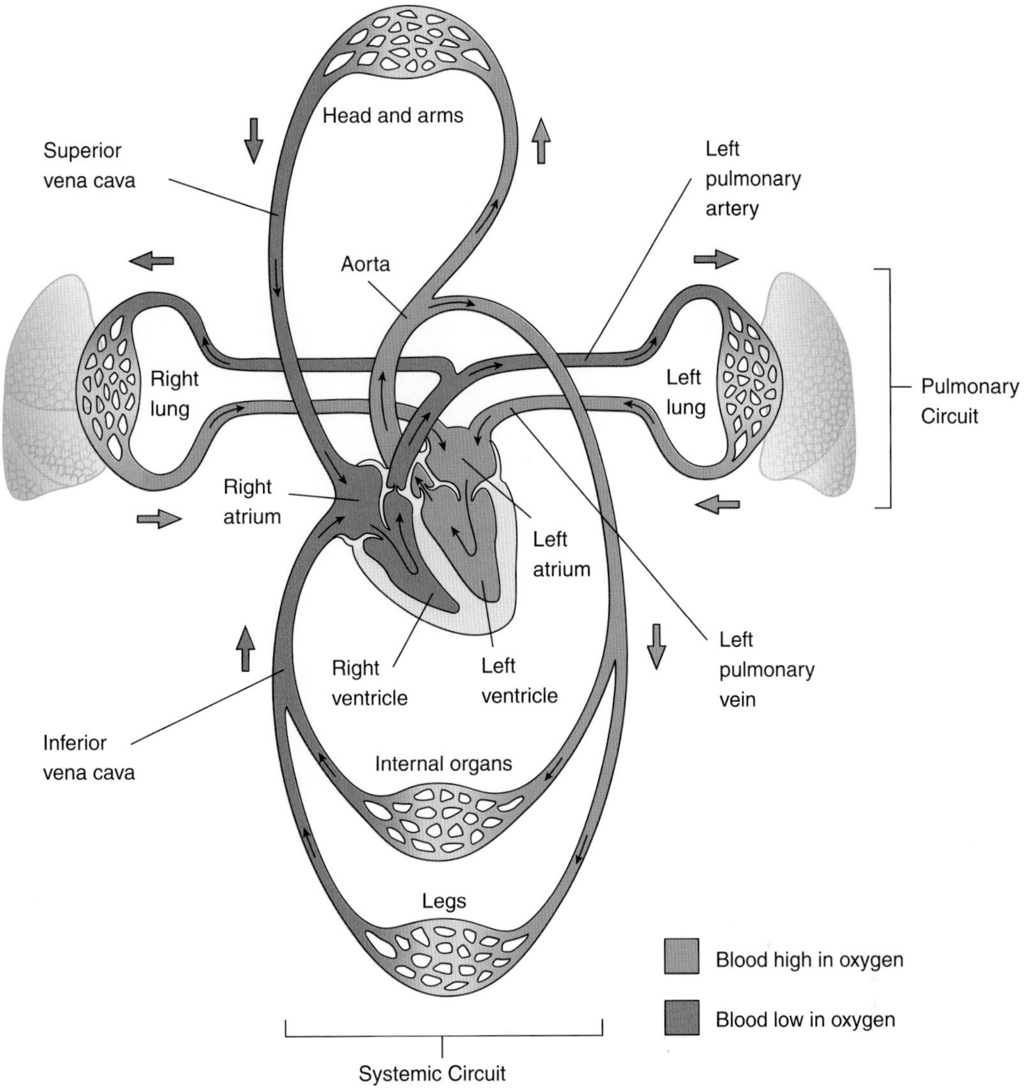


**FIGURE 10-1** The cardiovascular system. The cardiovascular system consists of blood flow in a closed system of vessels. The pulmonary circuit carries blood to and from the lungs, and the systemic circuit carries blood to and from all other parts of the body. Blood that is low in oxygen leaves the right side of the heart and enters the lungs, whereas blood that is rich in oxygen leaves the lungs and is returned to the left side of the heart to be pumped out to the systemic circuit. The vessels depicted in *red* signify blood that is high in oxygen; the vessels depicted in *blue* signify blood that is low in oxygen.

## STRUCTURE AND FUNCTION

### The Heart

The heart is a four-chambered hollow organ with three layers. Its lowermost tip is called the **apex**. The innermost layer is called the **endocardium**. The middle layer, which is the actual heart muscle and the thickest of the three layers, is called the **myocardium**. The outer layer of the heart is called the **epicardium**, which is surrounded by the **pericardium**, a sac that surrounds the heart (see Figure 10-2).

TABLE 10-1 WORD PARTS RELATED TO THE CARDIOVASCULAR SYSTEM

| Word Part | Meaning |
|---|---|
| angi/o | vessel |
| aort/o | aorta |
| arteri/o | artery |
| ather/o | fatty |
| atri/o | atrium |
| brady- | slow |
| cardi/o | heart |
| coron/o | crown; encircling, such as in the coronary blood vessels encircling the heart |
| -ectasis | dilation, expansion |
| electr/o | electricity |
| -emia | blood |
| endo- | within, inner |
| -gram | written record |
| hem/o | blood |
| hemat/o | blood |
| isch | restricting, thinning |
| my/o | muscle |
| peri- | around, surrounding |
| phleb/o | vein |
| -stenosis | a narrowing |
| tachy- | fast |
| thromb/o | clot |
| valv/o | valve |
| valvul/o | valve |
| varic/o | dilated |
| vas/o | vessel |
| ven/o | vein |
| ventricul/o | ventricle |



## Word Parts Exercise

After studying Table 10-1, write the meaning of each of the word parts.

| WORD PART | MEANING |
|---|---|
| 1. root meaning vein | 1. ______________ |
| 2. root meaning heart | 2. ______________ |
| 3. root meaning vessel | 3. ______________ |
| 4. root meaning within, inner | 4. ______________ |

## Word Parts Exercise (continued)

| WORD PART | MEANING |
|---|---|
| 5. prefix meaning fast | 5. ______ |
| 6. root meaning clot | 6. ______ |
| 7. prefix meaning around, surrounding | 7. ______ |
| 8. root meaning fatty | 8. ______ |
| 9. root meaning atrium | 9. ______ |
| 10. suffix meaning written record | 10. ______ |
| 11. suffix meaning blood | 11. ______ |
| 12. root meaning muscle | 12. ______ |
| 13. suffix meaning a narrowing | 13. ______ |
| 14. root meaning blood | 14. ______ |
| 15. root meaning artery | 15. ______ |
| 16. root meaning vein | 16. ______ |
| 17. root meaning valve | 17. ______ |
| 18. root meaning aorta | 18. ______ |
| 19. prefix meaning slow | 19. ______ |
| 20. root meaning dilated | 20. ______ |
| 21. root meaning crown | 21. ______ |
| 22. suffix meaning dilation or expansion | 22. ______ |
| 23. root meaning vessel | 23. ______ |
| 24. root meaning electricity | 24. ______ |
| 25. root meaning ventricle | 25. ______ |
| 26. root meaning restricting, thinning | 26. ______ |

The heart acts as a double pump whose chambers are separated by a wall called the **septum**. Remember anatomic position when thinking about blood flow and how it relates to the figures. The right side of the heart is the right side of the patient and will be shown on the left in figures on the book pages, just as anatomic position states it should be. The right side of the heart pumps

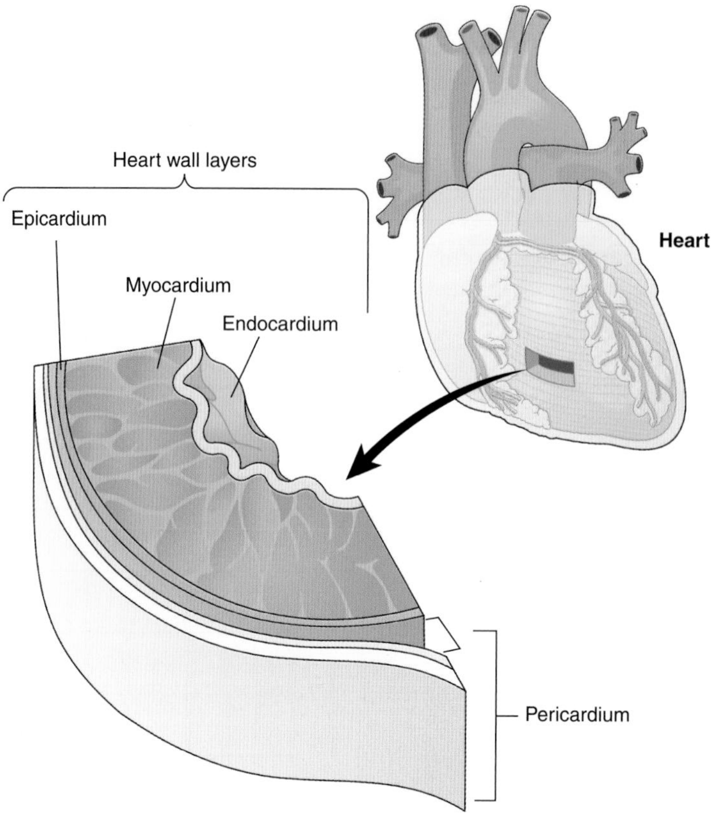


**FIGURE 10-2** Layers of the heart and pericardium. The heart wall is composed of three layers: the epicardium, myocardium, and endocardium. Note the thickness of the myocardium or "muscle" layer. The pericardium is composed of two layers and has fluid in the space between the layers. This fluid helps to reduce friction when the heart beats.

deoxygenated blood to the **lungs** where the blood picks up oxygen. Because the right side is pumping a shorter distance, the muscle in this side of the heart is thinner. The left side of the heart receives blood that has been oxygenated in the lungs, and it pumps the oxygenated blood through the entire body. In the heart, blood travels through four distinct chambers. The atria are the superior (top) chambers and the ventricles are the inferior (bottom) chambers. The four chambers are as follows:

- **Right atrium:** upper right chamber that receives blood from all body parts except the lungs; the **interatrial septum** separates the right and left **atria** (plural of *atrium*).
- **Right ventricle:** lower right chamber that receives blood from the right atrium and pumps it to the lungs; the **interventricular septum** separates the right and left ventricles.
- **Left atrium:** upper left chamber that receives oxygen-rich blood as it returns from the lungs.
- **Left ventricle:** lower left chamber that pumps blood out the aorta (large artery) to all parts of the body.

### *Blood Flow Through the Heart*

Blood first enters the heart from either the **superior vena cava** or **inferior vena cava**. Both of these veins drain into the right atrium. Blood leaves the heart at the left ventricle by way of a large artery called the **aorta**. Blood flow through the heart is directed by one-way valves located at the entrance and exit to each of the ventricles. The **atrioventricular (AV) valves** are found at the entrance to the ventricles and are so named because they come between the atria and ventricles. The **right AV valve** is also known as the **tricuspid valve** because it has three cusps (flaps) that open and close. It controls the opening between the right atrium and right ventricle. The **left AV** valve is located between the left atrium and left ventricle and is called the **bicuspid valve** or **mitral valve**. It has two cusps that control blood flow.

Why is the left AV valve also called the mitral valve? This name comes from the valve's similarity to a miter, which is a tall ceremonial hat that is tapered to a point and worn by some clergymen as a symbol of their office.

The exit valves separate the ventricles from the lungs on the right side and the rest of the body on the left side. These valves are named **semilunar** because the flaps resemble half moons. The exit point at the right ventricle is called the **pulmonary valve** (*pulmonary semilunar valve*), and it is located between the right ventricle and the **pulmonary arteries**, the vessels that lead to the lungs. The **aortic valve** (*aortic semilunar valve*) is located between the left ventricle and the aorta, the vessel that leads to the rest of the body. The pathway of blood through the heart is illustrated in Figure 10-3.

Use the adjective "ventricular" only when you are absolutely sure of the meaning of the phrase you are uttering. The reason for caution is that the brain, as well as the heart, contains ventricles.



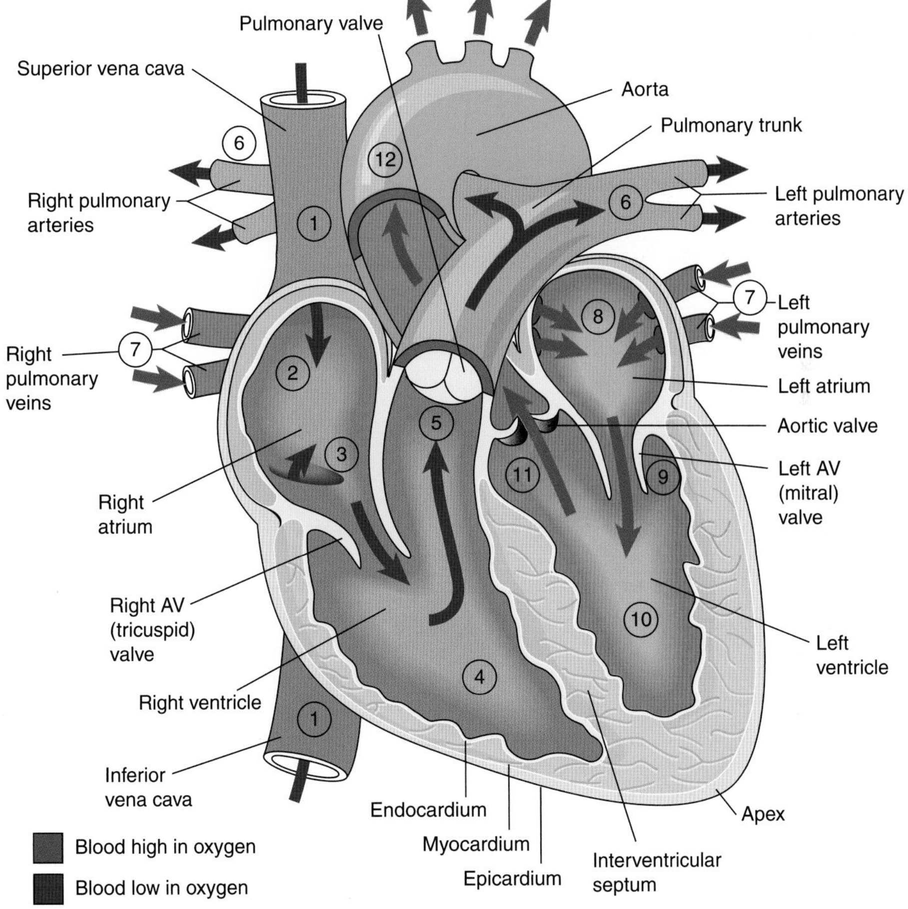


**FIGURE 10-3** The heart and pathway of blood flow. Deoxygenated blood returns from the body into the heart through the superior and inferior venae cavae. The pathway of the blood through the heart begins when blood is returned to the vena cava (#1) and exits the heart through the aorta (#12) to the rest of the body. Note: The right side of the heart is colored in *blue*, signifying deoxygenated blood. The left side of the heart is colored in *red* because it carries oxygenated blood.

## The Heartbeat

To pump blood effectively throughout the body, the heart must contract and relax in a rhythmic cycle known as a **heartbeat**. The **conducting system of the heart** generates and transmits signals that stimulate the myocardium of the heart to contract and relax in sequence. The conducting system of the heart includes the following (see Figure 10-4):

- **Sinoatrial node (SA node):** located in the upper posterior wall of the right atrium; action potential is generated here and distributed to other cells of the conducting system; conducting cells form **intermodal pathways** that distribute the impulse across the atria as it travels toward the ventricles; also called the pacemaker of the heart.
- **Atrioventricular node (AV node):** located at the junction between the atria and ventricles; continues to generate impulses toward the atrioventricular bundle.
- **Atrioventricular bundle (AV bundle** or **bundle of His)** and **right and left bundle branches:** AV bundle is located at the top of the interventricular septum; right and left bundle branches travel down each side of the septum toward the apex; transmit impulses to the Purkinje fibers.
- **Purkinje fibers:** peripheral fibers extending from the bundle branches that end in the right and left ventricles; stimulation from the AV bundle causes excitation of the ventricular muscles, resulting in contraction.

The electrical activity of the heart can be recorded on an **electrocardiogram (ECG, EKG)**. The machine that does the recording is called an **electrocardiograph**.

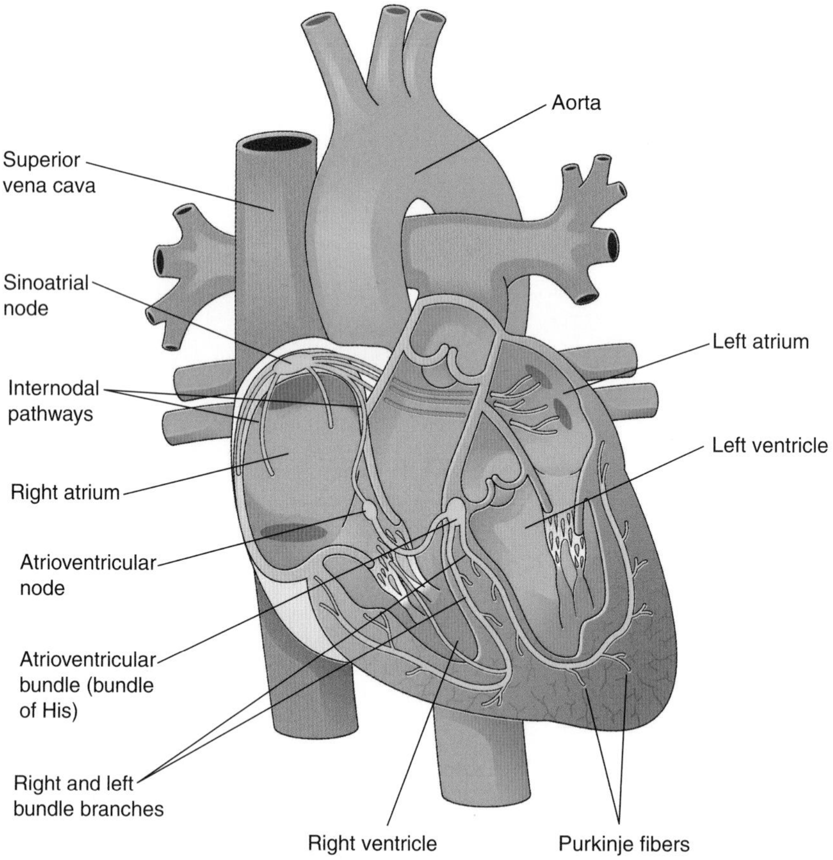


**FIGURE 10-4** Conducting system of the heart. The electrical stimulus begins in the sinoatrial node. The electrical stimulus moves from the sinoatrial node, through the internodal pathways, to the atrioventricular node, through the atrioventricular bundle, through the right and left bundle branches, and terminates in the Purkinje fibers where excitation of the ventricles occurs.

Why bundle of His? Why not "bundle of His or Hers"? In 1893, German physician, Wilhelm His, figured out that a heartbeat starts in a particular group of AV fibers, which were, subsequently, named for him. A Czech anatomist/physiologist, Jan Evangelista Purkyně, likewise discovered the Purkinje (or Purkyne) fibers. Born in 1787, Purkyně contributed many other scientific discoveries to the world. For example, he was the first to show that fingerprints could be used to establish identity, and his studies of the human eye foreshadowed motion pictures.

Each heart contraction, called **systole**, is followed by a relaxation called **diastole**. These complete rounds of cardiac systole and diastole make up the **cardiac cycle** and are illustrated in Figure 10-5.

**Heart rate (HR)** is the number of times the heart beats per minute. The blood that is forced through the vessels by contraction creates an increase darterial pressure that can be felt as a pulse. The radial artery on the thumb side of the anterior wrist is a common location for feeling an arterial pulse.

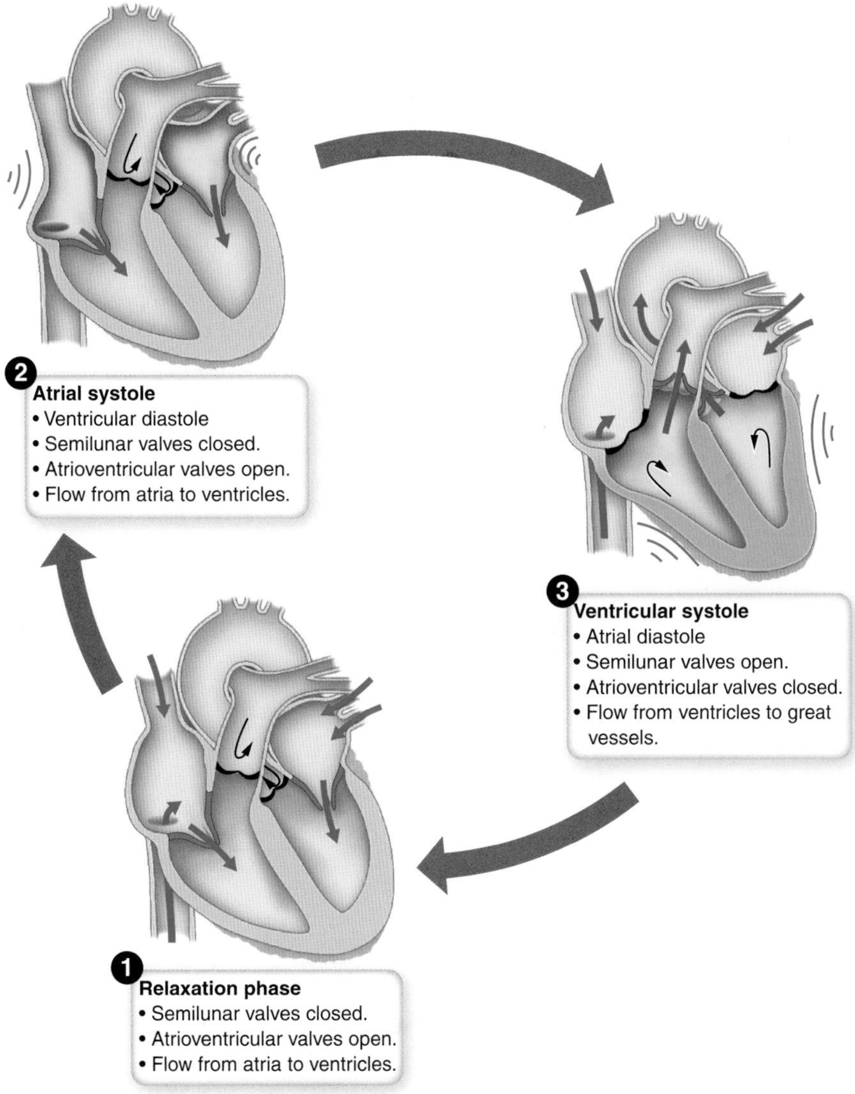
2 Atrial systole
• Ventricular diastole
• Semilunar valves closed.
• Atrioventricular valves open.
• Flow from atria to ventricles.
3 Ventricular systole
• Atrial diastole
• Semilunar valves open.
• Atrioventricular valves closed.
• Flow from ventricles to great vessels.
1 Relaxation phase
• Semilunar valves closed.
• Atrioventricular valves open.
• Flow from atria to ventricles.

**FIGURE 10-5** The three phases of the cardiac cycle.

## Blood Vessels

Blood vessels are tubular structures that convey blood. The types of blood vessels include arteries, arterioles, capillaries, venules, and veins (see Figure 10-6).

- **Arteries:** thick-walled, muscular, elastic blood vessels that carry blood away from the heart. With the exception of pulmonary and umbilical arteries, arteries contain oxygenated blood.
- **Arterioles:** branches of the arteries that carry blood to the capillaries.
- **Capillaries:** blood vessels that connect the arterial and venous systems; they are only one cell thick and allow for the exchange of nutrients, gases, and wastes.
- **Venules:** vessels that are continuous with capillaries and transport blood to the veins.
- **Veins:** blood vessels that carry blood toward the heart. With the exception of pulmonary and umbilical veins, veins contain deoxygenated blood.

The **lumen** of a blood vessel is the tubular space through which blood flows. The nervous system can stimulate the lumen to be opened, known as **vasodilation**, or closed, which is called **vasoconstriction**. Vasodilation and vasoconstriction each can have an effect on blood pressure (BP).

BP is a measurement of the amount of pressure exerted against the walls of blood vessels. BP is recorded as a fractional number, **systolic** over **diastolic**. For example, 120/80 means the systolic pressure is 120 and the diastolic pressure is 80. Systolic pressure occurs when the highest pressure is exerted against the vessel walls, and diastolic pressure occurs when the lowest pressure is exerted against the vessel walls. BP can be measured by several methods, but the most common is with an instrument called a **sphygmomanometer**, commonly called a BP cuff.

## Blood

Blood is a fluid connective tissue made up of plasma (55%) and formed elements (45%). **Plasma** is a clear, straw-colored fluid that is composed mostly of water (91%), along with proteins and other nutrients in solution. The formed elements in blood consist of **red blood cells** (**RBCs**), also called

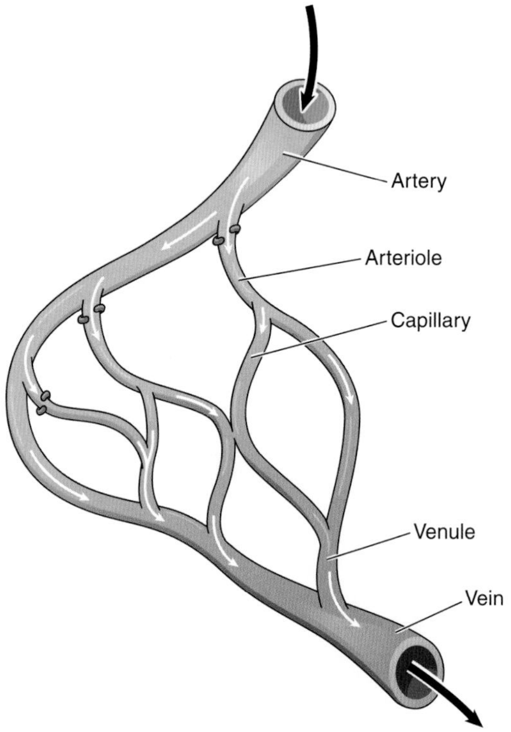


**FIGURE 10-6** The five types of blood vessels.

**TABLE 10-2 BLOOD TYPES AS DONORS AND RECIPIENTS**

| Blood Type | Can Donate to | Can Receive from |
|---|---|---|
| A | A or AB only | A or O only |
| B | B or AB only | B or O only |
| AB (universal recipient) | AB only | A, B, AB, O |
| O (universal donor) | A, B, AB, O | O only |

**erythrocytes**; **white blood cells** (**WBCs**), also called **leukocytes**, and **platelets**, also called **thrombocytes**. Each element has an important role, ranging from the transportation of oxygen (erythrocytes), to defense of the body against harmful organisms (leukocytes), to blood clotting (platelets). The following list identifies the structure and function of each element:

- **RBCs:** The main function of RBCs is to transport oxygen. The oxygen binds to **hemoglobin** (**Hb**), a protein.
- **WBCs:** WBCs are the body's main defense against harmful organisms; there are five types of leukocytes: **neutrophils**, **eosinophils**, **basophils**, **lymphocytes**, and **monocytes**. Owing to the role leukocytes play in the body's defense, they will be discussed again in Chapter 11, which covers the lymphatic system and immunity.
- **Platelets:** These cell fragments play an important role in the blood-clotting process. They are the smallest of the formed elements, roughly half the size of erythrocytes.

### *Blood Groups*

The four major blood groups (types) are **A**, **B**, **AB**, and **O**. Blood type compatibility is an important consideration when blood is transfused from one person to another. Table 10-2 lists the blood type compatibilities for donors and recipients.

The presence or absence of a protein on the surface of an RBC is responsible for what is known as the **Rh factor**. The Rh factor is named for the first two letters in the word *rhesus*, a reference to the rhesus macaque, the blood of which was used in early experiments. A person whose blood contains the Rh factor is **Rh positive ($Rh^+$)**. People with blood that does not contain the Rh factor are **Rh negative (Rh)**.

### Quick Check

**Fill in the blanks.**

1. Arteries transfer blood to ______________________.
2. ______________________ are blood vessels that return blood to the heart.
3. Erythrocyte is another term for ______________________.

## DISORDERS RELATED TO THE CARDIOVASCULAR SYSTEM

Heart disease includes numerous problems and is a leading cause of death. This section discusses disorders related to the cardiovascular system.

### Coronary Artery Disease

**Coronary artery disease (CAD)** is narrowing of the lumen of one or more of the coronary arteries, usually due to atherosclerosis. Normal blood vessels have a smooth lumen. When there is a progressive buildup of plaque or fatty deposits on inner arterial walls, the lumen narrows, creating **atherosclerosis.** One cause of plaque buildup in the coronary arteries is a condition of increased blood fat (lipid) called **hyperlipidemia**. Common types of lipids are high-density lipoproteins (HDLs) and low-density lipoproteins (LDLs). When there is a hardening and loss of elasticity in the artery, impeding blood flow to the heart muscle, the condition is called **arteriosclerosis** (see Figure 10-7). An inadequate supply of blood and oxygen to tissues is called **ischemia**. In the heart, the myocardium is the tissue that suffers from a lack of blood flow and oxygen.

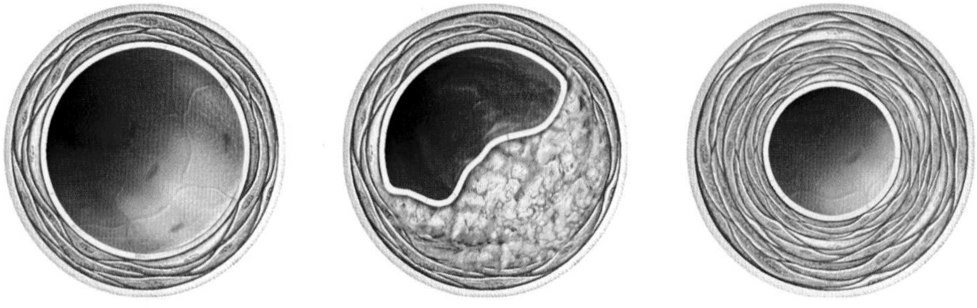


**FIGURE 10-7** A comparison between atherosclerosis and arteriosclerosis.



## Blood Clots

A **thrombus** is a blood clot in a blood vessel, which can impede blood flow to the myocardium and cause ischemia. **Thrombosis** is the formation of a thrombus. An **embolus** is a blood clot that moves throughout the bloodstream.

## Myocardial Infarction and Congestive Heart Failure

A **myocardial infarction** (**MI**), commonly called a *heart attack*, results from a lack of oxygen supply to the myocardium. Various diagnostic tests are used to identify abnormal cardiac function. Among these are an ECG; **echocardiography** (ultrasonic examination of the heart); **cardiac catheterization** (insertion of a catheter and contrast dye into the coronary arteries to detect blockage); and a stress test.

A simple blood test to discover the presence of *troponin* may confirm a diagnosis of MI. **Troponin** is a muscle protein released into the bloodstream when an MI occurs.

**Congestive heart failure (CHF)** occurs when the heart cannot pump enough blood to meet the body's needs for oxygen and nutrients. This leads to edema (swelling) in the legs and fluid buildup in the lungs.

> The acronym MONA is sometimes used to refer to standard emergency treatment for a suspected heart attack. M stands for morphine, O for oxygen, N for nitroglycerin, and A for aspirin.

## Arrhythmias

A normal heart rhythm is called **sinus rhythm**. An **arrhythmia** is any irregularity of the heart's rhythm, such as a slow or fast rate or extra beats. **Bradycardia** (less than 50 beats/minute) is a slower than normal HR, and **tachycardia** (more than 90 beats/minute) is a faster than normal rate. **Fibrillation** describes rapid, random, and ineffective contractions of the heart. Some arrhythmias are more serious than others. **Atrial fibrillation**, commonly shortened to "A-fib," occurs when the atria beat faster than the ventricles. This condition causes a quivering motion of the atria, which is usually not life threatening, although it can predispose the atria to thrombi formation. It affects many people and can often be controlled with drugs. Sustained **ventricular fibrillation**, a condition in which the ventricles ineffectively pump blood, can be fatal.

### Hypertension

The term for high BP is **hypertension (HTN)**. It occurs when the systolic reading exceeds 140 mm Hg or the diastolic is >90 mm Hg. Over time, HTN may lead to arteriosclerosis (hardening of the arteries) and/or **left ventricular hypertrophy** (oversized left ventricle). When HTN is related to another medical problem, such as a kidney disorder, it is called **secondary hypertension**.

Are atherosclerosis and arteriosclerosis the same ailment? Not exactly. Both conditions exhibit similar symptoms; however, these symptoms occur for different reasons. A patient who has arteriosclerosis has hardening of the arteries caused by continuous high BP. A patient with atherosclerosis has similar symptoms because his or her arteries have been narrowed by plaque buildup. So, a patient can have arteriosclerosis and not have atherosclerosis and vice versa. Both have the same symptoms, however, and some patients have both conditions.



### Blood Disorders

Any abnormality of the blood may be called a **dyscrasia**. There are three major types: **anemia**, **leukemia**, and **clotting disorders**:

- **Anemia** is a condition marked by a deficiency of RBCs or a low level of Hb.
- **Leukemia** is characterized by an increased number of WBCs.
- **Clotting disorders** include **hemophilia** (hereditary bleeding disorder), **thrombocytopenia** (an insufficient number of thrombocytes), and **disseminated intravascular coagulation (DIC)** (extreme clotting caused by trauma or disease).

## DIAGNOSTIC TESTS, TREATMENTS, AND SURGICAL PROCEDURES

Medications and surgical procedures are used to treat arrhythmias. **Antiarrhythmic** medications, such as amiodarone, affect calcium channels in the heart to regulate rhythm. Other medications that are used in patients with atrial fibrillation may include blood thinners, such as Coumadin, Xarelto, and Eliquis, because these patients are at a higher risk of developing a blood clot due to blood pooling in the heart and not continuously flowing as it should. **Cardioversion**, a treatment for fibrillation, involves applying an electric current to restore a normal heart rhythm. **Ablation therapy**, applying radiofrequency waves to the heart, is used to cure a variety of cardiac arrhythmias, such as some tachycardias and atrial fibrillation.

Surgical procedures for treating blockages in blood vessels include the following:

- **Percutaneous transluminal coronary angioplasty (PTCA)** involves the insertion of a balloon-tipped catheter to open a blocked coronary artery (see Figure 10-8).

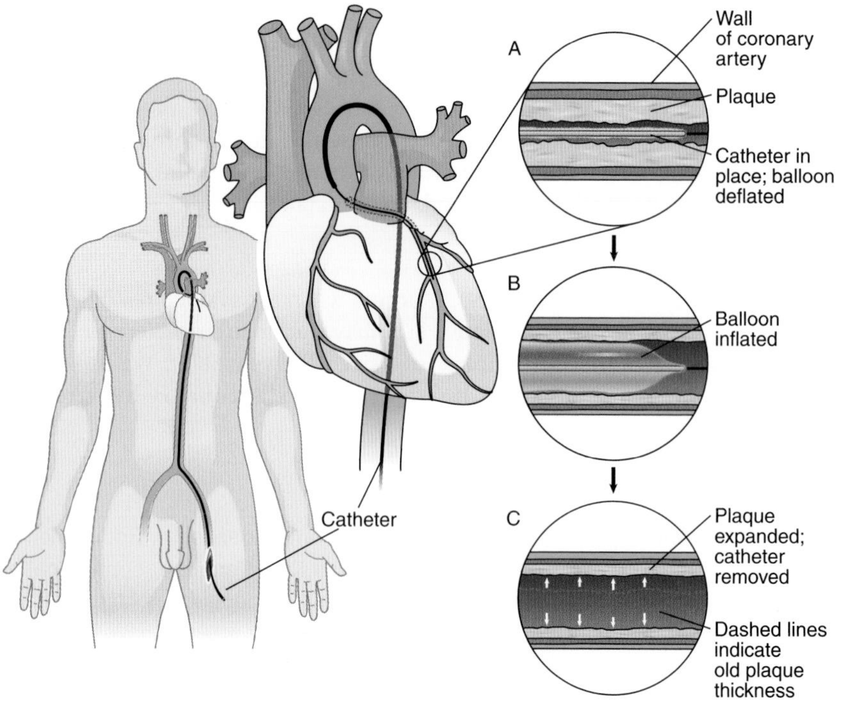


FIGURE 10-8 Percutaneoustransluminal coronary angioplasty (PTCA). **A.** Plaque deposits in the artery. **B.** Plaque buildup narrows the coronary vessel, impeding blood flow to the myocardium. **C.** The rough interior edges encourage clot formation in the artery.



- **Arterial stent** includes the implantation of a stent, which is a mesh tube that is implanted into an artery to provide support (see Figure 10-9).
- **Coronary artery bypass graft (CABG)** is a surgical procedure in which a damaged section of a coronary artery is replaced or bypassed with a graft vessel (see Figure 10-10).
- **Endarterectomy** is the removal of the inner lining of a blocked artery.

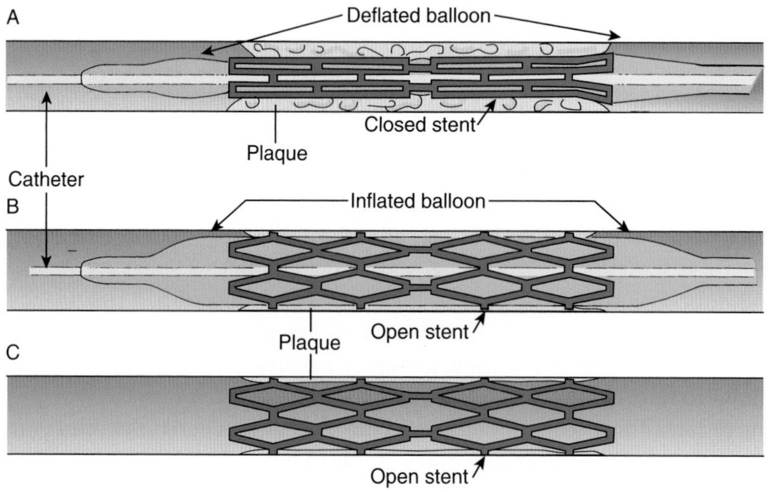


FIGURE 10-9 Arterial stent. **A.** A balloon-tipped catheter is placed into the artery with the balloon deflated and the stent closed. **B.** When the stent is in the proper position of the narrowed artery, the balloon is inflated, causing the stent to open. **C.** The catheter is removed, and the stent remains in place.

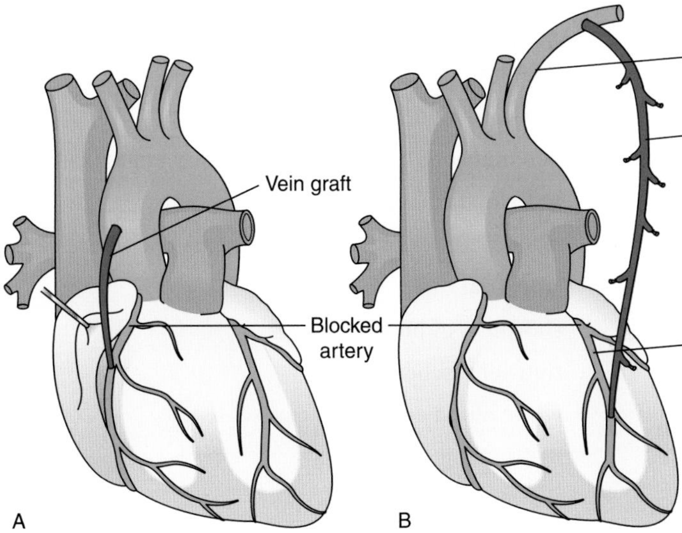


**FIGURE 10-10** Coronary artery bypass graft (CABG). **A.** A segment of the saphenous vein extracted from the leg is used to carry blood from the aorta to a part of the right coronary artery that is distal to the occlusion. **B.** The internal thoracic artery from the chest is used to bypass an obstruction in the left anterior descending artery. The graft redirects the blood flow or "bypasses" the blocked artery.

## PRACTICE AND PRACTITIONERS

The specialists who treat disorders of the cardiovascular system include cardiologists, cardiovascular surgeons, and hematologists. **Cardiologists** diagnose and treat heart disorders. **Cardiovascular surgeons** surgically correct disorders of the cardiovascular system. **Hematologists** treat disorders of the blood.

**Abbreviation Table** THE CARDIOVASCULAR SYSTEM

| ABBREVIATION | MEANING |
|---|---|
| A-fib | atrial fibrillation |
| AV | atrioventricular |
| BP | blood pressure |
| CABG | coronary artery bypass graft |
| CAD | coronary artery disease |
| CCU | cardiac care unit |
| CHF | congestive heart failure |
| DIC | disseminated intravascular coagulation |
| EKG or ECG | electrocardiogram, electrocardiograph, electrocardiography, cardiogram |
| Hb | hemoglobin (protein in the blood that carries oxygen) |
| HDL | high-density lipoprotein |
| HR | heart rate |
| HTN | hypertension |
| LDL | low-density lipoprotein |

*(continued)*

**Abbreviation Table** THE CARDIOVASCULAR SYSTEM (*continued*)

| ABBREVIATION | MEANING |
|---|---|
| MI | myocardial infarction |
| PTCA | percutaneous transluminal coronary angioplasty |
| RBC | red blood cell |
| $Rh^+$, $Rh^-$ | symbol for Rh blood group; Rh positive, Rh negative |
| SA | sinoatrial |
| SOB | shortness of breath |
| TIA | transient ischemic attack |
| WBC | white blood cell |



**Study Table** THE CARDIOVASCULAR SYSTEM

| TERM AND PRONUNCIATION | ANALYSIS | MEANING |
|---|---|---|
| **Structure and Function** | | |
| aorta (ay-OR-tah) | from the Greek word *aeirein* (to lift up or to be hung) | the main trunk of the systemic arterial system |
| aortic valve (ay-ORT-ikvalv) | from the Greek word *aeirein* (to lift up or to be hung); from the Latin word *valva* (that which turns) | valve between the left ventricle to the aorta; also called *aortic semilunar valve* |
| apex (A-peks) | from the Latin for summit or tip | the pointed inferior portion of the heart |
| arteries (AR-tuh-rees) | from the Greek word *arteria* (windpipe) | the largest of the blood vessels that carry blood away from the heart |
| arterioles (ar-TEER-ee-oles) | from the Greek word *arteria* (windpipe) | the smallest arteries that connect with the capillaries |
| atria (singular: atrium) (AY-tree-ah; AY-tree-uhm) | a Latin word meaning "entry hall" | upper two of the four heart chambers, composed of the right atrium and left atrium |
| atrioventricular node (AY-tree-oh-ven-TRIK-u-lahr); AV node | from the Latin word meaning "entry hall"; from the Latin *venter* (belly) | fibers located at the base of the right atrium near the ventricle that carry electrical stimulation to the AV bundle |
| atrioventricular valve (ay-tree-oh-ven-TRIK-yoo-ler valv) | from the Greek word *arteria* (windpipe); from the Latin word *venter* (belly) | a valve between an atria and a ventricle; there are two AV valves, a right and a left |
| basophil (BAY-soh-fil) | from the Greek *basis* and *philein* (to love) | a WBC with granules that stain with basic dyes |

**Study Table** THE CARDIOVASCULAR SYSTEM (*continued*)

| TERM AND PRONUNCIATION | ANALYSIS | MEANING |
|---|---|---|
| bicuspid valve (by-KUSS-pidvalv) | *bi*-(two); from the Latin *cuspidem* (cusp or point); from the Latin word *valva* (that which turns) | flap (valve) between the left atrium and left ventricle; also called *mitral valve* |
| bundle of His (BUHN-dl ov-hiz) | named for Swiss cardiologist Wilhelm His, Jr., who discovered the function of these cells in 1893 | located at the top of the interventricular septum; carries electrical impulses from the AV node to Purkinje fibers |
| capillaries (KAP-ih-layr-ees) | from the Latin word *capillus* (hair) | the smallest of the blood vessels where gas and nutrient exchange occurs |
| cardiac cycle (KAR-dee-ak SIGH-kuhl) | *cardi/o* (heart); *-ac* (adjective ending) | a complete round of systole and diastole |
| conducting system of the heart | common English words | The system of muscle fibers comprising the SA node, internodal pathways, AV node and bundle, right and left bundle branches, and Purkinje fibers |
| diastole (dye-AS-toh-lee) | from the Greek word *diastole* (dilation) | relaxation phase of the heart |
| endocardium (en-doh-KAR-dee-uhm) | *endo-* (within); *cardi/o* (heart) | the inner lining of the heart |
| eosinophil (ee-oh-SIHN-oh-fil) | from the Greek words *eos* (dawn); *philein* (to love) | a WBC that stains with certain dyes |
| epicardium (ep-ih-KAR-dee-uhm) | *epi-* (on, upon); *cardi/o* (heart) | the outer covering of the heart |
| erythrocytes (er-RITH-ro-sites) | *erythr/o* (red); *-cyte* (cell) | RBCs that carry oxygen |
| heartbeat (HART-beet) | common English word | a complete cycle of heart contraction and relaxation |
| heart rate (HART REYT) | common English words | the number of times per minute the heart contracts |
| hemoglobin (Hb) (hee-mo-GLO-bihn) | *hem-* (blood); from the Latin *globus* (globe) | the protein that gives blood its red color |
| inferior vena cava (in-FEER-ee-er VEE-nah KAV-ah) | *inferior*, a Latin word meaning "lower"; from the Latin words *vena* (vein); *cava* (hollow) | large vein that collects blood from the smaller veins of the lower body |
| left atrium (left AY-tree-uhm) | a Latin word meaning "entry hall" | upper left heart chamber |
| left ventricle (left VEN-tri-kul) | from the Latin word *venter* (belly) | lower left heart chamber |

(*continued*)

**Study Table** THE CARDIOVASCULAR SYSTEM *(continued)*

| TERM AND PRONUNCIATION | ANALYSIS | MEANING |
|---|---|---|
| leukocytes (LUKE-o-sytes) | *leuk/o* (white); *-cyte* (cell) | WBCs that play a role in immunity |
| lumen (LOO-muhn) | Latin for "light"; in anatomy used to describe an opening or passageway | the space in the interior of a hollow tubular structure like an artery |
| lymphocyte (LIM-foh-site) | from the Latin *lympho-* (lymph); *-cyte* (cell) | one of five types of WBC; distributed throughout lymphatic tissue |
| mitral valve (MY-trahlvalv) | from the Latin word *mitra* (turban); from the Latin word *valva* (that which turns) | flap (valve) between the left atrium and the left ventricle; also called *bicuspid valve* |
| monocyte (MON-oh-site) | *mon/o* (single); *-cyte* (cell) | a relatively large WBC |
| myocardium (my-oh-KAR-dee-uhm) | *my/o* (muscle); *cardi/o* (heart) | the heart muscle, which includes nerves and blood vessels |
| neutrophil (NU-troh-fil) | from the Latin word *neuter* (neither); from the Greek word *philein* (to love) | a mature WBC normally constituting more than half of the total number of leukocytes |
| pericardium (pehr-ih-KAR-dee-uhm) | *peri-* (surrounding); *cardi/o* (heart) | sac that surrounds the heart |
| plasma (PLAZ-muh) | a Greek word meaning "something molded" or "created" | the fluid portion of blood consisting mainly of water |
| platelets (PLATE-lets) | from the English word plate and the diminutive suffix *-let* | smallest of the formed elements; important in the clotting process; also called *thrombocytes* |
| pulmonary artery (PULL-moh-nahr-ee AHR-tuh-ree) | *pulmon/o* (lung); from the Greek word *arteria* (windpipe) | vessel that carries deoxygenated blood from the right ventricle to the lungs |
| pulmonary circuit (PULL-moh-nahr-ee SER-kit) | *pulmon/o* (lung); from the Latin word *circuitus* (going around) | passage of blood from the right ventricle through the pulmonary arteries to the lungs and back through the pulmonary veins to the left atrium |
| pulmonary valve (PULL-moh-nahr-eevalv) | *pulmon/o* (lung); from the Latin word *valva* (that which turns) | valve between the right ventricle and lungs; also called *pulmonary semilunar valve* |
| pulmonary veins (PULL-moh-nahr-eevayns) | *pulmon/o* (lung); from the Latin word *vena* (blood vessel) | vessels that carry oxygenated blood from the lungs to the left atrium |

## Study Table THE CARDIOVASCULAR SYSTEM (*continued*)

| TERM AND PRONUNCIATION | ANALYSIS | MEANING |
|---|---|---|
| pulse (puhls) | from the Latin word *pulsum* (push, knock, drive) | rhythmic expansion and contraction of an artery produced by pressure of the blood moving through the artery |
| Purkinje fibers (per-KIN-jee FIGH-berz) | named after Jan Evangelista Purkinje, who discovered them in 1839 | fibers that carry stimulation throughout the ventricles |
| red blood cells (red blud selz) | common English words | erythrocytes that contain Hb for carrying blood |
| Rh factor (AR-h FAK-ter) | from rh(esus), so-called because the blood group was discovered in rhesus monkeys | an antigen, first discovered in the rhesus monkey; a person is either Rh positive or Rh negative |
| right atrium (rite AY-tree-uhm) | a Latin word meaning "entry hall" | upper right heart chamber |
| right ventricle (rite VEN-trik-al) | from the Latin word *venter* (belly) | lower right heart chamber |
| semilunar valve (sem-ee-LOO-ner valv) | *semi-* (half); from the Latin word *luna* (moon) | a heart valve at the exit of a ventricle; pulmonary semilunar valve and aortic semilunar valve |
| septa (singular: septum) (SEPP-tah; SEPP-tuhm) | from the Latin word *saeptum* (a fence) | thin wall that separates cavities or masses; in the heart, septa separate the right atrium from the left atrium and the right ventricle from the left ventricle |
| sinoatrial node (SA node) (SYE-noh-AY-tree-ahl nohd) | from the Latin words *sinus* (bend, fold, curve) and *atrium* (entry hall) | known as the pacemaker of the heart; electrical impulse originates here |
| sinus rhythm (SYE-nus RITH-uhm) | *sinus*, a Latin word meaning "bend," "fold," "curve"; from the Greek word *rhythmos* (measured flow or movement) | normal rhythm of the heartbeat |
| superior vena cava (suh-PEER-ee-er VEE-nah KAV-ah) | *superior*, a Latin word meaning "higher"; from the Latin words *vena* (vein) and *cava* (hollow) | large vein that collects blood from the smaller veins of the upper body |
| systemic circuit (sis-TEM-ik SER-kit) | from the Greek word *systema* (an organized whole); from the Latin word *circuitus* (going around) | circulation of blood through the arteries, capillaries, and veins of the general system, from the left ventricle to the right atrium |
| systole (SIS-toh-lee) | a Greek word meaning "contraction" | contraction phase of the heart |

(*continued*)

**Study Table** THE CARDIOVASCULAR SYSTEM *(continued)*

| TERM AND PRONUNCIATION | ANALYSIS | MEANING |
|---|---|---|
| thrombocyte (THROM-boh-site) (also called platelet) | from the Greek word *thrombos* (clot of blood); *-cyte* (cell) | smallest of the formed elements; important in the coagulation process |
| tricuspid valve (try-KUSS-pidvalv) | *tri-*(three); from the Latin *cuspidem* (cusp or point) | valve between the right atrium and the right ventricle; also called *right AV valve* |
| troponin (TROH-poh-nihn) | from the Greek word *trepein* (to turn) | a muscle protein that is released into the bloodstream when a heart attack occurs |
| vascular (VASS-cue-lahr) | *vascul/o* (blood vessel); *-ar* (adjective suffix) | adjectival form of *vessel* |
| veins (VAYNS) | from the Latin word *vena* (vein) | the blood vessels that return blood from the tissues to the heart |
| venous (VEE-nuhs) | from the Latin word *vena* (vein) | adjectival form of *vein* |
| venules (VEEN-yuhlz) | from the Latin *venula* (diminutive form of *vena* [vein]) | small veins |
| ventricle (VEN-tri-kul) | from the Latin word *venter* (belly) | lower two of the four heart chambers, composed of the right ventricle and left ventricle |
| white blood cells (wite blud selz) | common English words | formed element in the blood that protects the body against harmful bacteria |
| **Disorders** | | |
| anemia (ah-NEE-mee-a) | from the Greek word *anaimia* (without blood) | abnormally low RBC count |
| aneurysm (AN-yur-iz-um) | from the Greek word *aneurysmos* (to dilate) | a localized dilation of an artery, cardiac chamber, or other vessel |
| angina pectoris (an-JY-nuh PEK-tor-is) | from the Greek word *agkhone* (a strangling); also *angere* (anguish); *pectoris*, a Latin word meaning "chest" | pain in the chest due to ischemia |
| angiospasm (AN-jee-o-spaz-uhm) | *angi/o* (blood vessel); from the Greek word *spasmos* (spasm) | spasm in blood vessels |
| angiostenosis (AN-jee-o-steh-NO-siss) | *angi/o* (blood vessel); *-stenosis* (a narrowing) | narrowing of a blood vessel |

**Study Table** THE CARDIOVASCULAR SYSTEM (*continued*)

| TERM AND PRONUNCIATION | ANALYSIS | MEANING |
|---|---|---|
| arrhythmia (ah-RITH-mee-ah) | *a-* (without); from the Greek word *rhythmos* (measured flow or movement); *-ia* (condition) | abnormal rhythm; irregular heartbeat |
| arteriosclerosis (ar-TEER-ee-o-sklu-RO-sis) | from the Greek word *arteria* (windpipe); *scler/o* (hardness); *-osis* (abnormal condition of) | hardening of the arteries |
| arteriospasm (ar-TEER-ee-o-spaz-uhm) | from the Greek word *arteria* (windpipe); from the Greek word *spasmos* (a spasm or convulsion) | spasm of an artery |
| arteriostenosis (ar-TEER-ee-oh-steh-NO-sihs) | from the Greek word *arteria* (windpipe); *-steno* (narrow); *-osis* (abnormal condition) | narrowing of an artery |
| atheroma (ath-er-OH-mah) | from the Greek word *ather* (groats, porridge); *-oma* (tumor) | fatty deposit or plaque within the arterial wall |
| atherosclerosis (ath-er-oh-skleh-ROH-sis) | *ather/o* (fatty); *scler/o* (hardening); *-osis* (abnormal condition of) | hardening and narrowing of the arteries |
| atrial fibrillation (A-fib) (fih-brih-LAY-shun) | from the Latin word *atrium* (entry hall) *-al* (adjective suffix); from the Latin word *fibra* (fiber, string, thread) | rapid, random, ineffective contractions of the atrium |
| atriomegaly (AY-tree-oh-MEG-ah-lee) | from the Latin word *atrium* (hall); *-megaly* (enlargement) | enlargement of an atrium |
| bradycardia (bray-dee-KAR-dee-ah) | *brady-* (slow); *cardi/o* (heart); *-ia* (condition) | abnormally slow heartbeat |
| cardiac arrest (KAR-dee-ak) | *cardi/o* (heart); from the Latin words *ad* and *restare* (to stop, remain behind) | cessation of heart activity |
| cardiomegaly (kar-dee-oh-MEG-ah-lee) | *cardi/o* (heart); *-megaly* (enlargement) | enlargement of the heart |
| cardiomyopathy (kar-dee-oh-my-AWP-uh-thee) | *cardi/o* (heart); *my/o* (muscle); *-pathy* (disease) | disease of the heart muscle (myocardium) |
| cardiopathy (kar-dee-AWP-uh-thee) | *cardi/o* (heart); *-pathy* (disease) | any heart disease |
| cardiorrhexis (kar-dee-oh-REX-ihs) | *cardi/o* (heart); *-rrhexis* (rupture) | rupture in the heart wall |
| carditis (kar-DY-tiss) | *cardi/o* (heart); *-itis* (inflammation) | inflammation of the heart |

(*continued*)

**Study Table** THE CARDIOVASCULAR SYSTEM *(continued)*

| TERM AND PRONUNCIATION | ANALYSIS | MEANING |
|---|---|---|
| congestive heart failure (CHF) (kuhn-JEST-iv hart FEYL-yer) | from the Latin word *congerere* (to bring together, pile up) | syndrome where the heart is unable to pump enough blood to meet the body's needs for oxygen and nutrients; as a result, fluid is retained and accumulates in the ankles and legs |
| coronary artery disease (CAD) (KAWR-u-ner-ee AHR-tuh-ree dih-ZEEZ) | from the Latin *coronarius* (of a crown); from the Greek word *arteria* (windpipe) | narrowing of the lumen of one or more coronary arteries, usually due to atherosclerosis |
| disseminated intravascular coagulation (DIC) (dih-SEMM-ihn-ay-ted ihn-tra-VASS-kyu-lahr koh-AG-yu-LAY-shun) | from the Latin *dis-* (in every direction); *seminare* (to plant, propagate); *intra-* (within); *vascul/o* (vessel); *-ar* (adjective suffix); coagulation (from the Latin verb *coagulo* [curdle]) | widespread clotting and obstruction of blood flow to the tissues |
| dyscrasia (dys-KRAY-sha) | *dys-* (bad, difficult); from the Greek word *krasis* (mingling) | general term for a blood disorder |
| embolus (EM-bow-lus) | from the Greek word *embolus* (plug or stopper) | a blood clot that is carried in the bloodstream |
| endocarditis (en-doh-kar-DY-tiss) | *endo-* (within); *cardi/o* (heart); *-itis* (inflammation) | inflammation of the endocardium |
| fibrillation (fib-ruh-LEY-shun) | from the Latin word *fibrilla* (little fiber) | exceedingly rapid contractions or twitching of muscle fibers |
| hemolysis (hee-MAWL-ih-sihs) | *hem/o* (blood); *-lysis* (destruction) | change or destruction of RBCs |
| hemophilia (hee-mo-FEEL-ee-ya) | *hem/o* (blood); *-phil(ia)* (attraction) | congenital disorder impeding the coagulation process |
| hemorrhage (HEM-o-rij) | *hem/o* (blood); *-rrhage* (burst forth) | discharge of blood; bleeding |
| hyperlipidemia (high-per-LIP-ih-DEE-mee-ah) | *hyper-* (above normal); *lip/o* (fat); *-demia* (from hema [blood]) | elevated cholesterol, triglycerides, and lipoproteins in the blood |
| hypertension (high-per-TEN-shun) | *hyper-* (above normal); from the Latin word *tendere* (to stretch) | elevated BP (>140/90 mm Hg) |
| hypertrophy (high-PUR-troh-fee) | *hyper-* (above normal); *-trophy* (nourishment) | increase in size of a part or organ |

10 | Cardiovascular System

**Study Table** THE CARDIOVASCULAR SYSTEM (*continued*)

| TERM AND PRONUNCIATION | ANALYSIS | MEANING |
|---|---|---|
| ischemia (is-KEE-mee-ah) | from the Greek word *iskhaimos* (a stopping of the blood); *-ia* (condition) | deficiency in blood supply and oxygen to the tissues |
| leukemia (loo-KEE-mee-uh) | leukos (Greek word for "white"); *-emia* (blood) | progressive proliferation of abnormal leukocytes |
| myocardial infarction (MI) (my-oh-KAR-dee-ahl in-FARK-shun) | *my/o* (muscle); *cardi/o* (heart); *-al* (adjective suffix); from the Latin word *infractionem* (a breaking) | heart attack |
| myocarditis (my-oh-kar-DY-tiss) | *my/o* (muscle); *cardi/o* (heart); *-itis* (inflammation) | inflammation of the heart muscle |
| pericarditis (pehr-ih-kar-DY-tiss) | *peri-* (surrounding); *cardi/o* (heart); *-itis* (inflammation) | inflammation of the pericardium |
| secondary hypertension (SEK-uhn-der-ee high-per-TEN-shun) | *hyper-* (above normal); from the Latin word *tendere* (to stretch) | hypertension due to a known cause |
| tachycardia (tak-ih-KAR-dee-ah) | *tachy-* (fast); *cardi/o* (heart); *-ia* (condition) | abnormally rapid heartbeat |
| thrombocytopenia (THROM-boh-sigh-toh-PEE-nee-ah) | *thromb/o* (blood clot); *cyt/o* (cell); *-penia* (deficiency) | abnormal decrease in the number of thrombocytes (platelets) |
| transient ischemic attack (TIA) (TRAN-see-ent is-KEE-mik uh-TAK) | isch: root from the Greek word for restricting or thinning; *-emia*, suffix referring to blood | sudden loss of neurologic function with complete recovery usually within 24 h; mini-stroke |
| thrombus (THROM-bus) | *thromb/o* (blood clot) | blood clot attached to an interior wall of a vein or artery |
| thrombosis (throm-BOH-sis) | Greek word for "a clumping or curdling" | formation or presence of a thrombus (blood clot) |
| valvulitis (valv-yu-LY-tiss) | from the Latin word *valva* (that which turns); *-itis* (inflammation) | inflammation of a heart valve |
| vasculitis (also angiitis) (VAS-kyu-ligh-tis) | *vascul/o* (blood vessel); *-itis* (inflammation) | inflammation of a vessel |
| vasoconstriction (VAZE-oh-kon-STRIK-shun) | *vas/o* (duct, blood vessel); from the Latin word *constingere* (to draw tight) | narrowing of blood vessels |
| vasodilation (VAZE-oh-dy-LAY-shun) | *vas/o* (vessel); from the Latin word *dilitare* (to make wider) | widening of blood vessels |

(*continued*)

**Study Table** THE CARDIOVASCULAR SYSTEM *(continued)*

| TERM AND PRONUNCIATION | ANALYSIS | MEANING |
|---|---|---|
| ventricular fibrillation (ven-TRIK-yoo-ler fib-ruh-LAY-shun) | from the Latin word *venter* (belly); from the Latin word *fibrilla* (little fiber) | exceedingly rapid contractions or twitching of ventricular heart muscle that replaces normal contraction |
| **Diagnostic Tests, Treatments, and Surgical Procedures** | | |
| ablation (ah-BLAY-shun) | from the Latin words *ab-* (away); and *latus* (brought) | partial destruction of the pathway of the electrical conducting system of the heart to treat irregular heart rhythms |
| angiogram (AN-jee-oh-gram) | *angi/o* (blood vessel); *-gram* (record or picture) | printed record obtained through angiography |
| angiography (an-jee-AWG-ruff-ee) | *angi/o* (blood vessel); *-graphy* (process of recording) | radiography of a blood vessel after injection of a contrast dye |
| angioplasty (AN-jee-oh-plass-tee) | *angi/o* (blood vessel); *-plasty* (surgical repair) | surgical repair of a blood vessel |
| antianginals (an-tee-AN-jih-nulz) | *anti-* (against); from the Greek *ankhone* (strangling); *-al* (adjective suffix) | drugs used to treat chest pain |
| antiarrhythmics (an-tee-uh-RITH-micks) | *anti-* (against); *a-* (without); from the Greek word *rhythmos* (measured flow or movement) | drug used to treat rhythm abnormalities |
| arterial stent (ar-TEER-ee-ul stent) | English word *stenting* refers to the process of stiffening | a device implanted into an artery to open and provide support to the arterial wall |
| atrioseptoplasty (AY-tree-oh-SEP-toh-plass-tee) | from the Latin words *atrium* (entry hall) and *saeptum* (fence); *-plasty* (surgical repair) | surgical repair of an atrial septum |
| cardiac catheterization (KAR-dee-ak KATH-eh-ter-eye-zay-shun) | *cardi/o* (heart); *-ac* (pertaining to); from the Greek word *kathienai* (to let down, thrust in) | procedure where a catheter is inserted into an artery and guided into the heart; may be used for diagnosis of blockages or for treatment |
| cardiac glycosides (KAR-dee-ak GLYE-koh-sides) | *cardi/o* (heart); *-ac* (pertaining to); *glyc/o* (sugar) + *-ide* | drugs used to improve heart output by increasing the muscular contraction |
| cardiogram (KAR-dee-oh-gram) | *cardi/o* (heart); *-gram* (record or picture) | a graphic trace of electrical activity in the heart |

**Study Table** THE CARDIOVASCULAR SYSTEM (*continued*)

| TERM AND PRONUNCIATION | ANALYSIS | MEANING |
|---|---|---|
| cardiotomy (kar-dee-AW-tuh-mee) | *cardi/o* (heart); *-tomy* (cutting operation) | incision into the heart or incision into the cardia of the stomach |
| cardioversion (KAR-dee-oh-VER-zhun) | *cardi/o* (heart); from the Latin word *vertere* (to turn) | use of electrical shock to restore the heart's normal rhythm |
| coronary artery bypass graft (CABG) (KAWR-uh-ner-ee AHR-tuh-ree BYE-pas graft) | from the Latin *cor* (heart); from the Greek word *arteria* (windpipe); common English words | through an open chest, a graft (piece of vein or other heart artery) is implanted on the heart to bypass a blockage |
| diuretic (DYE-ur-eh-tik) | from the Greek word *diouretikos* (prompting urine) | a drug used to increase urination and thereby decrease water content in blood to decrease BP |
| echocardiography (EK-oh-KAR-dee-AH-grah-fee) | from the Greek word *ekhe* (sound); *cardi/o* (heart); *-graphy* (process of recording) | ultrasonic procedure used to evaluate the structure and motion of the heart |
| electrocardiogram (ee-LEK-troh-KAR-dee-oh-gram) | *electro-* (electricity); Greek *kardia* (heart); *gramma* (drawing) | graphic record of the heart's action currents |
| electrocardiograph (ee-LEK-troh-KAR-dee-oh-graf) | *electro-* (electricity); *kardia* (heart); *graph* (instrument for recording) | an instrument for recording the electrical currents that traverse the heart |
| endarterectomy (end-art-er-ECK-toh-mee) | *endo-* (within); *arteri/o* (artery); *-ectomy* (excision) | surgical removal of the lining of an artery |
| nuclear stress test (NOO-klee-er stres test) | common English words | assessment of blood flow through the heart through the use of a nuclear element injection while the patient exercises |
| percutaneous transluminal coronary angioplasty (PTCA) (pur-kyoo-TEY-nee-uhs trans-LOO-min-uhl KAWR-uh-ner-ee AN-jee-uh-plas-tee) | *per-* (through); *cutane/o* (skin); *trans-* (across, through); *lumen* (passage); *coron/o* (crown); *angi/o* (blood vessel); *-plasty* (surgical repair) | an operation for enlarging the narrowed lumen of a coronary artery by inflating and withdrawing a balloon on the tip of an angiographic catheter |
| pericardiotomy (PEHR-ih-car-dee-AW-toh-mee) | *peri-* (surrounding); *cardi/o* (heart); *-tomy* (cutting operation) | incision into the pericardium |
| sphygmomanometer (SFIG-moh-mah-NOM-eh-ter) | from the Greek words *sphygmos* (pulse), *manos* (thin), *metros* (measure) | instrument used to measure BP |

(*continued*)

**Study Table** THE CARDIOVASCULAR SYSTEM (*continued*)

| TERM AND PRONUNCIATION | ANALYSIS | MEANING |
|---|---|---|
| statins (STAT-inz) | from lovastatin, from *lo* + *vastatin* (stuff) | a class of cholesterol-lowering drug |
| valvoplasty (VALV-oh-plass-tee); also valvuloplasty (VALV-yu-loh-plass-tee) | from the Latin word *valva* (that which turns); *-plasty* (surgical repair) | surgical repair of a heart valve |
| valvotomy (valv-AW-toh-mee) | from the Latin word *valva* (that which turns); *-tomy* (cutting operation) | surgical removal of a blocked heart valve (stenosis of a heart valve) by cutting into it; also called *valvulotomy* |
| **Practice and Practitioners** | | |
| cardiologist (kar-dee-AWL-oh-jist) | *cardi/o* (heart); *-logist* (one who specializes) | heart specialist |
| cardiology (kar-dee-AWL-oh-jee) | *cardi/o* (heart); *-logy* (study of) | medical specialty dealing with the heart |
| cardiovascular surgeon (kar-dee-oh-VAS-kyoo-ler SUR-jun) | *cardi/o* (heart); *vas/o* (vessel) | a medical practitioner who surgically corrects disorders of the cardiovascular system |
| hematologist (HEE-mah-tah-lo-gist) | *hemat/o* (blood); *-logist* (one who specializes) | blood specialist |
| hematology (HEE-mah-TAH-lo-jee) | *hemat/o* (blood); *-logy* (study of) | medical specialty dealing with blood |

## END-OF-CHAPTER EXERCISES

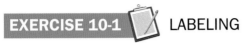

### EXERCISE 10-1 LABELING

**Using the following list, choose the correct terms to label the diagram correctly.**

| | | |
|---|---|---|
| aorta | left AV (mitral) valve | right atrium |
| aortic valve | pulmonary arteries | right ventricle |
| left atrium | pulmonary valve | superior and inferior vena cava |
| left ventricle | pulmonary veins | right AV (tricuspid) valve |

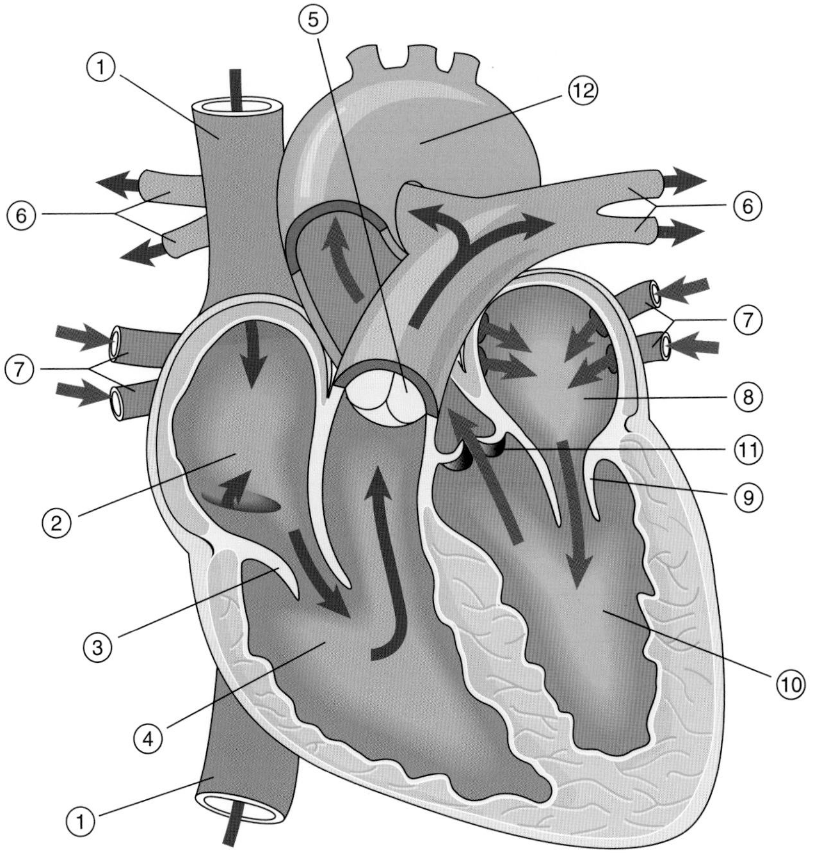


1. ______________________ 5. ______________________ 9. ______________________

2. ______________________ 6. ______________________ 10. ______________________

3. ______________________ 7. ______________________ 11. ______________________

4. ______________________ 8. ______________________ 12. ______________________

## EXERCISE 10-2 WORD PARTS

**Break each of the following terms into its word parts: prefix, root, or suffix. Give the meaning of each word part and then define the term.**

1. erythrocyte

   root: ______________________________

   suffix: ______________________________

   definition: ______________________________

2. atherosclerosis

   root: ______________________________

   root: ______________________________

   suffix: ______________________________

   definition: ______________________________

3. cardiomyopathy

   root: ______________________________

   root: ______________________________

   suffix: ______________________________

   definition: ______________________________

4. endocarditis

   prefix: ______________________________

   root: ______________________________

   suffix: ______________________________

   definition: ______________________________

5. thrombocytopenia

   root: ______________________________

   root: ______________________________

   suffix: ______________________________

   definition: ______________________________

6. angiogram

   root: ______________________________

   suffix: ______________________________

   definition: ______________________________

7. hematology

   root: ______________________________

   suffix: ______________________________

   definition: ______________________________

8. pericardiotomy

   prefix: ______________________________

   root: ______________________________

   suffix: ______________________________

   definition: ______________________________

## EXERCISE 10-3 WORD BUILDING

**Use the word parts listed to build the terms defined.**

| | | | | |
|---|---|---|---|---|
| a-, an- | -dilation | inter- | peri- | valv/o |
| angio/o | -ectomy | leuk/o | -philia | vas/o |
| arteri/o | -emia | -lysis | -rhythm | ven/o |
| ather/o | erythr/o | -megaly | -spasm | ventricul/o |
| atri/o | -genic | my/o | -stenosis | |
| cardi/o | hem/o; hemat/o | -oma | thromb/o | |
| -cyte | -ic, -ia, -ac, -al, -ar, -ary -ous, -um | -penia | -tomy | |

1. originating in the heart ______________________
2. an incision into the atrium ______________________
3. an RBC ______________________
4. hereditary bleeding disorder caused by a deficiency of a clotting factor ______________________
5. spasm of a vein ______________________
6. removal of a blood clot ______________________
7. dilation of a vessel ______________________
8. enlargement of the heart ______________________
9. narrowing of an artery ______________________
10. fatty plaque ______________________
11. a WBC ______________________
12. the surgical removal of a valve ______________________
13. pertaining to the heart ______________________
14. destruction of RBCs ______________________
15. between the ventricles ______________________
16. an abnormally low level of Hb ______________________
17. heart muscle ______________________
18. removal of a fatty plaque ______________________
19. abnormal heart rhythm ______________________

## EXERCISE 10-4 MATCHING

**Match the term with its definition.**

| | | |
|---|---|---|
| 1. ______________ | ischemia | a. pacemaker of the heart |
| 2. ______________ | anemia | b. electric current used to restore normal sinus rhythm |
| 3. ______________ | cardioversion | c. surgical removal of the inner lining of an artery |
| 4. ______________ | SA node | d. abnormality of the blood |
| 5. ______________ | Hb | e. thrombocytes |
| 6. ______________ | vasoconstriction | f. a protein in the RBC |
| 7. ______________ | tricuspid valve | g. deficiency of blood flow to an organ |
| 8. ______________ | endarterectomy | h. vessels are narrowed |
| 9. ______________ | platelets | i. low level of Hb in the blood |
| 10. ______________ | dyscrasia | j. between the right atrium and right ventricle |



## EXERCISE 10-5 MULTIPLE CHOICE

**Choose the correct answer for the following multiple choice questions.**

1. Which of the following is a type of WBC?
   a. thrombocyte
   b. eosinophil
   c. erythrocyte
   d. platelet

2. What is the term that describes the destruction of bacteria by special WBCs?
   a. phagocytosis
   b. leukocytosis
   c. erythrocytosis
   d. neutrophilosis

3. Platelets are also referred to as ______________________.
   a. erythrocytes
   b. thrombocytes
   c. basophils
   d. neutrophils

4. Oxygen-carrying pigment of RBCs is called ______________________.
   a. hematocrit
   b. Hb
   c. leukemia
   d. gamma globulin

5. Which of the following is a malignant disease of the blood?
   a. leukemia
   b. leukopenia
   c. erythropenia
   d. thrombosis

6. Which of the following terms describes hardened tissue?
   a. sclerotic
   b. thrombotic
   c. occluded
   d. fibrillated

7. The heart muscle is supplied with blood vessels called ________________.
   a. capillaries
   b. coronary arteries
   c. corpuscles
   d. carpals

8. What is the function of a leukocyte?
   a. transports $O_2$
   b. manufactures Hgb
   c. initiates coagulation
   d. defends against disease

9. Which is the smallest blood vessel?
   a. artery
   b. arteriole
   c. vein
   d. capillary

10. Which of the following is characteristic of the artery in arteriostenosis?
   a. hardened
   b. soft
   c. dilated
   d. narrowed



## EXERCISE 10-6 FILL IN THE BLANK

**Fill in the blank with the correct answer.**

1. The term for low BP is ________________.

2. The term for a rapid pulse rate is ________________.

3. A ________________ is medical specialist who deals with blood.

4. The artery that carries blood out of the heart to the lung is the ________________ artery.

5. The "universal donor" is the blood type ________________ while the "universal recipient" is the blood type ________________.

6. The study of the heart and heart conditions is ________________.

7. An incision into a vein is a ________________.

8. Elevated blood fat is called ________________.

9. The mitral valve is also called the left AV valve and the ________________ valve.

10. The two veins that carry blood into the right atrium are the ________________ and the ________________.

## EXERCISE 10-7 ABBREVIATIONS

**Write out the term for the following abbreviations.**

1. ________________ BP
2. ________________ A-fib
3. ________________ LDL
4. ________________ SOB
5. ________________ WBC
6. ________________ AV
7. ________________ CAD
8. ________________ CHF
9. ________________ HR
10. ________________ Hb
11. ________________ MI
12. ________________ TIA

**Write the abbreviation for the following terms.**

13. ________________ hemoglobin
14. ________________ atrial fibrillation
15. ________________ red blood cell
16. ________________ sinoatrial
17. ________________ congestive heart failure

18. ______________________ electrocardiogram

19. ______________________ coronary artery bypass graft

20. ______________________ hypertension

21. ______________________ disseminated intravascular coagulation

22. ______________________ high-density lipoprotein

23. ______________________ percutaneous transluminal coronary angioplasty

## EXERCISE 10-8 SPELLING

**Select the correct spelling of the medical term.**

1. The ______________________ BP reflects the arterial pressure during relaxation of a cardiac chamber.
   a. distolic
   b. diastolic
   c. diatolic
   d. diastollic

2. An adjective meaning "related to the myocardium" is ______________________.
   a. myocardial
   b. mycardial
   c. myocardal
   d. miocardial

3. A deficiency in blood supply to the tissues is ______________________.
   a. ichemia
   b. iscemia
   c. ischemia
   d. ishemia

4. The condition that exhibits both hardening and narrowing of the arteries is called ______________________.
   a. athrosclersis
   b. atheroclerosis
   c. atheroscleris
   d. atherosclerosis

5. A ______________________ is a WBC.
   a. leukocyte
   b. lukocyte
   c. luekocyte
   d. leukosite

6. An abnormal decrease in the number of thrombocytes or platelets is called ______________________.
   a. thrombocytpenia
   b. thrombocytopenia
   c. throbcytopenia
   d. thombecytpenia

7. The smallest blood vessel that connects the arterial and venous systems is known as a ______________________.
   a. capilary
   b. cappilary
   c. capillarie
   d. capillary

8. An abnormally rapid heartbeat is called ______________________.
   a. tachicardia
   b. tachycardia
   c. tacycardia
   d. tachycarda

9. A blood disorder characterized by an excessive increase in the number of WBCs is ______________________.
   a. lukemia
   b. lukimia
   c. leukemia
   d. luekemia

10. A drug used to treat heart rhythm abnormalities is called an ______________________.
    a. antiarrhythmic
    b. antarhythmic
    c. antiarhythmic
    d. antiarythmic

## EXERCISE 10-9 CASE STUDY

**Read the case and answer the questions that follow.**

**BRIEF HISTORY:** The patient is a 56-year-old male who had been complaining of recurrent chest pain when performing mild activities at home. The chest pain subsides when he lies down. He also has experienced shortness of breath (SOB) when carrying in the groceries and climbing up one set of stairs. He has a history of high BP.

**EMERGENCY ROOM VISIT:** The patient arrives at the emergency room with angina pectoris that is relieved by rest, a BP of 180/110 mm Hg, and SOB. An EKG is performed, which indicates that the patient is having atrial arrhythmias and an MI. He is given aspirin and started on antiarrhythmics, diuretics, vasodilators, and oxygen. He is admitted to the CCU for observation and treatment.

**DIAGNOSIS:** Hypertension, an MI, and atrial fibrillation.

1. Define angina pectoris. ______________________________

2. What does the acronym SOB stand for? ______________________________

3. What is hypertension? ______________________________

4. What is an EKG? ______________________________

5. What type of pharmacologic intervention is used with this patient? Define each drug classification.
______________________________
______________________________
______________________________
______________________________

6. What is an MI? What are the two roots in myocardial, and what do they mean?
______________________________
______________________________

7. Define atrial fibrillation. ______________________________

# 11 The Lymphatic System and Immunity

## LEARNING OUTCOMES

***Upon completion of this chapter, you should be able to:***

- Name the organs that make up the lymphatic system.
- Understand the relationship between the cardiovascular system and the lymphatic system.
- Name the types of immunity.
- Pronounce, spell, and define medical terms related to the lymphatic system and its disorders.
- Pronounce, spell, and define medical terms related to immunity and immune disorders.
- Interpret abbreviations associated with the lymphatic system.

## INTRODUCTION

The lymphatic system and immunity are considered together because each supports the other. The **lymphatic system** is a network of tissues, organs, nodes, and lymphatic vessels (*lymphatics*) spread throughout the body. Fluid called **lymph** is found within lymphatic vessels, and this lymph empties from the *right lymphatic duct* and the *thoracic duct* into specific veins in the thorax to reenter the bloodstream. These veins are the *left subclavian vein* and the *right subclavian vein* (see Figure 11-1). Lymph contains a type of white blood cells called **lymphocytes**, which are groups of B cells (*B lymphocytes*) and T cells (*T lymphocytes*) important to immune function. Medically speaking, **immunity** refers to the body's ability to resist disease, and we gain immunity either actively (through contact with a disease or by vaccinations) or passively (from our mothers while in utero, from breast milk, or through injection of antibodies). **Vaccines** are substances used to stimulate the production of antibodies and to provide immunity against disease without inducing the disease.

What is lymph? Like plasma, which is the fluid part of blood, lymph is a fluid that consists mostly of water. It also contains a low concentration of proteins in solution and, of course, lymphocytes. The word lymph is also used as an adjective in naming lymph vessels and lymph nodes. A second adjective, lymphatic, is most often used when referring either to the whole system or to some specific part of the system, such as the "right lymphatic duct." Either adjective, however, is acceptable.

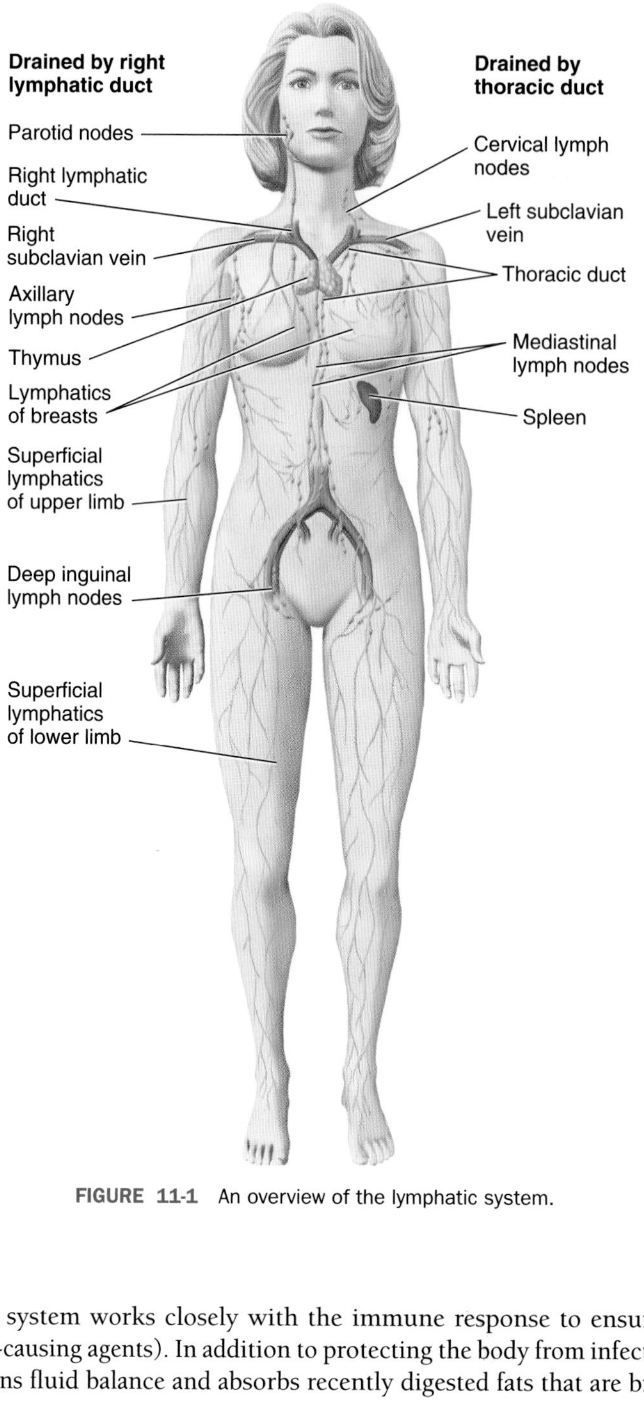


**FIGURE 11-1** An overview of the lymphatic system.



The lymphatic system works closely with the immune response to ensure defense against **pathogens** (disease-causing agents). In addition to protecting the body from infection, the lymphatic system also maintains fluid balance and absorbs recently digested fats that are broken down in the digestive tract.

## WORD PARTS RELATED TO THE LYMPHATIC SYSTEM AND IMMUNITY

*Lymph* is actually a Latin word meaning "water" or "clear water." The roots that come from this word are lymph/o and lymphat/o. The root word immun/o comes from the Latin word *immunis*, which means exempt from. In the medical sense, immun/o means the body is "exempt" from illness. Table 11-1 lists word parts that make up lymphatic system and immunity terms.

**TABLE 11-1** WORD PARTS RELATED TO THE LYMPHATIC SYSTEM AND IMMUNITY

| Word Part | Meaning |
|---|---|
| an- | without |
| immun/o | immune system |
| lymph/o | lymph or lymphatic system |
| lymphaden/o | lymph nodes |
| lymphangi/o | lymph vessels |
| lymphat/o | lymph or lymphatic system |
| -megaly | enlargement |
| -oid | resembling |
| path/o | disease |
| phag/o | ingest or engulf |
| -phylaxis | protection |
| splen/o | spleen |
| thym/o | thymus |
| tonsill/o | tonsil |

## Word Parts Exercise

After studying Table 11-1, write the meaning of each of the word parts.

| WORD PART | MEANING |
|---|---|
| 1. immun/o | 1. ______ |
| 2. phag/o | 2. ______ |
| 3. -phylaxis | 3. ______ |
| 4. -megaly | 4. ______ |
| 5. tonsill/o | 5. ______ |
| 6. splen/o | 6. ______ |
| 7. an- | 7. ______ |
| 8. lymphaden/o | 8. ______ |
| 9. lymphangi/o | 9. ______ |
| 10. lymph/o, lymphat/o | 10. ______ |
| 11. thym/o | 11. ______ |
| 12. -oid | 12. ______ |
| 13. path/o | 13. ______ |

## STRUCTURE AND FUNCTION

Lymphatic tissues include *tonsils*, the *thymus*, *spleen*, *lymph nodes*, *lymphoid nodules of the small intestine* (Peyer's patches), and the *appendix*. **Tonsils** are masses of lymphatic tissue in the pharynx that filter bacteria. The **thymus** is a lymphatic organ located in the chest deep to the sternum. The **spleen** is a large mass of lymphatic tissue in the upper left quadrant of the abdomen involved with destroying bacteria by **phagocytosis** (ingestion by lymphocytes) and removing old blood cells by **hemolysis** (red blood cell rupture). Cells able to complete phagocytosis are called **phagocytes** and include **macrophages**, **microphages**, **neutrophils**, and **monocytes**.

Bean-shaped masses of lymphatic tissue distributed along lymphatic vessels are called **lymph nodes**. Collections of closely packed lymphoid nodules in the wall of the small intestine, known as **Peyer's patches**, are involved with intestinal immunity. The **appendix**, a worm-like structure that extends from the intestine, contains immune system cells that protect the "good bacteria" living in the gut (see Figure 11-1).

Whereas the cardiovascular system circulates blood within a closed system, the lymphatic system distributes lymph on a one-way path via lymphatic vessels. Lymphatic vessels, which run alongside blood vessels, begin where lymphatic capillaries interlace with the blood capillaries of the cardiovascular system, forming networks. Recall that lymph is similar to blood in that it contains special cells called *lymphocytes*, which are a type of white blood cell that fights disease and infection.

How does blood become lymph? Fluid travels from the arterioles to the venules. Some of the fluid that leaks out of the blood capillaries is left in the tissues (interstitial fluid). This fluid is picked up by the open-ended lymph capillaries and circulates in the lymphatic system as lymph. Lymph continues to flow in the lymphatic system until it is returned to the bloodstream at the (see Figure 11-2).

How does lymph return to the bloodstream? Lymph is picked up by the lymph vessels, filtered by the lymph nodes, propelled back into the venules, and then into the veins. The lymphatic vessels from bigger structures called lymphatic trunks, which merge into the thoracic duct on the left side of the body or the right lymphatic duct on the right sides of the body. These ducts then empty into the left or right subclavian vein (see Figure 11-1).

All of these structures play an important role in the body's immune responses. An immune response is the body's reaction to an **antigen** (a substance that induces an immune response in the body). An **antibody** is a soldier-like protein that protects the body and inactivates antigens.

Immunity is classified as innate immunity or adaptive immunity. **Innate immunity** (natural immunity) is genetically determined resistance that a person is born with. **Adaptive immunity** is a type of resistance that is acquired only after a person has been exposed to a particular antigen.

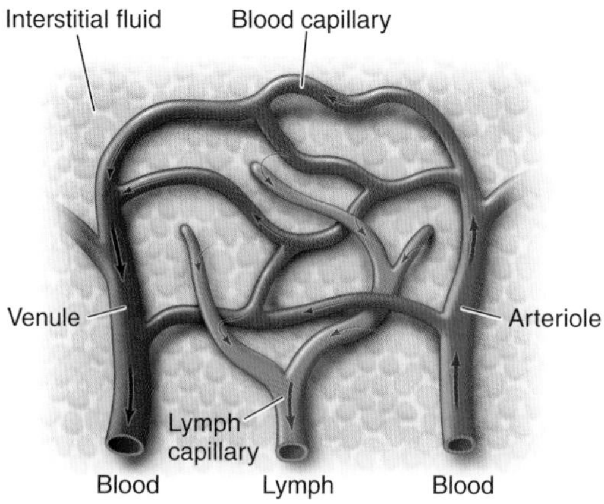


**FIGURE 11-2** Lymph flow. This figure shows the structural relationship between the blood capillaries and the lymph capillaries.

Adaptive immunity is then broken down into two categories, each with two subcategories. The two types of adaptive immunity are *active* (resistance that results from previous exposure to an antigen) and *passive* (resistance that results from the transfer of antibodies). The two types of active immunity are *naturally acquired* (results from contact with the disease) and *artificially acquired* (results from vaccination). The two types of passive immunity are *naturally acquired* (resistance that results through the placenta or from breast milk) and *artificially acquired* (resistance that results from injection of antibodies) (see Figure 11-3).

## Quick Check

**Fill in the blanks.**

1. Besides fighting infection, the lymphatic system maintains ________________ balance and absorbs recently digested ________________.
2. Name the tissues and organs of the lymphatic system. ________________ ____________________________
3. An ________________ is a substance that induces an immune response.

## DISORDERS RELATED TO THE LYMPHATIC SYSTEM AND IMMUNITY

A primary function of the lymphatic system is to filter out harmful organisms. When bacteria spread into the lymphatic system or when an injury to the body is not treated effectively, an infection can result causing **lymphadenitis**, which is swelling of a lymph node. Swelling of lymph tissue is called **lymphedema** (see Figure 11-4). Lymphedema is the result of infection or obstruction of the lymph vessels. **Lymphadenopathy**, any disease process affecting lymph nodes, is an indicator of possible infection. **Autoimmune diseases** are any disorders in which normal body tissues are destroyed by the immune response being directed against the body's own tissue. An **allergy** is a hypersensitivity

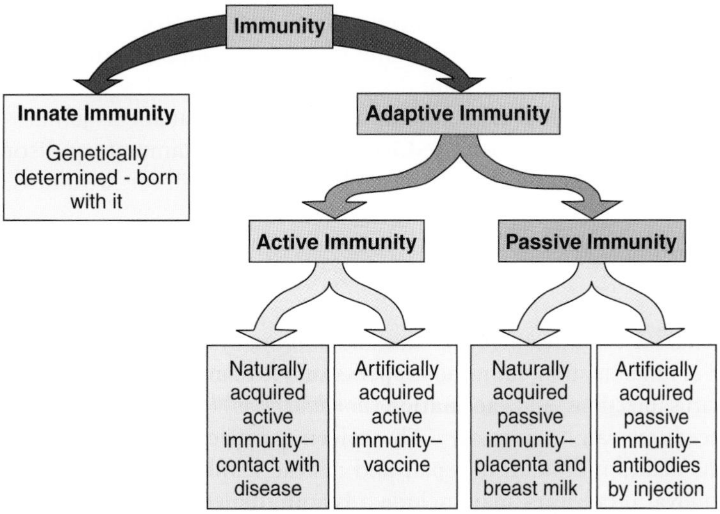


**FIGURE 11-3** The types of immunity.

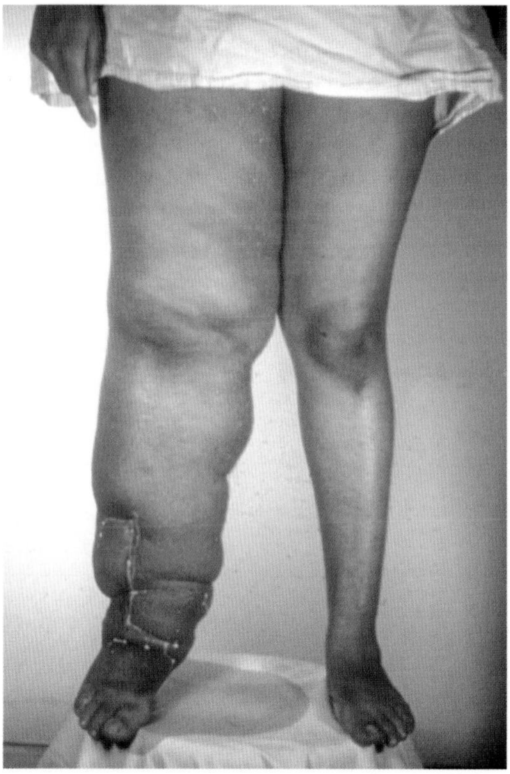

**FIGURE 11-4** Lymphedema of the right lower extremity in a patient with elephantiasis. Elephantiasis is a parasitic infection that causes lymphatic vessel obstruction.



reaction to a particular antigen (allergen), such as pollen, a particular food, or dust. Lymph and immune disorders include the following:

- **Acquired immunodeficiency syndrome (AIDS)** is caused by the human immunodeficiency virus (HIV) and is an infectious process characterized by swollen lymph glands or lymphadenopathy.
- **Infectious mononucleosis** is an acute infection caused by the Epstein-Barr virus (EBV) and is characterized by fever, enlarged cervical lymph nodes, and fatigue.
- **Splenomegaly**, enlargement of the spleen, is indicative of infectious disease.
- **Anaphylaxis** is a systemic, life-threatening reaction to a foreign substance.
- **Hodgkin's lymphoma** is a malignant disease of the lymph nodes.
- **Rheumatoid arthritis (RA)** is an autoimmune disorder that affects joints.
- **Systemic lupus erythematosus (SLE)** is a chronic inflammatory disorder that affects connective tissue throughout the body and is marked by fever, weakness, joint pain, and lymphadenopathy.

## DIAGNOSTIC TESTS, TREATMENTS, AND SURGICAL PROCEDURES

A range of treatments exists for treating lymphatic and immune system disorders. They include **corticosteroids** for relief of inflammation, **immunosuppressants** to dampen the immune response, **antiviral** agents to thwart virus infections, and **vaccination** (*immunization*) to offer artificially acquired immunity.

Surgical procedures can be necessary. The spleen is especially fragile, making it susceptible to rupturing. This makes it difficult to repair and instead a **splenectomy** (excision of the spleen) occurs. Other removal procedures may include a **lymphadenectomy** (removal of a lymph node), **lymphangiectomy** (removal of a lymph vessel), **thymectomy** (removal of the thymus), or **tonsillectomy** (removal of a tonsil).

## PRACTICE AND PRACTITIONERS

**Allergists** specialize in diagnosing and treating altered immunologic and allergic conditions, and **hematologists** provide diagnosis and treatment of blood and blood-forming tissue disorders. **Immunology** is the study of the immune system. An **immunologist** is a specialist who studies, diagnoses, and treats problems associated with immunity. **Oncologists** may become involved in the care of patients with tumors.

**Abbreviation Table** THE LYMPHATIC SYSTEM AND IMMUNITY

| ABBREVIATION | MEANING |
|---|---|
| AIDS | acquired immunodeficiency syndrome |
| EBV | Epstein-Barr virus |
| HIV | human immunodeficiency virus |
| RA | rheumatoid arthritis |
| SLE | systemic lupus erythematosus |

**Study Table** THE LYMPHATIC SYSTEM AND IMMUNITY

| TERM AND PRONUNCIATION | ANALYSIS | MEANING |
|---|---|---|
| **Structure and Function** | | |
| acquired immunity (uh-KWIRE-duh ih-MYOO-ni-tee) | common English words | resistance resulting from previous exposure to an infectious agent |
| allergen (AL-ur-jehn) | from the Greek word *allos* (other); *-gen* (producing) | an antigen that induces an allergic or hypersensitive response |
| antibody (AN-ti-bod-ee) | *anti-* (against) + body | a molecule generated in specific opposition to an antigen |
| antigen (AN-tuh-jehn) | *anti-* (against); *-gen* (producing) | agent or substance that provokes an immune response |
| appendix (ah-PEN-dicks) | from the Latin verb *appendum* (attach) | tube-shaped sac attached to an opening into the large intestine that plays a role in immunity |
| artificial immunity (ahr-tuh-FISH-uhlih-MYOO-ni-tee) | common English words | immunization; immunity acquired from a vaccination |
| autoimmunity (aw-toh-ih-MYOO-ni-tee) | *auto-* (self) + immunity | antibodies or lymphocytes produced against antigens normally present in the body; literally, immune to oneself |
| B cell (BEE sell) | B refers to the fact that these cells are derived from bone marrow | nonthymus dependent, short-lived lymphocyte; *B lymphocyte* |

(*continued*)

**Study Table** THE LYMPHATIC SYSTEM AND IMMUNITY *(continued)*

| TERM AND PRONUNCIATION | ANALYSIS | MEANING |
|---|---|---|
| B lymphocyte (BEE LIHM-foh-site) | B refers to the fact that these cells are derived from bone marrow; *lymph/o* (lymph); *-cyte* (cell) | nonthymus dependent, short-lived lymphocyte; *B cell* |
| immunity (ih-MYOO-ni-tee) | from the Latin word *immunis* (exempt) | protection against disease |
| inflammation (in-flah-MAY-shun) | common English word | redness and swelling caused by injury or abnormal stimulation by a physical, chemical, or biologic agent |
| leukocyte (LUKE-oh-site) | *leuk/o* (white); *-cyte* (cell) | white blood cell |
| lymph (LIMF) | *lymph/o* (lymph) | a fluid collected from tissues throughout the body that contains mostly white blood cells and flows through the lymphatic vessels |
| lymph node (LIMF NODE) | *lymph/o* (lymph); from the Latin word, *nodus* (knot) | small, bean-shaped mass of lymphatic tissue that filters bacteria and foreign material from the lymph; located on larger lymph vessels in the cervical, mediastinal, axillary, and inguinal regions |
| lymphatic system (lihm-FAT-tik SIS-tuhm) | *lymph/o* (lymph); *-atic* (adjective suffix) | collectively, the vessels, nodes, and capillaries that carry the lymph and its disease-fighting cells to the areas in which they are needed |
| lymphocyte (LIHM-foh-syte) | *lymph/o* (lymph); *-cyte* (cell) | white blood cell in the lymphatic system |
| lymphoid nodules of the small intestine (LIMF-oid NOD-yulz) | common English words | collections of spherical masses of lymphoid cells closely packed together; *Peyer's patches* |
| macrophage (MAK-roh-fayj) | *macro-* (large); *phag/o* (ingest or engulf) | large phagocyte |
| microphage (MIKE-roh-fayj) | *micro-* (small); *phag/o* (ingest or engulf) | small phagocyte |
| monocyte (MON-oh-site) | *mono-* (single); *-cyte* (cell) | a type of white blood cell that is also a phagocyte |

**Study Table** THE LYMPHATIC SYSTEM AND IMMUNITY (*continued*)

| TERM AND PRONUNCIATION | ANALYSIS | MEANING |
|---|---|---|
| natural immunity (NACH-er-uhl ih-MYOO-ni-tee) | common English words | resistance manifested by an individual who has not been immunized; immunity passed on from mother to fetus or from mother to baby in breast milk |
| neutrophil (NU-troh-fil) | *neutr/o* (neutral); *-phil* (love) | a type of white blood cell that is also a phagocyte |
| pathogen (PATH-oh-jehn) | *path/o* (disease); *-gen* (produce) | substance that produces disease |
| Peyer's patches (PEY-erz PACH-ez) | named after Swiss anatomist Johann Peyer | collections of spherical masses of lymphoid cells closely packed together; *lymphoid nodules of the small intestine* |
| phagocyte (FAG-oh-syte) | *phag/o* (ingest or engulf); *-cyte* (cell) | white blood cell that clears away pathogens and debris |
| phagocytosis (FAG-oh-sy-toh-sis) | *phag/o* (ingest or engulf); *cyt/o* (cell); *-osis* (condition of) | process of ingestion and digestion carried out by white blood cells |
| reaction (ree-AK-shun) | common English word | an action of an antibody on a specific antigen; also, in reference to immune responses, an abnormal or unwanted reaction |
| spleen (SPLEEN) | *splen/o* (spleen) | immune system organ that gets rid of damaged red blood cells and reclaims and stores iron |
| T cell (TEE SELL) | T (stands for thymus); | thymus dependent, long-lived lymphocyte; *T lymphocyte* |
| T lymphocyte (TEE LIHM-foh-syte) | T (stands for thymus); *lymph/o* (lymph); *-cyte* (cell) | thymus dependent, long-lived lymphocyte; *T cell* |
| thymus (THYE-muhs) | *thym/o* (thymus) | immune system gland located behind (deep to) the sternum |
| tonsil (TON-sihl) | *tonsill/o* (tonsil) | collection of lymph tissue; in common understanding, the lingual, pharyngeal, and (especially) palatine tonsils |
| **Disorders** | | |
| allergy (AL-er-jee) | From the Greek word, *allos* (other) + *ergon* (work) | extreme sensitivity reaction to a normally harmless substance |

(*continued*)

**Study Table** THE LYMPHATIC SYSTEM AND IMMUNITY (*continued*)

| TERM AND PRONUNCIATION | ANALYSIS | MEANING |
|---|---|---|
| anaphylaxis (an-ah-FIL-ax-ihs) | *ana-* (without); from the Greek word *phylaxis* (protection) | life-threatening reaction to a foreign substance; symptoms include blockage of air passages, decreased blood pressure, generalized edema |
| acquired immunodeficiency syndrome (uh-KWAHY-erd im-yoo-no-di-FISH-uhn-see SIN-drohm) | from the Latin word *acquirere* (gain); *immunis* (exempt); *deficere* (to desert, fail) | a deficiency of cellular immunity induced by infection with the HIV |
| autoimmune disease (aw-toh-ih-MEWN di-ZEEZ) | *auto-* (self) + *immunis* (exempt from) and from Old French *desaise* (lack of each) | disorder in which the immune response is directed against the body's own tissues |
| elephantiasis (el-eh-fan-TYE-uh-sis) | from the Greek word, *elephas* (elephant) and *-iasis* (suffix forming the name of the disease) | lymphatic disease caused by filaria (parasitic roundworm) that is characterized by swelling of the legs and male scrotum |
| hemolysis (hee-MAWL-ih-sihs) | *hem/o* (blood); *-lysis* (destruction) | change or destruction of red blood cells |
| Hodgkin's lymphoma (HODJ-kinz lim-FOH-mah) | named after English physician Thomas Hodgkin (1798–1866) who first described it; *lymph/o* (lymph or lymphatic system); *-oma* (tumor) | chronic malignant disease of the lymph nodes; *Hodgkin disease* |
| immunodeficiency (IM-yoo-noh-dee-FISH-ehn-see) | *immun/o* (immune system) + deficiency | impairment of the immune system |
| infectious mononucleosis (in-FEK-shus mon-uh-noo-klee-OH-sis) | from the Latin word *infectionem* (infection); *mono-* (one); Latin *nucleus* (kernel); *-osis* (abnormal condition) | an acute illness of young adults caused by the EBV; spread by saliva transfer; characterized by fever, sore throat, enlargement of lymph nodes and spleen |
| lymphadenitis (lim-FAD-eh-NYE-tiss) | *lymph/o* (lymph or lymphatic system); *aden/o* (gland); *-itis* (inflammation) | inflammation of a lymph node or lymph nodes |
| lymphadenopathy (lim-fah-deh-NOP-ah-thee) | *lymph/o* (lymph or lymphatic system); *aden/o* (gland); *-pathy* (disease) | chronic or excessively swollen lymph nodes; any disease of the lymph nodes |
| lymphangiitis (lim-FAN-jee-EYE-tiss) | *lymphangi/o* (lymph vessel); *-itis* (inflammation) | inflammation of lymph vessels; *lymphangitis; lymphatitis* |

**Study Table** THE LYMPHATIC SYSTEM AND IMMUNITY (*continued*)

| TERM AND PRONUNCIATION | ANALYSIS | MEANING |
|---|---|---|
| lymphangitis (lim-fan-JY-tiss) | *lymphangi/o* (lymph vessel); *-itis* (inflammation) | inflammation of lymph vessels; *lymphangiitis; lymphatitis* |
| lymphatitis (lim-fah-TY-tiss) | *lymph/o* (lymph or lymphatic system); *-itis* (inflammation) | inflammation of the lymph vessels or nodes; *lymphangiitis*; *lymphangitis* |
| lymphedema (lim-feh-DEE-mah) | *lymph/o* (lymph or lymphatic system); from the Greek word *oidema* (a swelling tumor) | swelling of the subcutaneous tissues due to obstruction of lymph vessels or nodes |
| lymphoma (lim-FOH-mah) | *lymph/o* (lymph or lymphatic system); *-oma* (tumor) | tumor of lymph tissue |
| lymphopathy (lim-FOP-ah-thee) | *lymph/o* (lymph or lymph gland); *-pathy* (disease) | disease of the lymph vessels or nodes |
| rheumatoid arthritis (ROO-mah-toid ar-THRY-tuhs) (RA) | from the Greek word *rheuma* (flux); *-oid* (resemblance of) | systemic disease that affects the connective tissue; involves many joints, especially those of the hands and feet |
| splenitis (splee-NY-tiss) | *splen/o* (spleen); *-itis* (inflammation) | inflammation of the spleen |
| splenomegaly (splee-noh-MEG-ah-lee) | *splen/o* (spleen); *-megaly* (enlargement) | enlargement of the spleen |
| splenopathy (splee-NOP-ah-thee) | *splen/o* (spleen); *-pathy* (disease) | any disease of the spleen |
| systemic lupus erythematosus (sis-TEM-ik LOO-pus er-ih-THEEM-uh-toh-sis) (SLE) | adjective form of the English word *system; lupus* (a Latin word meaning "wolf"); *erythematosus* (from the Greek word *erythema* meaning "flush") | an inflammatory, autoimmune connective tissue disorder with variable features; diffuse erythematous (red) butterfly rash on face |
| thymitis (thye-MY-tihs) | *thym/o* (thymus); *-itis* (inflammation) | inflammation of the thymus |
| tonsillitis (TAWN-sih-LY-tihs) | *tonsill/o* (tonsils); *-itis* (inflammation) | inflammation of a tonsil (commonly, the palatine tonsil) |
| **Diagnostic Tests, Treatments, and Surgical Procedures** | | |
| antiviral (an-tee-VAHY-ruhl) | *anti-* (against); from the Latin word *virus* (poison, sap of plants, slimy liquid) | drug used to treat various viral infections or conditions |
| chemotherapy (KEE-moh-ther-ah-pee) | *chem/o* (chemical) + therapy, a common English word | treatment of malignancies using chemical agents and drugs (usually reserved for treatment of cancer) |

(*continued*)

**Study Table** THE LYMPHATIC SYSTEM AND IMMUNITY (*continued*)

| TERM AND PRONUNCIATION | ANALYSIS | MEANING |
|---|---|---|
| corticosteroids (kor-tih-ko-STER-oyds) | from the Latin word *cortex* (bark); from the Greek *steros* (solid, stable) | hormone-like preparations used as anti-inflammatory agents; topical agents used for their immunosuppressive and anti-inflammatory properties |
| immunization (IM-yoo-nuh-zay-shun) | *immun/o* (immune system); *-ization* (noun suffix) | protection from communicable diseases by administration of a weakened or killed pathogen, or a protein of a pathogen, to cause the immune system to create antibodies for future protection; *vaccination* |
| immunosuppressant (IM-yoo-no-suh-PRESS-ant) | *immun/o* (immune system) + suppressant | something that interferes with the immune system |
| lymphangiography (lim-FAN-jee-OG-rah-fee) | *lymphangi/o* (lymph vessel); *-graphy* (process of recording) | radiography of the lymph vessels |
| lymphadenectomy (lim-fad-eh-NEK-tah-mee) | *lymphaden/o* (lymph gland); *-ectomy* (excision) | removal of lymph nodes |
| lymphangiectomy (lim-FAN-jee-EK-tah-mee) | *lymphangi/o* (lymph vessel); *-ectomy* (excision) | removal of a lymph vessel |
| lymphangiotomy (lim-FAN-jee-OT-oh-mee) | *lymphangi/o* (lymph vessel); *-tomy* (cutting operation) | incision of a lymph vessel |
| lymphography (lim-FOG-ruh-fee) | *lympho-* (lymph) + *grapho* (to write) | visualization of lymphatics (lymphangiography) and lymph nodes (lymphadenography) by radiography after injecting a contrast dye (usually iodized oil) into a lymphatic vessel |
| splenectomy (splee-NEK-toh-mee) | *splen/o* (spleen); *-ectomy* (excision) | removal of the spleen |
| splenorrhaphy (splee-NOR-ah-fee) | *splen/o* (spleen); *-rraphy* (rupture) | suture of a ruptured spleen |
| splenotomy (splee-NOT-oh-mee) | *splen/o* (spleen); *-tomy* (cutting operation) | incision of the spleen |
| thymectomy (thye-MEK-toh-me) | *thym/o* (thymus); *-ectomy* (excision) | removal of the thymus |
| tonsillectomy (TAWN-sih-LEK-toh-mee) | *tonsill/o* (tonsil); *-ectomy* (excision) | removal of a tonsil |

**Study Table** THE LYMPHATIC SYSTEM AND IMMUNITY (*continued*)

| TERM AND PRONUNCIATION | ANALYSIS | MEANING |
|---|---|---|
| vaccination (vak-sih-NAY-shun) | from the Latin word *vaccinus* (relating to a cow). So named because of its early use of the cowpox virus against smallpox | protection from communicable diseases by administration of a weakened or killed pathogen, or a protein of a pathogen, to cause the immune system to create antibodies for future protection; *immunization* |
| vaccine (VAK-seen) | from the Latin word *vaccinus*, from *vacca* (cow). So named because of its early use of the cowpox virus against smallpox | substance used to stimulate antibody production and to provide immunity against a disease without causing the disease |
| **Practice and Practitioners** | | |
| allergist (AL-er-jist) | from the Greek words *allos* (other, different, strange) and *ergon* (activity); *-ist* (one who specializes) | a medical practitioner who specializes in the diagnosis and treatment of allergies |
| hematologist (hee-mah-TAHL-oh-jist) | *hemat/o* (blood); *-logist* (one who specializes) | a medical practitioner who specializes in the diagnosis and treatment of blood disorders |
| immunologist (im-yoo-NOL-oh-jist) | *immun/o* (immune system); *-logist* (one who specializes) | a medical practitioner specializing in the immune system |
| immunology (IM-yoo-NOL-oh-jee) | *immun/o* (immune system); *-logy* (study of) | the medical specialty dealing with the immune system |
| oncologist (on-KOL-oh-jist) | from the Greek word *onkos* (mass, bulk); *-logist* (one who specializes) | a medical practitioner who specializes in the diagnosis and treatment of malignant tumors (cancer) |

# END-OF-CHAPTER EXERCISES

## EXERCISE 11-1 LABELING

**Using the following list, choose the correct terms to label the diagram correctly.**

| | | |
|---|---|---|
| axillary lymph nodes | mediastinal lymph nodes | superficial lymphatics of lower limb |
| cervical lymph nodes | spleen | thymus |

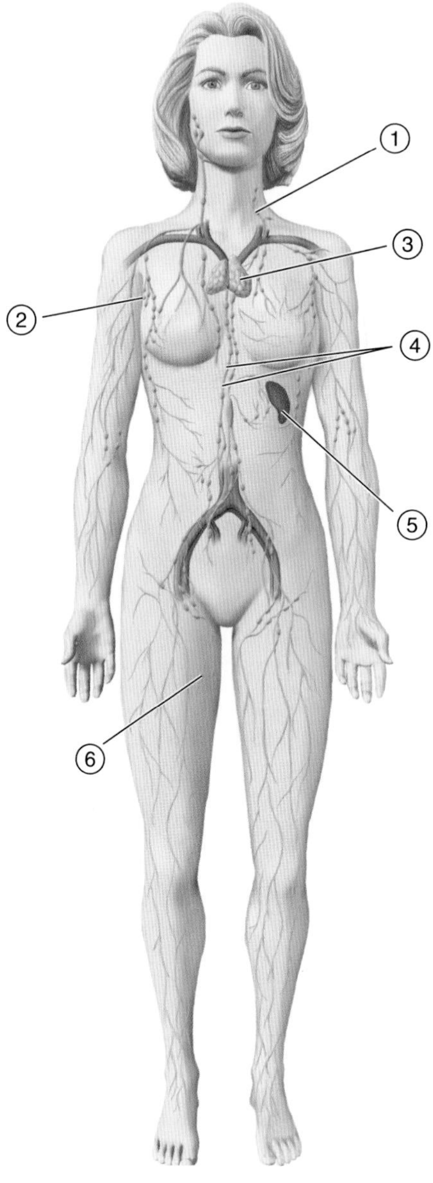


1. ______________________
2. ______________________
3. ______________________
4. ______________________
5. ______________________
6. ______________________

## EXERCISE 11-2 WORD PARTS

**Break each of the following terms into its word parts: prefix, root, or suffix. Give the meaning of each word part and then define the term.**

1. lymphocyte

   root: ______________________________

   suffix: ______________________________

   definition: ______________________________

2. phagocytosis

   root: ______________________________

   root: ______________________________

   suffix: ______________________________

   definition: ______________________________

3. anaphylaxis

   prefix: ______________________________

   root: ______________________________

   definition: ______________________________

4. hemolysis

   root: ______________________________

   suffix: ______________________________

   definition: ______________________________

5. lymphoma

   root: ______________________________

   suffix: ______________________________

   definition: ______________________________

6. splenectomy

   root: ______________________________

   suffix: ______________________________

   definition: ______________________________

7. thymectomy

   root: ______________________________

   suffix: ______________________________

   definition: ______________________________

8. immunology

   root: ______________________________

   suffix: ______________________________

   definition: ______________________________

## EXERCISE 11-3 WORD BUILDING

**Use the word parts listed to build the terms defined.**

| | | | |
|---|---|---|---|
| aden/o | immun/o | lymph/o | -pathy |
| angi/o | -itis | -megaly | phag/o |
| -cytosis | -logist | -oma | thym/o |
| -graphy | | | |

1. inflammation of a lymph gland ____________________
2. tumor of a lymph gland ____________________
3. enlargement of the thymus ____________________
4. inflammation of a lymph vessel ____________________
5. disease of a lymph gland ____________________
6. specialist who studies and treats the immune system ____________________
7. radiographic procedure of the lymphatic system ____________________
8. process of a WBC engulfing a harmful organism ____________________

## EXERCISE 11-4 MATCHING

**Match the term with its definition.**

1. ______________ lymphadenopathy
2. ______________ lymphedema
3. ______________ phagocytosis
4. ______________ autoimmune
5. ______________ splenomegaly
6. ______________ lymphocyte
7. ______________ immunology
8. ______________ anaphylaxis
9. ______________ appendix
10. ______________ immunization

a. enlarged spleen
b. specialty that deals with immune disorders
c. artificially acquired immunity
d. life-threatening allergic reaction to a foreign substance
e. disease of the lymph glands
f. accumulation of fluid in the intercellular tissues
g. the process of engulfing foreign materials
h. protective lymph organ that is attached to the proximal end of the large intestine
i. the body reacts to its own tissues
j. specialized WBC of the immune system

## EXERCISE 11-5 MULTIPLE CHOICE

**Choose the correct answer for the following multiple choice questions.**

1. The lymphatic organ that removes old blood cells by means of hemolysis is the ______________.
   a. tonsils
   b. spleen
   c. thymus
   d. appendix

2. Peyer's patches are found in the ______________.
   a. respiratory system
   b. cardiovascular system
   c. digestive system
   d. muscular system

3. Immunizations are a type of ______________.
   a. naturally acquired immunity
   b. naturally acquired passive immunity
   c. artificially acquired immunity
   d. innate immunity

4. Lymphocytes are a type of ____________________.
   a. white blood cell
   b. red blood cell
   c. platelet
   d. thrombocyte

5. The tonsils are located in the ____________________.
   a. larynx
   b. abdomen
   c. lungs
   d. pharynx

6. A practitioner who specializes in blood disorders is a(n) ____________________.
   a. allergist
   b. hematoligist
   c. immunologist
   d. oncologist

7. A treatment used to treat inflammation is a(n) ____________________.
   a. antiviral
   b. chemotherapy
   c. corticosteroid
   d. immunosuppressant

8. A molecule that is generated in specific opposition to an antigen is a(n) ____________________.
   a. allergen
   b. antibody
   c. pathogen
   d. leukocyte

9. The type of immunity passed down from mother to child is called ____________________.
   a. naturally acquired active immunity
   b. artificially acquired active immunity
   c. naturally acquired passive immunity
   d. autoimmunity

10. The root lymphaden/o means ____________________.
   a. lymph
   b. immune
   c. lymph vessel
   d. lymph node

## EXERCISE 11-6 FILL IN THE BLANK

**Fill in the blank with the correct answer.**

1. Lymph contains white blood cells, called ____________________, that fight infection.
2. The functions of the immune system are to protect the body from infection, absorb fats that are broken down in the digestive tract, and ____________________.
3. After lymph is picked up by the lymph vessels and filtered by the ____________________, it is propelled into venules and then into veins.
4. ____________________ immunity is genetically determined.
5. The ____________________ are masses of lymphatic tissue located in the pharynx to filter out bacteria.
6. Swelling caused by obstruction of lymphatic vessels is called ____________________.
7. Surgical removal of the spleen is called a ____________________.
8. The medical professional who specializes in diagnosing and treating altered immunologic and allergic conditions is known as a(n) ____________________.
9. The "T" in T cell stands for ____________________.
10. Failure of the immune system to adequately protect the body from infection is known as ____________________.

## EXERCISE 11-7 ABBREVIATIONS

**Write out the term for the following abbreviations.**

1. ______________________________ SLE
2. ______________________________ RA
3. ______________________________ EBV

**Write the abbreviation for the following terms.**

4. ____________________ acquired immunodeficiency syndrome
5. ____________________ human immunodeficiency virus

## EXERCISE 11-8 SPELLING

**Select the correct spelling of the medical term.**

1. A ____________________ is a type of white blood cell that is distributed throughout lymphatic tissue.
   a. lymphocyte
   b. limphocyte
   c. lymfocyte
   d. lymphosite

2. A ____________________ is a type of mature, phagocytic white blood cell.
   a. nuetrophil
   b. nutrophil
   c. neutrophil
   d. neutraphil

3. ____________________ is the process of ingestion and digestion by white blood cells.
   a. Pagocytosis
   b. Phagecytosis
   c. Phagocytosis
   d. Phageocytosis

4. Protection against infectious disease is called ____________________.
   a. immunity
   b. imunity
   c. imunnity
   d. ammunity

5. Some signs of the life-threatening reaction to a foreign substance called ____________________ are blockage of air passages, decreased blood pressure, and generalized edema.
   a. anephylaxis
   b. anaphilaxis
   c. aniphylaxis
   d. anaphylaxis

6. An impairment of the immune system is called an ____________________.
   a. imunodeficiency
   b. immunodeficiency
   c. immunedeficiency
   d. immunodeficency

7. ____________________ is the process by which resistance to an infectious disease is induced.
   a. Imunization
   b. Immunisation
   c. Immunizasion
   d. Immunization

8. Treatment of malignancies using chemical agents and drugs is called ____________________.
   a. kemotherapy
   b. cemotherapy
   c. chemotherapy
   d. chematherapy

9. A ____________________ is a medical practitioner who specializes in the diagnosis and treatment of blood disorders.
   a. hemtologist
   b. hematologist
   c. hemetologist
   d. hemitologist

10. An ____________________ is a substance that induces sensitivity or an immune response in the form of antibodies.
    a. antigen
    b. antugen
    c. antegin
    d. antegen

## EXERCISE 11-9 CASE STUDY

**Read the case and answer the questions below.**

**BRIEF HISTORY:** A 16-year-old male complained to his parents of being extremely fatigued. He was not able to keep up with his school schedule or after school sports. His throat was sore and he noticed "lumps" in his neck and groin. He had a fever and loss of appetite. He recently began to complain of pain in his upper left belly.

**OFFICE VISIT:** A physician examined the patient and ordered blood tests. He noted lymphadenopathy in the cervical, axillary, and inguinal areas. He also observed an erythematous throat and determined that the spleen was enlarged.

**DIAGNOSIS AND TREATMENT PLAN:** The diagnosis was mononucleosis, an infectious disease caused by a virus. The prescribed treatment consisted of over-the-counter analgesics to reduce the abdominal pain, along with fluids and rest. Throat lozenges were prescribed to ease sore throat discomfort.

1. What does "lymphadenopathy" mean? ____________________

2. What is the medical term for an "enlarged spleen"? ____________________

3. What is mononucleosis? ____________________

# The Respiratory System

12

**LEARNING OUTCOMES**

***Upon completion of this chapter, you should be able to:***

- Name the structures that make up the respiratory system.
- Pronounce, spell, and define medical terms related to the respiratory system and its disorders.
- Interpret abbreviations associated with the respiratory system.

## INTRODUCTION

The respiratory system is all the air passages from the nose to the pulmonary alveoli in the lungs. It is divided into an *upper respiratory tract* and a *lower respiratory tract*. The upper respiratory tract is made up of the **paranasal sinuses**, **nasal cavity**, **nose**, and **pharynx**. The lower respiratory tract is made up of the **larynx**, **lungs**, **trachea**, **bronchi**, **bronchioles**, and **alveoli** (see Figure 12-1). The respiratory system allows us to inhale oxygen ($O_2$) and exhale carbon dioxide ($CO_2$). Oxygen is a gas needed by our cells, and carbon dioxide is a gaseous metabolic waste that needs to be eliminated. Figure 12-2 shows the process of this gas exchange, which is accomplished through external and internal respiration. **External respiration** is the process in which air is brought into the lungs, and oxygen and carbon dioxide are exchanged in the bloodstream at the capillaries surrounding the alveoli. **Internal respiration** is the process where oxygen and carbon dioxide move between the bloodstream and the body's cells.

## WORD PARTS RELATED TO THE RESPIRATORY SYSTEM

The word part *spir/o* (which is a root) and the suffix *–pnea* are both used to describe breathing. Pulmon/o means lung, and is the root of the word **pulmonary** (an adjective used to describe the lungs). Similarly, nas/o means nose and provides the root for **nasal** (an adjective used to describe the nose). Another root meaning nose is rhin/o. Nasal comes from the Latin word for nose, *nasus*, while rhin/o comes from the Greek word for nose, *rhis*. Pneum/o comes from the Greek word *pneumon* (lung) and can refer to the lungs or air. Pneum/o is the root for the well known infection pneumonia. Table 12-1 shows common word parts related to the respiratory system.

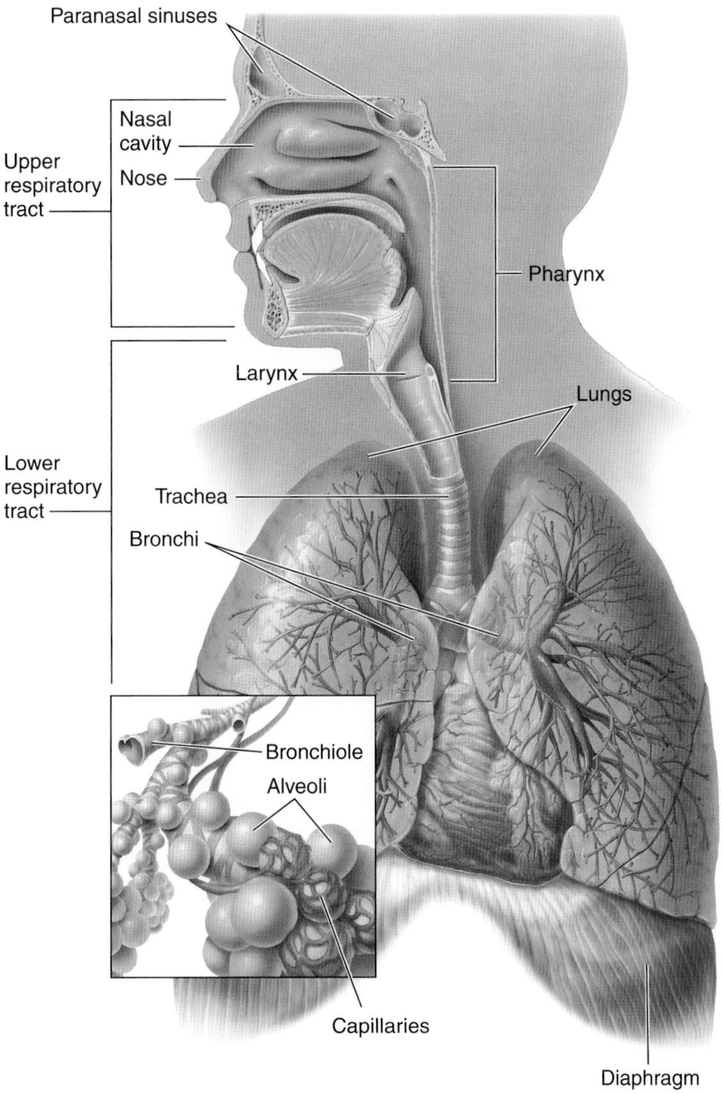


**FIGURE 12-1** The structures of the upper and lower respiratory system.

## STRUCTURE AND FUNCTION

The respiratory system begins with the paranasal sinuses, nasal cavity, and nose and then descends to the pharynx, larynx, and trachea. Inferior to the trachea, the system splits into the right and left side. This inferior portion consists of the bronchi and bronchioles that branch in the lungs, and the tiny air sacs called alveoli. A dome-shaped muscle important for breathing, called the **diaphragm**, is located at the base of the lungs.

### The Nose, Nasal Cavity, and Paranasal Sinuses

Air enters the nose through openings called **nostrils**. The **nose** is lined with small hairs that trap particles and prevent them from entering the respiratory tract. Air then passes into the **nasal cavity**, a space on either side of a wall called the **nasal septum** that divides the nose into left and right halves. Here, the air is warmed and moistened. **Mucus**, a clear sticky secretion, coats the lining of

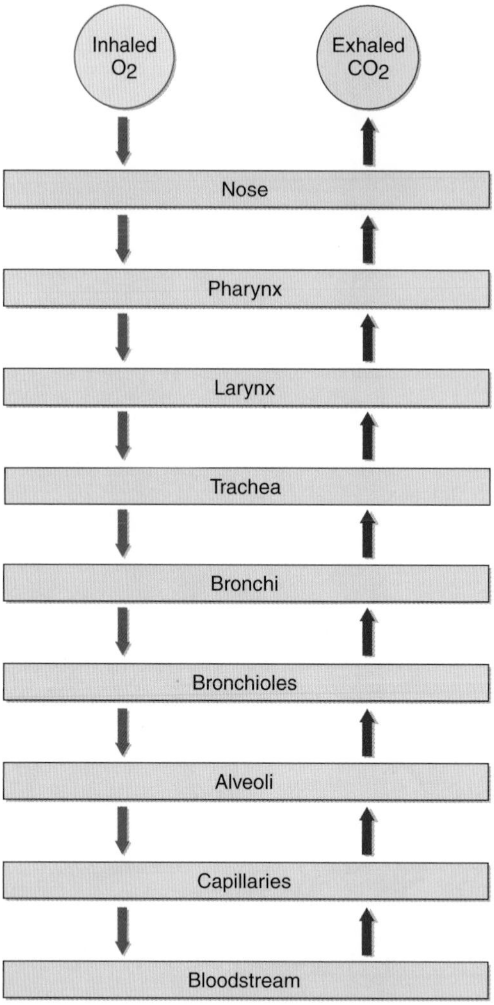


**FIGURE 12-2** Pathway of inhaled/exhaled air. *Red arrows* indicate oxygenated air and *blue arrows* represent deoxygenated air. Oxygen ($O_2$) enters the respiratory system through the nose and travels down through the pharynx and larynx and into the bronchi, bronchioles, and alveoli of the lungs where a gas exchange takes place. Oxygen moves into the bloodstream where it is carried to the cells and is exchanged with carbon dioxide ($CO_2$). The carbon dioxide passes back up through the respiratory structures and is exhaled.

**TABLE 12-1 COMMON WORD PARTS RELATED TO THE RESPIRATORY SYSTEM**

| **Word Part** | **Meaning** |
| --- | --- |
| adeno- | glandlike |
| spir/o | breathing |
| bronch/o, bronchi/o | bronchus |
| laryng/o | larynx |
| lob/o | lobe |
| nas/o | nose |
| or/o | mouth, opening |
| -oxia | oxygen |
| pharyng/o | pharynx |

**TABLE 12-1** COMMON WORD PARTS RELATED TO THE RESPIRATORY SYSTEM (*continued*)

| Word Part | Meaning |
|---|---|
| -phonia | voice |
| phren/o | diaphragm |
| pleur/o | rib, side, pleura |
| -pnea | breathing |
| pneumo-, pneumon/o | lungs, air |
| pulmon/o | lung |
| rhin/o | nose |
| sinus/o | sinus cavity |
| spir/o | breathing |
| thorac/o, thorac/i, thoracic/o | thorax, chest |
| tonsill/o | tonsil |
| trache/o | trachea |

## Word Parts Exercise

After studying Table 12-1, write the meaning of each of the word parts.

| WORD PART | MEANING |
|---|---|
| 1. -phonia | 1. ______________ |
| 2. trache/o | 2. ______________ |
| 3. thorac/o, thorac/i, thoracic/o | 3. ______________ |
| 4. bronch/o, bronchi/o | 4. ______________ |
| 5. -pnea | 5. ______________ |
| 6. laryng/o | 6. ______________ |
| 7. sinus/o | 7. ______________ |
| 8. pleur/o | 8. ______________ |
| 9. pneumo-, pneumon/o | 9. ______________ |
| 10. nas/o | 10. ______________ |
| 11. -oxia | 11. ______________ |
| 12. pharyng/o | 12. ______________ |
| 13. phren/o | 13. ______________ |
| 14. pulmon/o | 14. ______________ |
| 15. or/o | 15. ______________ |

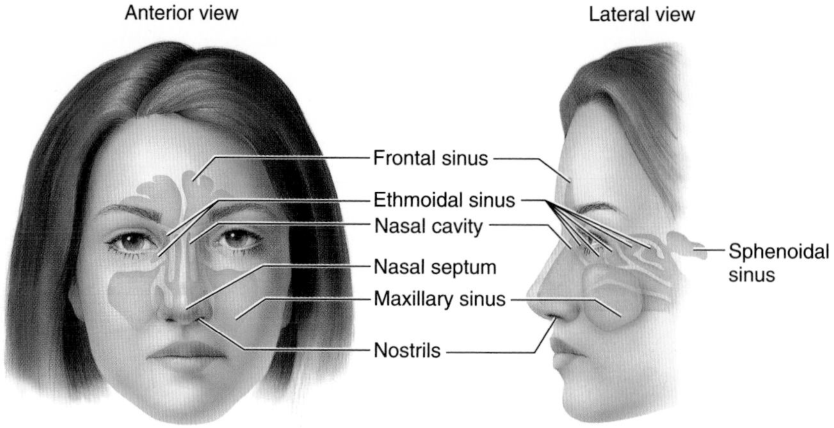


**FIGURE 12-3** The nasal cavity and paranasal sinuses.

the nasal cavity to filter out particles. The **paranasal sinuses** are air-filled cavities in the bones of the face that are connected to the nasal cavity. These sinuses include the frontal, ethmoidal, maxillary, and sphenoidal (see Figure 12-3).

## The Pharynx and Tonsils

The **pharynx**, also known as the throat, has three divisions: the *nasopharynx*, *oropharnyx*, and *laryngopharynx*. The **nasopharynx** is posterior to the nasal cavity, the **oropharynx** is the middle portion located posterior to the oral cavity (mouth), and the **laryngopharynx** is the lower portion posterior to the larynx (see Figure 12-4). Lymphatic tissue called **tonsils** that aid in filtering bacteria are associated with the pharynx. The **pharyngeal tonsil**, also known as the **adenoids**, is located in the nasopharynx; the **palatine tonsil** is in the oropharynx; and the **lingual tonsil** is at the base of the

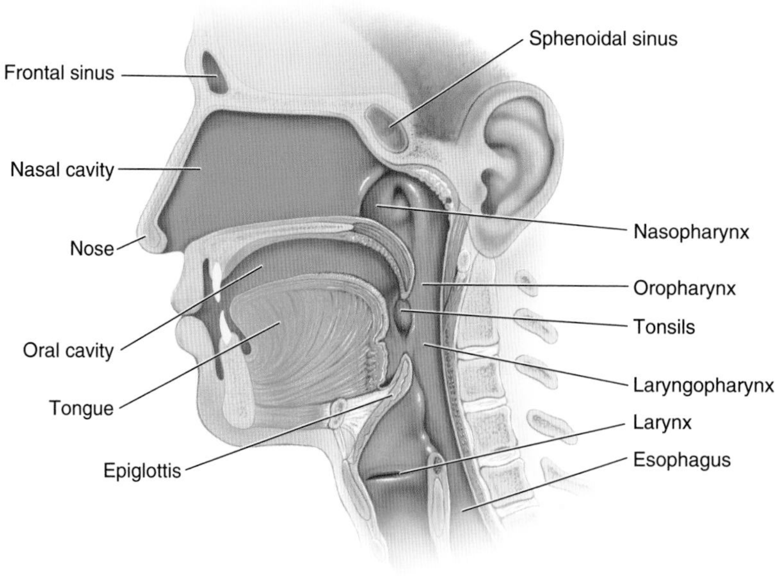


**FIGURE 12-4** The regions of the pharynx.

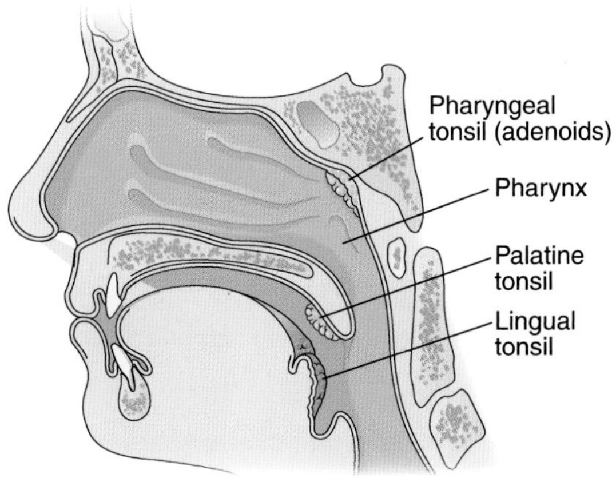


FIGURE 12-5 The pharynx and tonsils.

posterior portion of the tongue (see Figure 12-5). Removal of the tonsils and adenoids is referred to as a *tonsillectomy* and *adenoidectomy*; this is abbreviated as T and A.

## The Larynx and Trachea

The **larynx**, or *voice box*, is the organ that produces sound. Located between the pharynx and trachea, it is made up of cartilages and elastic membranes that house the vocal cords (vocal folds) and the muscles that control them (see Figure 12-4 and 12-6). Air enters the larynx through a slit-like opening called the **glottis**. A flap of cartilage known as the **epiglottis** protects the glottis during swallowing to prevent food or liquids from entering the respiratory tract. As air flows over the **vocal cords**, they vibrate to produce sound (see Figure 12-6).

## The Trachea, Bronchi, Bronchioles, and Alveoli

The **trachea** (windpipe) is a cartilaginous tube that conducts air from the larynx to the bronchial tree. The **bronchial tree** consists of air-passage tubes that lead from the trachea to the lungs. It begins with two major airways called the **left bronchus** and **right bronchus**. The plural form of *bronchus* is

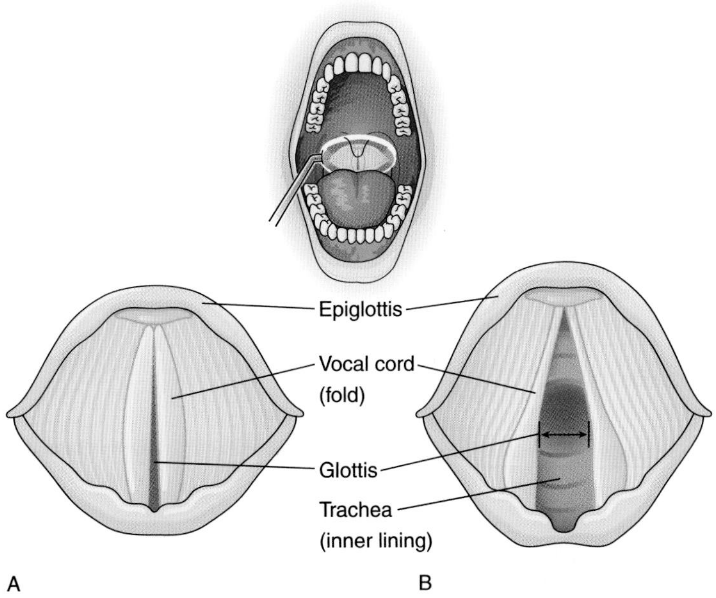


FIGURE 12-6 The vocal cords with **(A)** glottis closed and **(B)** glottis open.

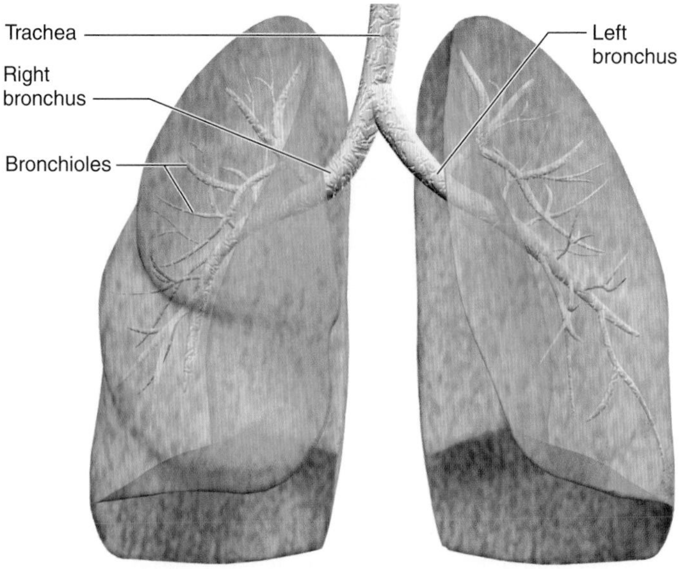


FIGURE 12-7 The trachea and bronchial tree.

*bronchi*. Air passes through the bronchi, which subdivide into increasingly smaller branches called **bronchioles**. The flow of air terminates in the bronchial tree in tiny air sacs called **alveoli**. Alveoli are structures where gas exchange of oxygen and carbon dioxide occurs (see Figure 12-1 and 12-7).

## The Lungs

The **lungs** are paired, spongy organs of breathing located in the thoracic (chest) cavity. They are enclosed in the **pleura**, which is a membrane composed of two layers called the **parietal pleura** and the **visceral pleura** (see Figure 12-8). The parietal (outer) pleura line the thoracic cavity and form

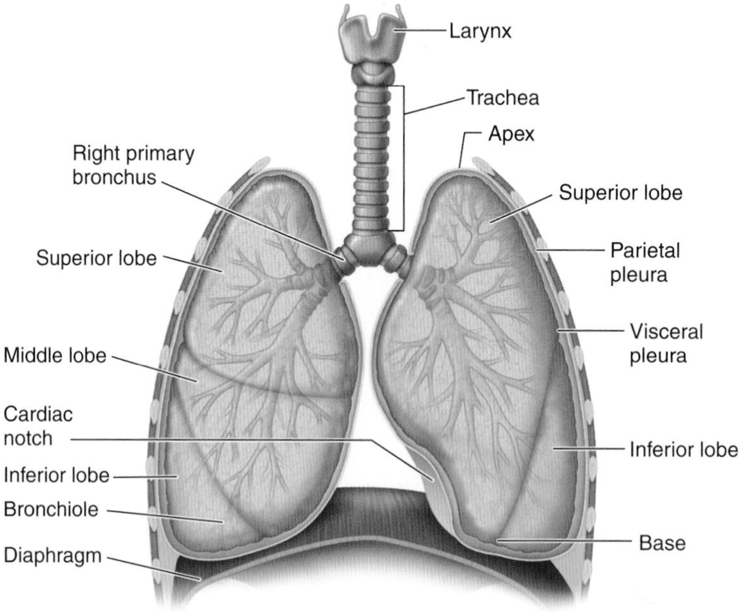


FIGURE 12-8 The lungs are paired organs of breathing located in the thoracic cavity. They are enclosed by an outer parietal pleura and an inner visceral pleura.

the sac containing each lung. The visceral (inner) pleura closely surround each lung. The right lung is slightly larger than the left and has three lobes called the **superior lobe**, **middle lobe**, and **lower lobe**. The left lung has only two lobes, the **superior lobe** and **inferior lobe**. The left lung also has a medial indentation called the **cardiac notch**, which provides room for the heart. Each cone-shaped lung has an upper **apex** and a lower **base**, which rests on the diaphragm. The lungs and airways bring in fresh, oxygen-enriched air and get rid of waste carbon dioxide made by the cells in the body.

## The Diaphragm

The **diaphragm** is a sheet of muscle that separates the thoracic cavity (which houses the lungs) from the lower abdominal cavity. The diaphragm is a major muscle used in breathing. When the diaphragm contracts, it moves inferiorly, the chest expands, and inhalation (inspiration or breathing in) occurs. When the diaphragm relaxes, it moves superiorly, the chest contracts, and exhalation (expiration or breathing out) occurs (see Figure 12-9). Two adjectives that mean the same thing and are used to describe the *diaphragm, are diaphragmatic and phrenic.*

### Quick Check

1. Another name for the voice box is the ____________________.
2. Another name for the windpipe is the ____________________.
3. Another name for the throat is the ____________________.

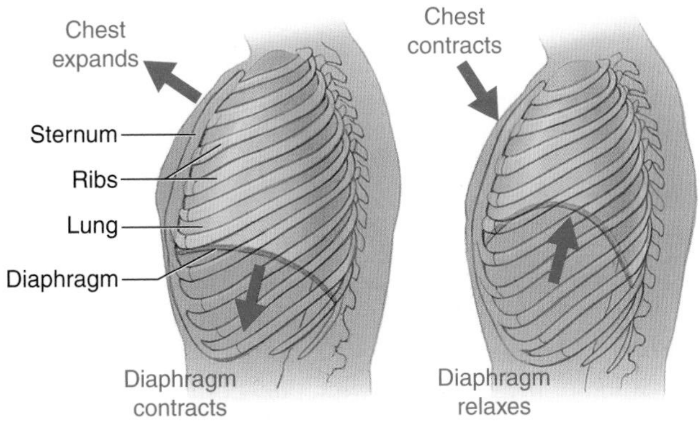


**FIGURE 12-9** The process of breathing.

## DISORDERS RELATED TO THE RESPIRATORY SYSTEM

The pathway through which air moves in and out of the lungs needs to remain **patent** (a common English word that when used as a medical term means "physically open") in order for proper oxygen and carbon dioxide exchange to take place. When this pathway becomes partially blocked, the body's normal response is a sneeze or cough, which may produce **sputum** (mucus from the lower respiratory system); **hemoptysis**, which is spitting or coughing up blood; or other secretions that need to be removed for optimal airway **patency** (state of being freely open).

Abnormal breath sounds are another indication of respiratory disease. **Rales**, also known as crackles, are high-pitched popping sounds usually originating in the smaller airways. **Rhonchi** (singular, *rhonchus*) are low-pitched sounds that come from the larger airways. **Wheezing** or whistling sounds may indicate excessive secretions or partially obstructed airways. **Stridor** is a high-pitched squeaking sound that occurs when one breathes in, which is a sign of respiratory obstruction, especially in the trachea or larynx. Respiratory diseases may also alter breathing patterns and rates. Normal breathing, **eupnea**, should be regular and effortless. The following is a list of abnormalities in breathing:

**Tachypnea:** rapid breathing rate (it is normal to have tachypnea during exercise)

**Bradypnea:** abnormally slow breathing rate

**Apnea:** cessation of breathing; short periods of apnea may occur during sleep

**Dyspnea:** difficult or labored breathing

**Orthopnea:** discomfort or difficulty in breathing while lying flat; difficulty is relieved by sitting up

**Cheyne Stokes:** a cyclical breathing pattern in which breathing gradually decreases to a complete stop and then returns to normal

**Kussmaul breathing:** rapid, deep breathing; characteristic of diabetic acidosis or other causes of acidosis

A number of disorders affect the respiratory system. Some result in **rhinitis**, inflammation of the nasal mucous membrane, or **dysphonia**, altered voice production, which is usually painful or difficult (seen commonly in laryngitis). Disorders are discussed under the following broad categories: infectious disorders, obstructive lung diseases, and expansion disorders.

## Infectious Disorders

Infectious disorders are diseases that are capable of being transmitted from person to person without actual contact. An upper respiratory infection is commonly called a URI. Here are some common respiratory system infectious disorders:

**Common cold virus:** any virus strain associated with the common cold, chiefly rhinoviruses

**Sinusitis:** inflammation of any sinus mucous membrane

> Although rhinoviruses most frequently cause the common cold, there are over 200 other viruses, including the human coronavirus and the respiratory syncytial virus, that can also cause the common cold. Coronaviruses also cause bird bronchitis, mouse hepatitis, and newborn calf diarrhea.

**Croup:** acute obstruction of the upper respiratory tract (upper airway) in infants and children resulting in a barking cough with difficult and noisy breathing; also called **laryngotracheobronchitis**

**Epiglottitis:** inflammation of the epiglottis, which may cause respiratory obstruction

**Influenza (flu):** acute infectious respiratory disease caused by influenza viruses

**Pneumonia:** inflammation of the lung parenchyma (lung tissue of bronchioles, bronchi, blood vessels, and alveoli); may be caused by infection of a bacteria or a virus

**Laryngitis:** inflammation of the larynx mucous membrane

**Pertussis (whooping cough):** acute inflammation of the larynx, trachea, and bronchi caused by *Bordetella pertussis*

**Tuberculosis (TB):** infection caused by *Mycobacterium tuberculosis*; symptoms include fatigue, anorexia, weight loss, fever, chronic cough, and hemoptysis

## Obstructive Lung Diseases

Obstructive disease impairs airflow through the bronchial tree. The obstruction may be caused by an increased production of secretions or actual destruction of the lung tissues. Well-known disorders that fall into this category include:

**Asthma:** lung disease characterized by reversible inflammation and constriction

**Cystic fibrosis (CF):** genetic disorder in which the lungs become clogged with excessive amounts of abnormally thick mucus

**Chronic obstructive pulmonary disease (COPD):** an umbrella term that includes both emphysema and chronic bronchitis (described next)

**Emphysema:** condition in which the alveoli are enlarged and inefficient, leading to shortness of breath (SOB)

**Chronic bronchitis:** inflammation of the mucous membrane of the bronchi

### Expansion Disorders

Adequate lung expansion is necessary for proper gas exchange to take place. Some disease conditions cause restrictions on the lung's capacity, thereby causing inadequate exchange between the atmosphere and the lungs. **Atelectasis** (collapsed lung) and **pneumothorax** (accumulation of air in the pleural cavity) are two such disorders.

## DIAGNOSTIC TESTS, TREATMENTS, AND SURGICAL PROCEDURES

Both noninvasive and invasive procedures are used to diagnose respiratory system disorders. The noninvasive procedures include chest X-rays (CXRs), lung scans, pulse oximetry, arterial blood gases (ABGs), and computed tomography scans. **Pulse oximetry** measures the oxygen saturation of arterial blood, whereas an **ABG** measures the amount of oxygen and carbon dioxide dissolved in arterial blood. Invasive procedures may include thoracentesis and bronchoscopy. A **thoracentesis** (*pleural tap*) is an insertion of a needle into the pleural cavity to withdraw fluid. A **bronchoscopy** is an examination of the trachea and bronchial tree through a viewing instrument called a bronchoscope (see Figure 12-10). Respiratory therapists perform **pulmonary function tests (PFTs)** on patients to assess breathing. A **spirometer** is an instrument used for measuring the air capacity of the lungs. Examples of air volumes and lung capacities measured by spirometry are presented in Table 12-2.

Treatment of lung conditions commonly includes medication. **Antihistamines** are drugs used to treat acute allergic reactions, like the symptoms seen in common pollen allergies. **Decongestants** are used to treat congestion. There are multiple types of drugs that one inhales. For example, a **bronchodilator** is used to expand the bronchi. Another example is an inhaled corticosteroid, which is used to reduce inflammation in the respiratory system.

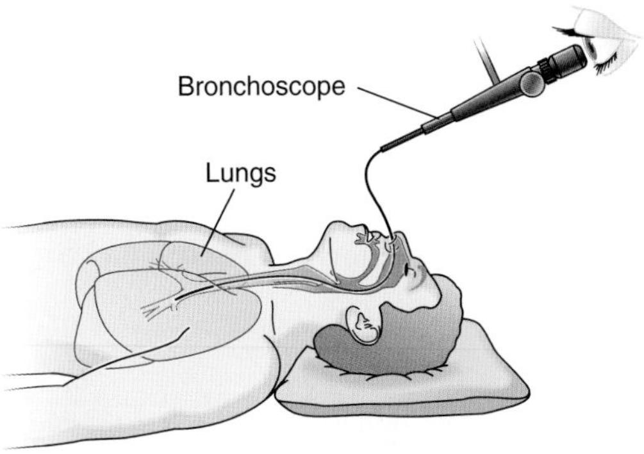


**FIGURE 12-10** Bronchoscopy. Introduction of a bronchoscope through the nose that is then guided down into the bronchi. Visual examination (suffix -scopy means "visual examination") can be made of the bronchial tree, biopsies may be taken from the bronchi, and secretions may be removed for analysis or to reduce respiratory distress.

**TABLE 12-2 PULMONARY VOLUMES AND CAPACITIES**

| Volume | Description | Average Value |
|---|---|---|
| tidal volume (TV) | volume of air entering or exiting the lungs during normal breathing | 500 mL |
| inspiratory reserve volume (IRV) | volume of air entering the lungs plus the tidal volume during forced inhalation | 300 mL |
| expiratory reserve volume (ERV) | volume of air exiting the lungs plus the tidal volume during forced exhalation | 1000 mL |
| vital capacity (VC) | maximum volume of air that can be exhaled after taking the deepest possible breath | 4500 mL |
| residual volume (RV) | volume of air in the lungs at all times | 1500 mL |
| total lung capacity (TLC) | volume of air that the lungs can hold | 6000 mL |

## PRACTICE AND PRACTITIONERS

Several different health care professionals diagnose and treat respiratory system disorders. A **pulmonologist** is a physician who specializes in **pulmonology**, which is the study of the lungs and their related structures. Both **otolaryngologists** and **otorhinolaryngologists** diagnose and treat disorders of the ears, nose, and throat. **Respiratory therapists** are allied health care professionals who specialize in airway management, mechanical ventilation (breathing), and blood acid–base balance.

**Abbreviation Table THE RESPIRATORY SYSTEM**

| ABBREVIATION | MEANING |
|---|---|
| ABG | arterial blood gas |
| BP | blood pressure |
| CF | cystic fibrosis |
| c/o | complains of |
| $CO_2$ | carbon dioxide |
| COPD | chronic obstructive pulmonary disease |
| CXR | chest X-ray |
| ERV | expiratory reserve volume |
| F | fahrenheit |
| ICU | intensive care unit |
| IRV | inspiratory reserve volume |
| $O_2$ | oxygen |
| P | pulse |
| PFT | pulmonary function test |
| R | respiration |
| RV | residual volume (as measured with test equipment) |
| SOB | shortness of breath |

## Abbreviation Table THE RESPIRATORY SYSTEM (*continued*)

| ABBREVIATION | MEANING |
|---|---|
| T | temperature |
| T and A | tonsillectomy and adenoidectomy |
| TB | tuberculosis |
| TLC | total lung capacity |
| TV | tidal volume |
| URI | upper respiratory infection |
| VC | vital capacity |
| WBC | white blood cell |

## Study Table THE RESPIRATORY SYSTEM

| TERM AND PRONUNCIATION | ANALYSIS | MEANING |
|---|---|---|
| **Structure and Function** | | |
| adenoids (AD-en-oidz) | from the Greek word *adenoeides* (gland) | epithelial and lymphatic structure located on the posterior wall of the nasopharynx; also called pharyngeal tonsil |
| alveoli (al-VEE-oh-lye); singular: alveolus (al-VEE-oh-luss) | diminutive of the Latin word *alveus* (cavity, hollow) | tiny air sacs in the lungs where the exchange of oxygen and carbon dioxide occurs between the lungs and blood |
| apex (AY-pex) | a Latin word meaning "summit," "peak," "tip" | upper tip of each lung |
| base (beys) | common English word | word used to describe the bottom of each lung |
| bronchi (BRON-kye); singular: bronchus (BRON-kuss) | *bronch/o-*, *bronch/i-* (bronchus) | tubes (right and left) branching off from the trachea and into the lungs |
| bronchiole (BRON-kee-ole) | *bronch/o-*, *bronch/i-* (bronchus) | very small branches of bronchi that extend into the lungs |
| cilia (SIHL-ee-ah) | plural of the Latin word *cilium* (eyelash, eyelid) | small hairs in the upper respiratory tract that sweep foreign matter and mucus out of the respiratory tract |
| diaphragm (DY-uh-fram) | from the Greek word *diaphragma* (partition, barrier) | the dome-shaped major muscle of breathing located at the base of the thoracic cavity |

**Study Table** THE RESPIRATORY SYSTEM (*continued*)

| TERM AND PRONUNCIATION | ANALYSIS | MEANING |
| --- | --- | --- |
| epiglottis (ep-ih-GLOT-ihs) | *epi-* (upon) + the Greek *glottis* (tongue, mouth of the windpipe) | a mucous membrane-covered, leaf-shaped piece of cartilage at the root of the tongue |
| external respiration (eks-TUR-nuhl res-puh-REY-shun) | from the Latin words *externus* (outside) and *respirationem* (breathing) | process in which air is brought into the lungs and oxygen and carbon dioxide are exchanged in the bloodstreamat the capillaries surrounding the alveoli |
| glottis (GLOT-is) | a Greek word meaning "tongue," "mouth of the windpipe" | part of the larynx consisting of the vocal folds (vocal cords) and the slit-like opening between the folds |
| internal respiration (in-TUR-nuhl res-puh-REY-shun) | from the Latin words *internus* (internal) and *respirationem* (breathing) | process where oxygen and carbon dioxide move between the bloodstream and the body's cells |
| laryngopharynx (LAYN-in-go-FAYR-inx) | *laryng/o* (larynx); *-al* (adjective suffix); *pharyng/o* (pharynx) | lower portion of the pharynx |
| larynx (LAYR-inx) | *laryng/o* (larynx) | air passageway between the pharynx and the trachea that holds the vocal cords; commonly called the voice box |
| lingual tonsils (LING-gwuhl TON-suhlz) | from the Latin words *lingua* (tongue) and *tonsillae* (tonsil) | collection of lymphatic tissue on the under surface of the tongue |
| lobe (lohb) | from the Latin word *lobus* (lobe) | a subdivision of the lung; the left lung has a *superior lobe*, *middle lobe*, and *lower lobe*; the right lung has a *superior lobe* and *inferior lobe* |
| lungs (luhngz) | from the German word *lunge* (lung) | organs of breathing located in the pulmonary cavities of the thorax |
| mediastinum (MEE-dee-ahs-TYN-um) | from the Latin word *mediastinus* (midway) | area between the lungs that houses the heart, aorta, trachea, esophagus, and bronchi |
| mucus (MYU-kus) | a Latin word meaning "slime," "mold" | clear secretion produced by the mucous membranes of the respiratory tract |

**Study Table** THE RESPIRATORY SYSTEM (*continued*)

| TERM AND PRONUNCIATION | ANALYSIS | MEANING |
|---|---|---|
| nasal (NAY-zuhl) | *nas/o* (nose); *-al* (adjective suffix) | adjective referring to the nose |
| nasal cavity(NAY-zuhl KAV-ih-tee) | from the Latin words *nasus* (nose) and *cavus* (hollow) | the space on either side of the nasal septum that extends from the nostril to the pharynx |
| nasal septum (NAY-zuhl SEP-tum) | *nas/o* (nose); *-al* (adjective); from the Latin word *saeptum* (partition) | the wall dividing the nasal cavity into halves |
| nasopharynx (NAY-zoh-FAYR-inx) | *nas/o* (nose); *pharyng/o* (pharynx) | upper portion of the pharynx |
| nose (nohz) | from the Latin word *nasus* (nose) | specialized organ at the entrance of the respiratory system |
| oropharynx (awr-oh-FAR-ingks) | from the Latin word *oris* (mouth); *pharyng/o* (pharynx) | middle portion of the pharynx |
| palatine tonsils (PAL-uh-tahyn TON-suhlz) | from the Latin word *tonsillae* (tonsil) | a mass of lymphatic tissue embedded in the lateral wall of the oral pharynx |
| paranasal sinuses (pair-uh-NAY-zul SIGH-nuh-sez) | *para-* (alongside); *nas/o* (nose); *-al* (adjective); from the Latin word *sinus* (cavity) | paired air-filled cavities in the bones of the face that are connected to the nasal cavity; these include the frontal, sphenoidal, maxillary, and ethmoidal sinuses |
| patency (PAY-tehn-see) | from the Latin word *patere* (lie open, be open) | the state of being open |
| patent (PAH-tehnt or PAY-tehnt) | from the Latin word *patere* (lie open, be open) | open; adjective form of patency |
| pharyngeal tonsils (fuh-RIN-jee-uhl TON-suhlz) | from the Latin words *pharyngeus* (pharyx) and *tonsillae* (tonsil) | epithelial and lymphatic structure located on the posterior wall of he nasopharynx; also called adenoids |
| pharynx (FAYR-inx) | a Greek word meaning "throat" | passageway just inferior to the nasal cavity and mouth |
| phrenic (FREN-ik) | from the Greek word *phren* (midriff, heart, mind) | adjective referring to the diaphragm; synonymous with diaphragmatic |
| pleura (PLU-rah) | a Greek word meaning "side of the body," "rib" | serous membrane that surrounds the lung; *parietal pleura* is the outer layer; *visceral pleura* is the inner layer |

(*continued*)

**Study Table** THE RESPIRATORY SYSTEM (*continued*)

| TERM AND PRONUNCIATION | ANALYSIS | MEANING |
|---|---|---|
| pulmonary (PULL-muhn-ayr-ee) | *pulmon/o* (lung); *-ary* (adjective suffix) | adjective meaning relating to the lungs |
| sputum (SPYOU-tum) | from the Latin word *spuere* (to spit) | thick mucus ejected through the mouth |
| tonsils (TON-silz) | from the Latin word *tonsillar* (a stake) | lymphatic structures including the pharyngeal tonsil (adenoids), palatine tonsil, and lingual tonsil |
| trachea (TRAY-kee-uh) | from the Greek word *trakheia* (windpipe) | air passage extending from the larynx itno the thorax; *windpipe* |
| ventilation (ven-ti-LAY-shun) | from the Latin word *ventilo* (the wind) | movement of gases into and out of the lungs |
| vocal cords (VO-kuhl kords) | from the Latin words *vocalis* (speaking) and *chorda* (string) | folds of mucus membranes that are used in speech production |
| **Disorders** | | |
| apnea (APP-nee-uh) | *a-* (without); *-pnea* (breathing) | absence of breathing |
| asthma (AZ-mah) | a Greek word meaning "a panting" | a lung disease characterized by reversible inflammation and constriction |
| atelectasis (at-eh-LEK-tah-sihs) | from the Greek word *ateles* (incomplete); *ectasis* (expansion) | collapse of a lung or part of a lung, leading to decreased gas exchange |
| bradypnea (BRAH-dip-NEE-ah) | *brady-* (slow); *-pnea* (breathing) | abnormally slow breathing |
| bronchial pneumonia (BRAWN-kee-uhl nu-MO- nee-ah); also called *bronchopneumonia* | *bronchi/o* (bronchus); *-al* (adjective suffix); *pneumon/o* (air, lung) | inflammation of the smaller bronchial tubes |
| bronchiectasis (BRON-kee-EK-tay-sis) | *bronchi/o* (bronchus); *-ectasis* (expansion) | chronic dilation of the bronchi |
| bronchiolitis (bron-kee-oh-LYE-tihs) | *bronchi/o* (bronchus); *-itis* (inflammation) | inflammation of the bronchioles |
| bronchiostenosis (BRON-kee-oh-steh-NOH-sis) | *bronchi/o* (bronchus); *sten/o* (narrowing); *-osis* (abnormal condition of) | narrowing of the bronchial tubes |
| bronchitis (bron-KYE-tihs) | *bronchi/o* (bronchus); *-itis* (inflammation) | inflammation of the mucous membrane of the bronchial tubes |

**Study Table** THE RESPIRATORY SYSTEM (*continued*)

| TERM AND PRONUNCIATION | ANALYSIS | MEANING |
|---|---|---|
| bronchoconstriction (BRON-koh-kon-STRIK-shun) | *bronch/o* (bronchus); from the Latin word *constrictus* (compress) | the bronchi become narrowed or constricted |
| bronchodilation (BRON-koh-DYE-lay-shun) | *bronch/o* (bronchus); from the Latin word *dilatare* (make wider, dilate) | the bronchi become more open or dilated |
| bronchopneumonia (BRON-koh-nu-MO-nee-uh); also called *bronchial pneumonia* | *bronch/o* (bronchus); *pneumon/o* (air, lung); *-ia* (condition) | inflammation of the smaller bronchial tubes |
| bronchospasm (BRON-koh-spaz-uhm) | *bronch/o* (bronchus); from the Latin word *spasmus* (a spasm) | abnormal contraction of bronchi |
| Cheyne-Stokes (SHAYN STOHKS) | named after John Cheyne, British physician, and William Stokes, Irish physician, who first described the disorder in the 19th century | a rhythmic respiratory pattern where there is a variation in depth of respirations alternating with periods of apnea |
| common cold virus (KOM-uhn kohld VYE-ruhs) | *virus* is the Latin word for poison | any virus associated with the common cold, chiefly rhinoviruses |
| croup (krupe) | obsolete English verb (to croak) | a viral infection that causes swelling of the larynx and epiglottis; a barking noise is characteristic; *laryngotracheobronchitis* |
| cyanosis (sigh-uh-NOH-sis) | from the Greek, *kyanos* (dark blue color) | dark bluish discoloration of the skin and mucous membranes due to deficient oxygenation of the blood |
| cystic fibrosis (SIS-tik FYE-broh-sis) | from the Greek word *kystis* (bladder, pouch); from the Latin word *fibra* (fiber); *-osis* (abnormal condition) | genetic disorder in which the lungs become clogged with excessive amounts of abnormally thick mucus |
| dysphonia (DIS-fohn-ya) | *dys-* (difficult); *phon/o* (sound); *-ia* (condition) | difficult or painful speech |
| dyspnea (DISP-nee-uh) | *dys-* (difficult); *-pnea* (breathing) | difficulty breathing |
| emphysema (ehm-fih-SEE-mah) | a Greek word meaning "swelling" | condition in which the alveoli are inefficient because of distension |
| epiglottitis (ep-i-GLOT-eye-tis) | *epiglottis* (Latin for epiglottis); *-itis* (inflammation) | inflammation of the epiglottis |
| eupnea (yoop-NEE-uh) | *eu-* (good, normal); *-pnea* (breathing) | normal breathing while resting |

(*continued*)

**Study Table** THE RESPIRATORY SYSTEM (*continued*)

| TERM AND PRONUNCIATION | ANALYSIS | MEANING |
|---|---|---|
| hemoptysis (HEE-mop-ti-sis) | *hem/o* (blood); *-ptysis* (spitting) | spitting or coughing up blood |
| influenza (IN-flew-EN-zah); flu (floo) | an Italian word meaning "influence" (of planets or stars) | highly contagious viral infection of the upper respiratory tract that is spread by droplets |
| Kussmaul (KUHS-mowl) | named after 19th century German physician who first noted it among patients with advanced diabetes mellitus | rapid deep respirations that are characteristic of an acid–base imbalance (frequently seen in uncontrolled diabetes) |
| laryngitis (LAYR-ihn-jye-tis) | *laryng/o* (larynx); *-itis* (inflammation) | inflammation of the larynx |
| laryngospasm (lah-RIHN-go-spaz-uhm) | *laryng/o* (larynx); from the Latin word *spasmus* (a spasm) | involuntary contraction of the larynx |
| laryngostenosis (lah-RIHN-go-steh-NO-sihs) | *laryng/o* (larynx); *sten/o* (narrowing); *-osis* (abnormal condition) | a narrowing of the larynx |
| laryngotracheobronchitis (LAHYR-ing-go-TRAY-kee-oh-brahn-KYE-tis) | *laryng/o* (larynx); *trache/o* (trachea); *bronchi/o* (bronchus) | a viral infection that causes swelling of the larynx and epiglottis; a barking noise is characteristic; *croup* |
| orthopnea (or-THOP-NEE-ah) | *ortho-* (straight, correct); *-pnea* (breathing) | discomfort or difficulty in breathing while lying flat; difficulty is relieved by sitting up |
| pertussis (per-TUSS-ihs) | from the Latin *per-* (through); *tussis* (cough) | an acute infectious inflammation of the larynx, trachea, and bronchi caused by *Bordetella pertussis* |
| pharyngitis (fair-in-JYE-tihs) | *pharyng/o* (pharynx); *-itis* (inflammation) | inflammation of the pharynx |
| pharyngospasm (fah-RIN-goh-spas-uhm) | *pharyng/o* (pharynx); from the Latin word *spasmus* (a spasm) | involuntary contraction of the pharynx |
| phrenoplegia (fren-oh-PLEE-jee-ah) | *phren/o* (diaphragm); *-plegia* (paralysis) | paralysis of the diaphragm |
| pleurisy (PLUR-ih-see) | from the Latin word *pleurisis* (side of the body) | inflammation of the pleura (membrane that surrounds the lungs and lines the walls of the thoracic cavity) |
| pneumolith (NOO-mo-lith) | *pneum/o* (air, lung); from the Greek word *lithos* (stone) | calculus (stone) in a lung |

**Study Table** THE RESPIRATORY SYSTEM (*continued*)

| TERM AND PRONUNCIATION | ANALYSIS | MEANING |
|---|---|---|
| pneumonia (noo-MONE-yah) | *pneumon/o* (air, lung); *-ia* (condition) | inflammation of a lung caused by infection, chemical inhalation, or trauma; *pneumonitis* |
| pneumonitis (noo-mo-NYE-tihs) | *pneumon/o* (air, lung); *-itis* (inflammation) | inflammation of a lung caused by infection, chemical inhalation, or trauma; *pneumonia* |
| pneumothorax (NOO-moh- thoh-rax) | *pneumon/o* (air, lung); from the Greek word *thorakos* (breastplate, chest) | accumulation of air in the pleural cavity |
| rales (RAHLZ) | from the French word *raler* (to make a rattling sound in the throat) | abnormal breath sound; crackles |
| rhinitis (rye-NYE-tiss) | *rhin/o* (nose); *-itis* (inflammation) | inflammation of the inner lining of the nasal cavity |
| rhinopathy (rye-NOH-path-ee) | *rhin/o* (nose); *-pathy* (disease) | any disease of the nose |
| rhinorrhea (rye-noh-REE-ah) | *rhin/o* (nose); *-rrhea* (discharge) | discharge from the nose |
| rhonchi (RON-kye) | from the Greek *rhonchos* (snore) | abnormal breath sound; low-pitched sonorous sounds |
| sinusitis (sy-nuh-SYE-tihs) | *sinus/o* (sinus); *-itis* (inflammation) | inflammation of the respiratory sinuses |
| stridor (STRYE-dohr) | a Latin word meaning "harsh, high pitched" | high-pitched squeaking sound frequently associated with croup |
| tachypnea (TAK-ip-NE-ah) | *tachy-* (rapid); *-pnea* (breathing) | abnormal rapid respiration |
| tracheitis (tray-kee-EYE-tiss) | *trache/o* (trachea); *-itis* (inflammation) | inflammation of the trachea |
| tracheostenosis (TRAY-kee-oh-sten-OH-siss) | *trache/o* (trachea); *sten/o* (narrowing); -sis (condition) | abnormal narrowing of the trachea |
| tuberculosis (tu-BURK-yu-loh-sihs) | from the Latin word- *tuberculum* (small swelling, pimple); *-osis* (abnormal condition) | disease caused by presence of *Mycobacterium tuberculosis*, most commonly affecting the lungs |
| wheezing (WEE-zing) | common English word; from Old Norse *hvaesa* (to hiss) | abnormal breath sounds; whistling sounds heard with upper airway obstruction |

(*continued*)

**Study Table** THE RESPIRATORY SYSTEM (*continued*)

| TERM AND PRONUNCIATION | ANALYSIS | MEANING |
|---|---|---|
| **Diagnostic Tests, Treatments, and Surgical Procedures** | | |
| antihistamine (an-tee-HISS-tah-MEEN) | *anti-* (against); from the Greek word *histos* (tissue); from the Latin *amine* (ammonia, compound) | drug used to treat acute allergic reactions |
| antipyretic (an-tee-PYE-reh-tik) | *anti-* (against); from the Greek *pyretos* (fever); *-ic* (adjective suffix) | drug used to reduce fever |
| arterial blood gas (ahr-TEER-ee-uhl BLUD GAS) | *arteri/o* (artery) + blood + gas, common English words | measures the partial pressures of oxygen and carbon dioxide in the arterial blood |
| bronchodilator (bron-koh-DYE-lay-tor) | *bronch/o* (bronchus); from the Latin word *dilatare* (make wider) | drug used to expand the bronchi |
| bronchoplasty (BRON-koh-plass-tee) | *bronch/o* (bronchus); *-plasty* (surgical repair) | surgical repair of a bronchus |
| bronchoscope (BRON-koh-skope) | *bronch/o* (bronchus); *-scope* (instrument for viewing) | a device for visually inspecting the interior of a bronchus |
| bronchoscopy (bron-KOSS-ko-pee) | *bronch/o* (bronchus); *-scopy* (use of instrument for viewing) | inspection of the bronchial tree using a bronchoscope |
| decongestant (DEE-kon-jes-tant) | *de-* (away from, cessation); from the Latin word *congerere* (to bring together) | drug used to reduce congestion |
| laryngectomy (LAYR-ehn-JEK-toh-mee) | *laryng/o* (larynx); *-ectomy* (excision) | excision of the larynx |
| laryngoscope (lah-RIHN-go-skope) | *laryng/o* (larynx); *-scope* (instrument for viewing) | instrument with a light at the tip to aid in visual inspection of the larynx |
| laryngoplasty (lah-RIHN-go-plass-tee) | *laryng/o* (larynx); *-plasty* (surgical repair) | surgical repair of the larynx |
| laryngoscopy (LAYR-ihn-GOSS-koh-pee) | *laryng/o* (larynx); *-scopy* (use of instrument for viewing) | visual inspection of the larynx with the aid of a laryngoscope |
| laryngotomy (layr-ihn-GOT-oh-mee) | *laryng/o* (larynx); *-tomy* (cutting operation) | incision into the larynx |
| pharyngoplasty (fah-RIHN-go-plass-tee) | *pharyng/o* (pharynx); *-plasty* (surgical repair) | surgical repair of the pharynx |
| pharyngoscope (fah-RIN-goh-skope) | *pharyng/o* (pharynx); *-scope* (instrument for viewing) | instrument with a light at the tip to aid in the visual inspection of the pharynx |

**Study Table** THE RESPIRATORY SYSTEM (*continued*)

| TERM AND PRONUNCIATION | ANALYSIS | MEANING |
|---|---|---|
| pharyngoscopy (FAH-rihn-GAW-skoh-pee) | *pharyng/o* (pharynx); *-scopy* (use of instrument for viewing) | visual inspection of the pharynx with aid of a pharyngoscope |
| pharyngotomy (FAYR-ihn-GOT-oh-mee) | *pharyng/o* (pharynx); *-tomy* (cutting operation) | surgical incision into the pharynx |
| pneumonectomy (NOO-mo-NEK-toh-mee) | *pneumon/o* (air, lung); *-ectomy* (excision) | removal of pulmonary lobes from a lung |
| pneumonorrhaphy (noo-mo-NOR-ah-fee) | *pneumon/o* (air, lung); *-rrhaphy* (surgical suturing) | suturing of a lung |
| pneumonotomy (noo-mo-NOT-ah-mee) | *pneumon/o* (air, lung); *-tomy* (cutting operation) | incision into a lung |
| postural drainage (PAHS-chu-ral DRAIN-ej) | common English words | a physical therapy technique where the patient lies on his or her side on a decline to help drain the lungs |
| pulmonary function test (PULL-muhn-ayr-ee FUHNGK-shuhn test) | *pulmon/o* (lung); *-ary* (adjective suffix); function tests, common English words | measurement of lung volumes to assess breathing and ventilation; instrument used is a spirometer |
| pulse oximeter (puhls ahk-SIM-eh-tuhr) | from the Latin word *pellere* (to push, drive); from the Greek words *oxys* (sharp) and *metron* (measure) | a device that measures the oxygen saturation of arterial blood by reference to light wave lengths |
| pulse oximetry (puhls ahk-SIM-eh-tree) | from the Latin word *pellere* (to push, drive); from the Greek words *oxys* (sharp) and *metron* (measure) | a small instrument is placed on a finger or thin body part that measures the oxygen saturation of arterial blood |
| rhinoplasty (RYE-noh-plass-tee) | *rhin/o* (nose); *-plasty* (surgical repair) | surgery performed on the nose |
| rhinoscope (RYE-noh-skope) | *rhin/o* (nose); *-scope* (instrument for viewing) | a small mirror with a thin handle; used in rhinoscopy |
| rhinoscopy (rye-NAW-skoh-pee) | *rhin/o* (nose); *-scopy* (use of instrument for viewing) | visual inspection of the nasal areas |
| rhinotomy (rye-NAW-toh-mee) | *rhin/o* (nose); *-tomy* (cutting operation) | surgical incision into the nose |
| sinusotomy (sy-nus-OT-oh-mee) | *sinus/o* (sinus); *-tomy* (cutting operation) | incision into a sinus |
| spirometer (spy-ROM-eh-ter) | from the Latin word *spirare* (breath, blow, live); from the Greek word *metron* (measure) | a device used to measure respiratory gases |

(*continued*)

**Study Table** THE RESPIRATORY SYSTEM (*continued*)

| TERM AND PRONUNCIATION | ANALYSIS | MEANING |
|---|---|---|
| thoracentesis (THOH-rah-sen-TEE-sihs) | *thorac/o* (thorax); *-centesis* (surgical puncture) | insertion of a needle into the pleural cavity to withdraw fluid for diagnostic purposes, to drain excess fluid, or to re-expand a collapsed lung |
| tracheoplasty (TRAY-kee-oh-plass-tee) | *trache/o* (trachea); *-plasty* (surgical repair) | surgical repair of the trachea |
| tracheostomy (tray-kee-OS-toh-mee) | *trache/o* (trachea); from the Greek *stoma* (mouth) | surgical creation of an opening into the trachea to form an airway or to prepare for the insertion of a tube for ventilation |
| tracheotomy (tray-kee-AH-toh-mee) | *trache/o* (trachea); *-tomy* (cutting operation) | incision into the trachea for purpose of restoring airflow to the lungs |
| **Practice and Practitioners** | | |
| otolaryngologist (oh-toh-LAYR-ihn-GAW-loh-jist) | *ot/o* (ear); *laryng/o* (larynx); *-logist* (one who specializes) | physician who specializes in diagnosis and treatment of ear, nose, and throat diseases |
| otolaryngology (oh-toh-LAYR-ihn-GAW-loh-jee) | *ot/o* (ear); *laryng/o* (larynx); *-logy* (study of) | branch of medical study concerned with the ear, nose, and throat and diagnosis and treatment of its diseases |
| otorhinolaryngologist (oh-toh-RYE-no-layr-ihn-GAW-loh-jist) | *ot/o* (ear); *rhin/o* (nose); *laryng/o* (larynx); *-logist* (one who specializes) | physician who specializes in diagnosis and treatment of ear, nose, and throat diseases |
| pulmonologist (PULL-muhn-AWL-oh-jist) | *pulmon/o* (lung); *-logist* (one who specializes) | physician who specializes in diagnosing and treating respiratory disorders |
| pulmonology (PULL-muhn-AW-loh-jee) | *pulmon/o* (lung); *-logy* (study of) | medical specialty of diagnosing and treating respiratory disorders |
| respiratory therapist (RES-per-uh-tawr-ee THER-uh-pist) | from the Latin word *respirare* (breathe, blow back, blow again); therapist | allied health care professional who specializes in airway management, mechanical ventilation, and blood acid–base balance |

# END-OF-CHAPTER EXERCISES

## EXERCISE 12-1 LABELING

**Using the following list, choose the correct terms to label the diagram correctly.**

| | | |
|---|---|---|
| alveoli | lungs | trachea |
| bronchi | paranasal sinuses | |

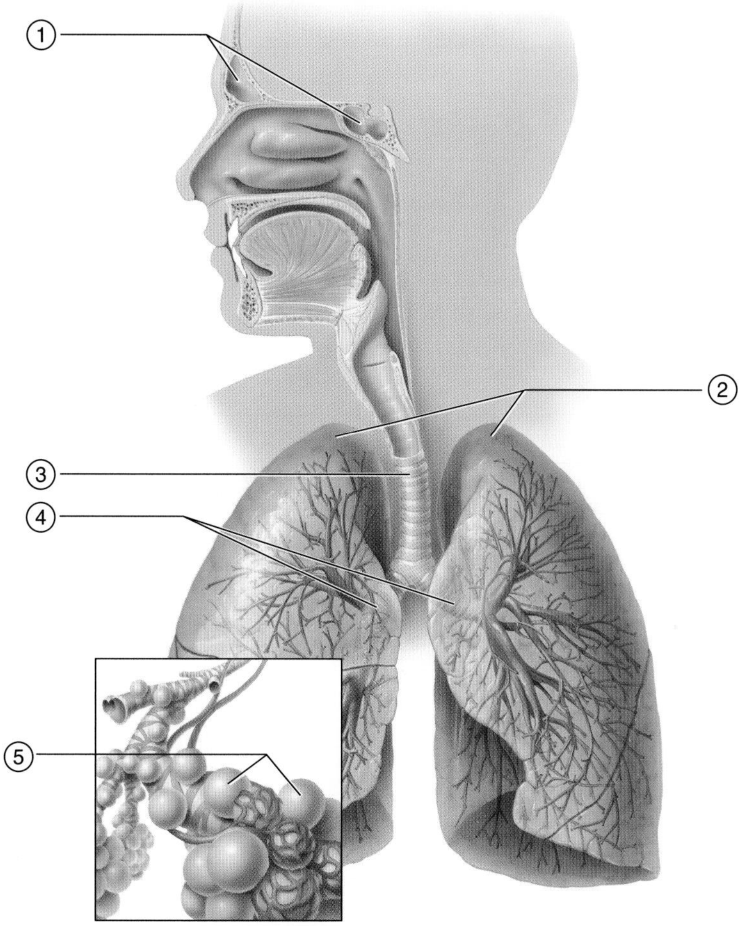


1. ____________ 3. ____________ 5. ____________

2. ____________ 4. ____________

## EXERCISE 12-2 WORD PARTS

**Break each of the following terms into its word parts: prefix, root, or suffix. Give the meaning of each word part and then define the term.**

1. *nasopharynx*

    root: ______________________________

    root: ______________________________

    definition: ______________________________

2. *pulmonary*

    root: ______________________________

    suffix: ______________________________

    definition: ______________________________

3. *dysphonia*

    prefix: ______________________________

    root: ______________________________

    suffix: ______________________________

    definition: ______________________________

4. *hemoptysis*

    root: ______________________________

    suffix: ______________________________

    definition: ______________________________

5. *laryngostenosis*

    root: ______________________________

    root: ______________________________

    suffix: ______________________________

    definition: ______________________________

6. *antipyretic*

    prefix: ______________________________

    root: ______________________________

    suffix: ______________________________

    definition: ______________________________

7. *rhinoplasty*

   root: ______________________________

   suffix: ______________________________

   definition: ______________________________

8. *otolaryngologist*

   root: ______________________________

   root: ______________________________

   suffix: ______________________________

   definition: ______________________________

## EXERCISE 12-3 WORD BUILDING

**Use *bronch/o* or *bronchi/o* to build the medical words meaning:**

1. inflammation of the bronchi ______________________

2. chronic dilation of the bronchioles ______________________

**Use the suffix –*itis* to build the medical words meaning:**

3. inflammation of the larynx ______________________

4. inflammation of a sinus ______________________

5. inflammation of the epiglottis ______________________

**Use the suffix -*pnea* to build the medical words meaning:**

6. rapid breathing ______________________

7. slow breathing ______________________

8. painful or difficulty breathing ______________________

9. difficulty breathing while lying down ______________________

## EXERCISE 12-4 MATCHING

**Match the term with its definition.**

| | | |
|---|---|---|
| 1. _____________ | alveoli | a. the lid or flap that helps prevent food and drink from entering the trachea |
| 2. _____________ | diaphragm | b. the "voice box" |
| 3. _____________ | pulmonary | c. indicating something in or associated with the lungs |
| 4. _____________ | trachea | d. the major muscle of the respiratory system |
| 5. _____________ | epiglottis | e. tiny "sacs" in the lungs that receive oxygen from the bronchioles and transfer it to the capillaries |
| 6. _____________ | pneumonia, pneumonitis | f. the "windpipe"; air flows through it to the bronchi |
| 7. _____________ | larynx | g. inflammation of a lung, caused by infection, chemical inhalation, or trauma |
| 8. _____________ | bronchioles | h. incision into the trachea |
| 9. _____________ | asthma | i. inner lining of the lung |
| 10. _____________ | pharynx | j. the smallest extensions of the bronchi, which pass air directly to the alveoli |
| 11. _____________ | emphysema | k. a lung disease characterized by reversible inflammation and constriction |
| 12. _____________ | bronchitis | l. throat |
| 13. _____________ | dyspnea | m. narrowing of a bronchial tube |
| 14. _____________ | tracheotomy | n. inflammation of the mucous membrane of the bronchial tubes |
| 15. _____________ | bronchiostenosis | o. difficulty breathing |
| 16. _____________ | apnea | p. inspection using a bronchoscope |
| 17. _____________ | visceral pleura | q. absence of breathing |
| 18. _____________ | bronchoscopy | r. condition in which the alveoli are inefficient due to distension |

## EXERCISE 12-5 MULTIPLE CHOICE

**Choose the correct answer for the following multiple choice questions.**

1. Pertussis is the medical term for ____________________.
   a. strep throat
   b. diphtheria
   c. whooping cough
   d. Lyme disease

2. What is the uppermost part of the pharynx?
   a. oropharynx
   b. laryngopharynx
   c. nasopharynx
   d. hypopharynx

3. What is the serous membrane that lines the walls of the pulmonary cavity?
   a. visceral pleura
   b. parietal pleura
   c. visceral peritoneum
   d. parietal peritoneum

4. Which procedure involves making an opening in the trachea to facilitate breathing?
   a. intubation
   b. tracheocentesis
   c. tracheoplasty
   d. tracheostomy

5. Which of the following would probably cause dysphonia?
   a. rhinitis
   b. laryngitis
   c. otitis
   d. ophthalmodynia

6. Which of the following is the same as pharyngitis?
   a. sore lung
   b. inflammation of the pharynx
   c. examination of the throat
   d. a fungal condition of the pharynx

7. Which term means the drawing of air into the lungs?
   a. respiration
   b. orthopnea
   c. inhalation
   d. hypoxia

8. What is another term for *pneumonia*?
   a. pleuropneumonia
   b. pneumonitis
   c. pulmonary edema
   d. pulmonary insufficiency

9. What is a collapse of part of a lung called?
   a. asthma
   b. atelectasis
   c. SIDS
   d. CF

10. What is a lobectomy?
    a. incision of the lung
    b. excision of a lung
    c. excision of a lobe of a lung
    d. bilateral incision of the skull

## EXERCISE 12-6 FILL IN THE BLANK

**Fill in the blank with the correct answer.**

1. Expectoration of blood is called ____________________.
2. The term for slow breathing is ____________________.
3. A surgical puncture of the lung is called a ____________________.
4. Pleurisy is ____________________.
5. The membrane that surrounds the lung is the ____________________.
6. The term for difficulty breathing while lying down is ____________________.
7. Chronic dilation of the bronchi is called ____________________.
8. Discharge from the nose is known as ____________________.
9. The abnormal breathing condition that describes alternating periods of apnea and dyspnea is ____________________.

## EXERCISE 12-7 ABBREVIATIONS

**Write out the term for the following abbreviations.**

1. ______________________________ COPD
2. ______________________________ ABG
3. ______________________________ TLC
4. ______________________________ CF
5. ______________________________ T and A
6. ______________________________ URI

**Write the abbreviation for the following terms.**

7. ____________________ tuberculosis

8. ____________________ oxygen

9. ____________________ carbon dioxide

10. ____________________ pulmonary function test

11. ____________________ residual volume

12. ____________________ shortness of breath

## EXERCISE 13-8 SPELLING

**Select the correct spelling of the medical term.**

1. The ____________________ is the major muscle responsible for breathing, located at the base of the thoracic cavity.
   a. diafram
   b. diaphram
   c. diagphram
   d. diaphragm

2. The ____________________ is more commonly known as the throat.
   a. pharinx
   b. pharynx
   c. pherinx
   d. pherynx

3. The ____________________, which is also called the windpipe, is the tube that connects the larynx to the bronchi.
   a. tracea
   b. trachia
   c. trachea
   d. traychea

4. Abnormally rapid breathing is called ____________________.
   a. tachypnea
   b. tachynea
   c. tachypnia
   d. tacypnia

5. Inflammation of a lung commonly caused by infection is called ____________________.
   a. pneumonia
   b. pnuemonia
   c. neumonia
   d. numonia

6. Discharge from the nasal mucous membrane is called ____________________.
   a. rinorea
   b. rhinorrhea
   c. rinoria
   d. rhinorhea

7. A ____________________ is a drug used to expand the bronchi.
   a. broncodilator
   b. bronchodilater
   c. bronkodilator
   d. bronchodilator

8. Inserting a needle into the pleural cavity to withdraw fluid, drain fluid, or re-expand a collapsed lung is called ____________________.
   a. thorcentesis
   b. thoracensis
   c. thoracentesis
   d. thoracenteesys

9. An ____________________ is a physician who specializes in the diagnosis and treatment of ear, nose, and throat diseases.
   a. otolaringologist
   b. otolaryngologist
   c. otolaryngolist
   d. otalaringologist

10. ____________________ is a Greek word that means "short breath" or "a panting."
    a. Asthma
    b. Asma
    c. Azma
    d. Azthma

## EXERCISE 12-9 CASE STUDY

**Analyze the following medical record and answer the questions below.**

**MEDICAL RECORD**

**HISTORY:** A 30-year-old female who c/o a nonproductive cough, dyspnea, and a fever of 3 days; patient has a negative history for smoking and has otherwise been in good health.

**PHYSICAL EXAM:** T 102°F, BP 104/65, R 26, P 108

Tachypnea is accompanied by mild cyanosis, and inspiratory rales are noted during a stethoscope exam. WBC is elevated, CXR shows diffuse infiltrates at the bases of both lungs. An ABG taken while the patient was breathing room air was abnormal and showed the patient had low oxygen content in the blood. A sputum specimen contained WBCs.

**DIAGNOSIS:** Pneumonia of unknown etiology.

**TREATMENT PLAN:** Admit patient to the ICU. Administer antibiotics and oxygen by face mask and monitor patient's status.

1. What are the findings on physical examination?
   a. Fast breathing, blue skin, and crackles heard in the lungs as the patient inhales
   b. Slow breathing, blue skin, and rales heard in the lungs as the patient holds her breath
   c. Slow breathing, blue skin, and rhonchi heard in the lungs as the patient exhales
   d. Fast heart rate, blue skin, and rales heard in the lungs as the patient inhales
   e. Fast breathing, blue skin, and wheezing heard in the lungs as the patient inhales

2. What is the patient's chief complaint? Circle the answer.
   a. Cannot breathe, fever, and coughing up material from lungs
   b. Dry cough and difficulty breathing
   c. Fever, coughing up sputum, and breathing fast
   d. Hoarse throat, dry cough, and fever
   e. Fever with a dry cough and difficulty breathing

# The Digestive System

13

## LEARNING OUTCOMES

***Upon completion of this chapter, you should be able to:***

- Name the major organs and accessory organs that make up the digestive system.
- Pronounce, spell, and define medical terms related to the digestive system and its disorders.
- Interpret abbreviations associated with the digestive system.

## INTRODUCTION

The digestive system is composed of organs whose job is to ingest food, change that food into a usable form, and then eliminate wastes. The **digestive tract** is a continuous tube beginning with the mouth and ending at the anus. This tract is also called the **gastrointestinal (GI) tract** or **alimentary canal**. Organs of the digestive system include the mouth, pharynx, esophagus, stomach, small intestine, and large intestine. Accessory organs of the digestive system include salivary glands, the liver, gallbladder, and pancreas (see Figure 13-1). The three main functions of the digestive system are digestion, absorption, and elimination. **Digestion** is the mechanical, chemical, and enzymatic processes in which ingested food is converted into substances the body can use. **Absorption** is taking in these substances by the body's cells. The removal of wastes from the body is called **elimination**.

The GI tract can be divided into an upper gastrointestinal (UGI) tract and a lower GI tract. The UGI consists of the mouth, esophagus, and the stomach. The pyloric sphincter at the distal end of the stomach marks the end of the upper GI tract. Past this point, the GI tract is called the lower GI tract. The lower GI tract consists of the small intestine and the large intestine. The small intestine is subdivided into three different parts. The large intestine is also divided into three different parts.

## WORD PARTS RELATED TO THE GASTROINTESTINAL SYSTEM

The term GI is made up of two words from two different languages. "Gastr/o" is the root word for stomach and comes from the Greek language, whereas *intestinum* is the Latin word for gut. The other name this tract is known by is alimentary canal. The root word "aliment/o" means nutrition. Eating or swallowing can be designated by either the root phag/o or the suffix –phagia, which both refer to eating. Many of the word parts related to the digestive system are listed in Table 13-1.

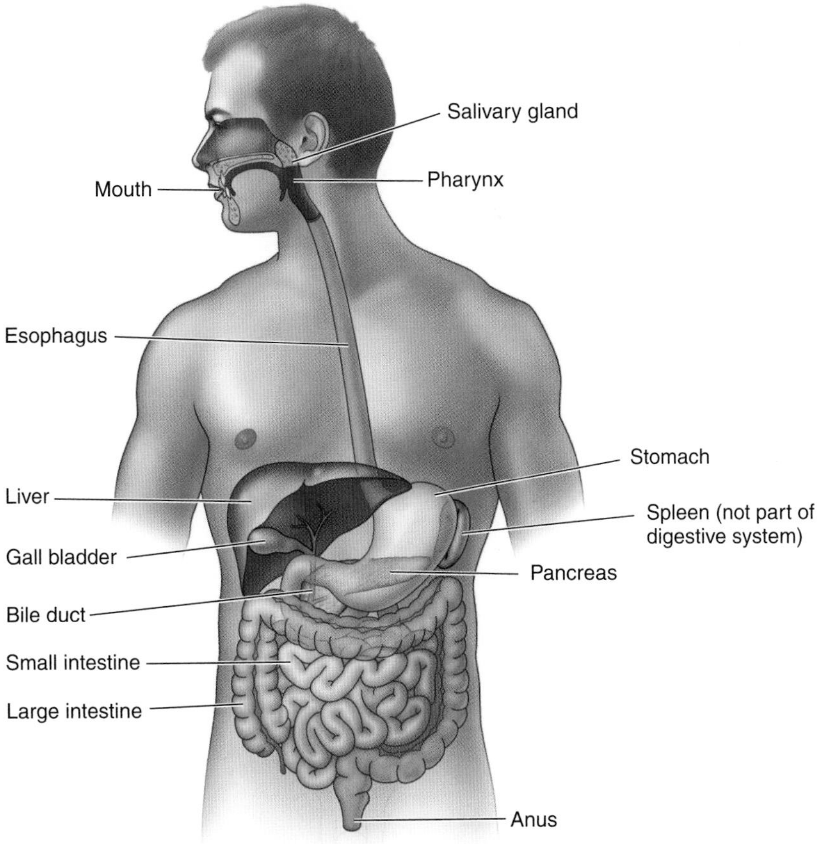


**FIGURE 13-1** Structures of the digestive system.

**TABLE 13-1 WORD PARTS RELATED TO THE DIGESTIVE SYSTEM**

| Word Part | Meaning |
|---|---|
| abdomin/o | abdomen |
| aliment/o | nutrition |
| bucc/o | cheek |
| cheil/o | lip |
| chol/e, chol/o | bile, gall |
| cholangi/o | bile duct |
| cholecyst/o | gallbladder |
| choledoch/o | common bile duct |
| col/o, colon/o | colon |
| dent/i, dent/o | teeth |
| diverticul/o | diverticulum |
| duoden/o | duodenum |
| -emesis | vomiting |
| enter/o | intestine |
| esophag/o | esophagus |

**TABLE 13-1 WORD PARTS RELATED TO THE DIGESTIVE SYSTEM (*continued*)**

| Word Part | Meaning |
|---|---|
| gastr/o | stomach |
| gingiv/o | gums |
| gloss/o | tongue |
| hepat/o | liver |
| ile/o | ileum |
| jejun/o | jejunum |
| lapar/o | abdomen |
| -lith | stone |
| pancreat/o | pancreas |
| -pepsia | digestion |
| phag/o | eating, swallowing |
| -phagia | eat or swallow |
| proct/o | anus and rectum |
| pylor/o | pylorus |
| rect/o | rectum |
| -scope | instrument used for viewing |
| -scopy | visual examination |
| sial/o | salivary glands |
| sigmoid/o | sigmoid colon |
| stomat/o | mouth |

## Word Parts Exercise

After studying Table 13-1, write the meaning of each of the word parts.

| WORD PART | MEANING |
|---|---|
| 1. -phagia | 1. ______________________ |
| 2. choledoch/o | 2. ______________________ |
| 3. stomat/o | 3. ______________________ |
| 4. sigmoid/o | 4. ______________________ |
| 5. abdomin/o | 5. ______________________ |
| 6. enter/o | 6. ______________________ |
| 7. lapar/o | 7. ______________________ |
| 8. rect/o | 8. ______________________ |
| 9. -lith | 9. ______________________ |

## Word Parts Exercise (continued)

| WORD PART | MEANING |
|---|---|
| 10. sial/o | 10. ______ |
| 11. hepat/o | 11. ______ |
| 12. pylor/o | 12. ______ |
| 13. chol/e, chol/o | 13. ______ |
| 14. cholangi/o | 14. ______ |
| 15. esophag/o | 15. ______ |
| 16. -emesis | 16. ______ |
| 17. -scope | 17. ______ |
| 18. gloss/o | 18. ______ |
| 19. jejun/o | 19. ______ |
| 20. gastr/o | 20. ______ |
| 21. cheil/o | 21. ______ |
| 22. ile/o | 22. ______ |
| 23. pancreat/o | 23. ______ |
| 24. bucc/o | 24. ______ |
| 25. cholecyst/o | 25. ______ |
| 26. -pepsia | 26. ______ |
| 27. col/o, colon/o | 27. ______ |
| 28. dent/i, dent/o | 28. ______ |
| 29. phag/o | 29. ______ |
| 30. duoden/o | 30. ______ |
| 31. proct/o | 31. ______ |
| 32. gingiv/o | 32. ______ |
| 33. -scopy | 33. ______ |
| 34. aliment/o | 34. ______ |

# STRUCTURE AND FUNCTION

The food we eat needs to be converted into a form our bodies can use. The digestive tract and associated organs are responsible for that conversion.

## Major Organs of the Digestive Tract

The major organs of the digestive tract are those that make up the one-way tube. These structures include mouth, pharynx, esophagus, stomach, small intestine, and large intestine.

### *The Mouth (Oral Cavity)*

Digestion begins in the mouth (oral cavity), where food is broken apart by **mastication**, which is a technical term for chewing. A slightly acidic fluid called *saliva* is produced by the salivary glands. Saliva moistens the food and forms a **bolus**, a small ball of masticated food that is pushed back and downward with the tongue.

> Why *bolus* and not simply *ball* or *mass*? That is a good question, especially as the Latin word *bolus*, which means ball, has a more common medical meaning that has no direct connection to the digestive system. Bolus can simply mean "a large pill" or a dose of medication given intravenously for a special purpose. Within the GI system, it refers to a ball of chewed food.

### *The Pharynx and Esophagus*

Next, the bolus enters the pharynx (throat), which, as you know from Chapter 12, is also part of the respiratory tract. From the pharynx, the bolus passes into the **esophagus**, a tube that connects the throat to the stomach. Here, the bolus is lubricated with mucus before being carried into the stomach by wavelike muscular contractions called **peristalsis**. The **lower esophageal sphincter (LES)**, also called the *cardiac sphincter*, is a ringlike muscle that controls the flow from the esophagus into the stomach (Figure 13-2).

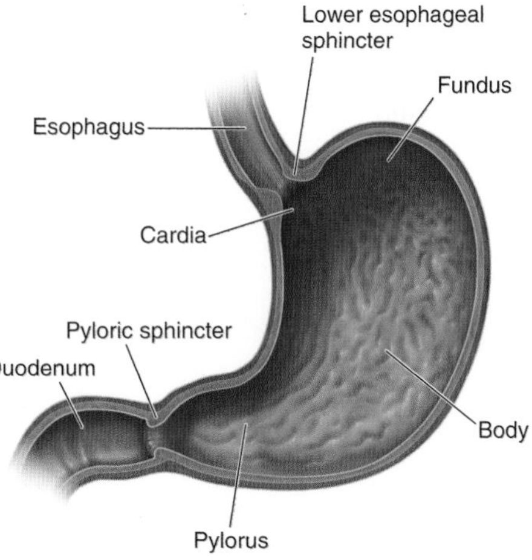


**FIGURE 13-2** The esophagus, stomach, and duodenum.

### *The Stomach*

The stomach is a J-shaped organ that physically and chemically digests food. The regions of the stomach include the *cardia*, *fundus*, *body*, and *pylorus*. Its first job is to act as a temporary storage place for the food while it does its second job: secreting hydrochloric acid and enzymes to help break down proteins, fats, and carbohydrates. Digestion includes physical changes, such as the reduction of particle size and liquefaction (converting solids to liquids), and chemical changes needed to produce fuel for the body's cells. After 3 or 4 hours, the stomach's contents, which by this stage consist of a liquid called **chyme** (pronounced kyme), begin to enter the small intestine. Chyme passes through the **pyloric sphincter**, a ring of muscle at the distal end of the stomach, and into the **duodenum**, the first part of the small intestine. At times, a *nasogastric tube*, which is a narrow tube passed into the stomach via the nose, is used short term to supply nutrition or it can be used to aspirate the stomach. Nutrition that is maintained entirely by central venous injection or by other non-GI route is termed *total parenteral nutrition* (TPN). Shorthand for "nothing by mouth" is NPO, derived from the Latin *non per os*. Figure 13-2 shows the esophagus, stomach, and duodenum.

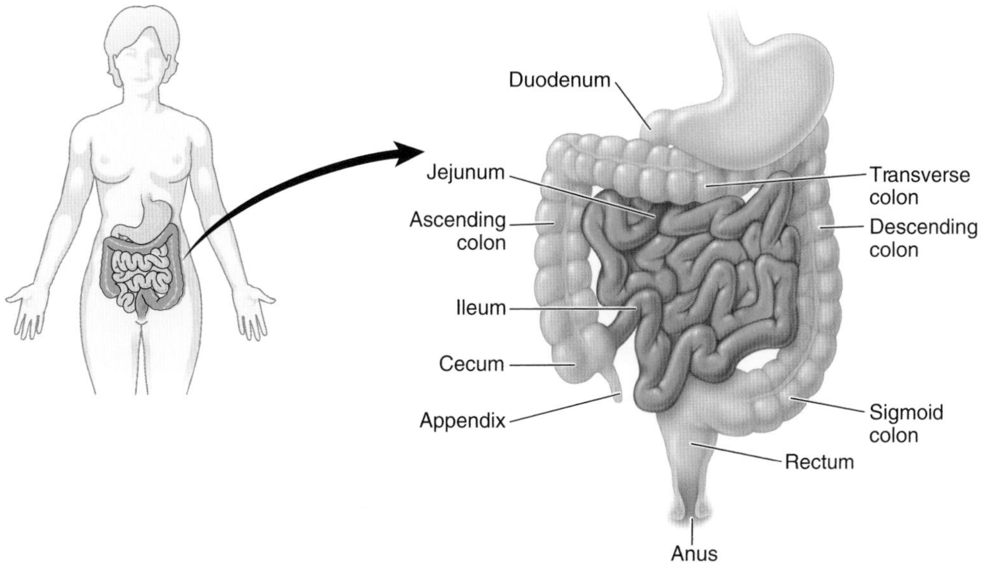


**FIGURE 13-3** The small and large intestines. The small intestine, illustrated in *dark pink*, is made up of the duodenum, jejunum, and ileum. The large intestine, illustrated in *light pink*, can be divided into the ascending colon, transverse colon, and the descending colon. The intestinal tract ends at the anus.

### *The Small Intestine*

The lower GI tract begins with the small intestine, which extends from the stomach's pyloric sphincter to the first part of the large intestine. Although it is about 20 feet in length, it is known as the small intestine because it is smaller in diameter than the large intestine. The small intestine is divided into three parts: the **duodenum**, **jejunum**, and **ileum**. From the duodenum, chyme moves into the jejunum and from there into the ileum. The **ileocecal sphincter** (not shown) controls the flow from the ileum into the cecum, the first part of the large intestine (see Figure 13-3).

> Isn't the ileum also the name of one of the three bones making up the hip? No, that's the ilium. Although both words are pronounced the same, they have one letter that is different. If you remember that hip and ilium both have an "i" in the middle, you will be able to distinguish these two terms, which have different roots.

### *The Large Intestine*

The large intestine extends from the ileocecal valve to the anus. It is divided into three parts: the **cecum**, **colon**, and **rectum**. The **cecum** is the beginning part of the large intestine. Attached to the cecum is a tube-shaped sac called the **appendix**. This structure is sometimes called the *vermiform appendix*. Vermiform, which means wormlike, is usually omitted, and the single word *appendix* is the preferred term. The appendix consists of lymphatic tissue and is, functionally speaking, part of the lymphatic system.

The colon is subdivided into four parts: the **ascending colon**, **transverse colon**, **descending colon**, and **sigmoid colon** (see Figure 13-3). The last part, the sigmoid colon, continues from the descending colon and connects to the rectum. The rectum takes up approximately the last 6 inches of the large intestine and terminates at the **anus**, through which wastes are eliminated. Figure 13-4 illustrates the pathway of food through the GI tract.

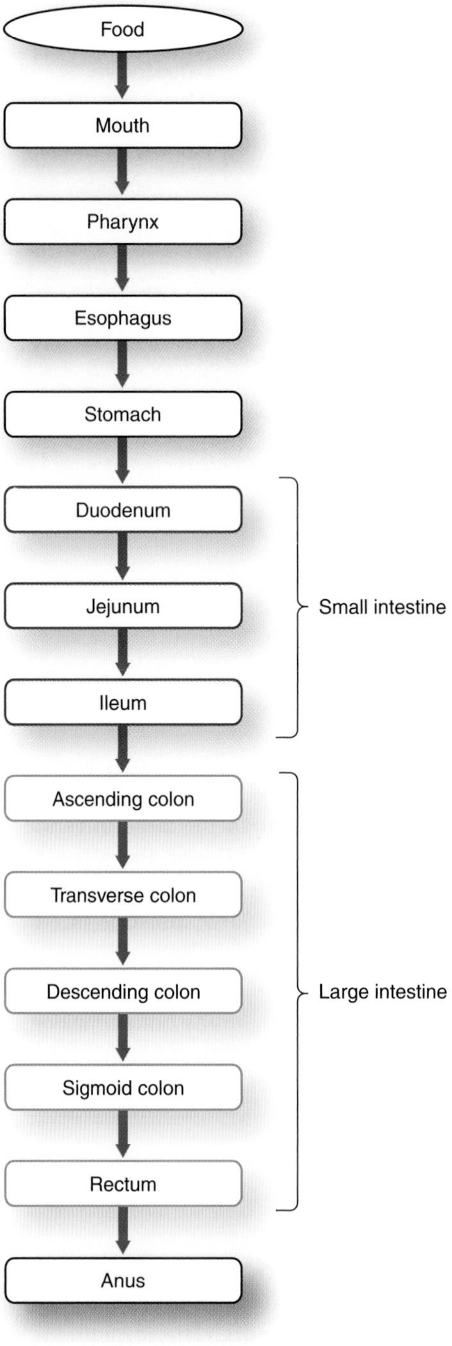


**FIGURE 13-4** Pathway of food through the gastrointestinal tract.

## Accessory Organs

Although the *salivary glands*, *liver*, *gallbladder*, and *pancreas* are not part of the GI tract, they play key roles in the digestive process. Because they are not part of the one-way canal, they are referred to as **accessory organs** of the digestive system (see Figure 13-5).

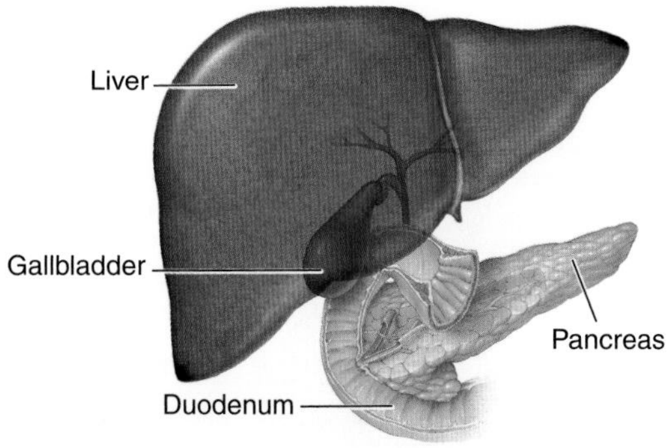


**FIGURE 13-5** Accessory organs of the digestive system.



### *Salivary Glands*

**Salivary glands** are any of the saliva-secreting glands (*parotid*, *submandibular*, and *sublingual*) of the oral cavity. The senses of taste and smell stimulate the salivary glands to secrete **saliva**, a watery liquid that contains enzymes that begin the digestive process. Saliva also helps flush bacteria in the mouth and keeps the teeth and tongue clean. Figure 13-1 shows the location of the salivary glands.

### *Liver*

The liver, located in the upper right quadrant of the abdomen deep to the diaphragm, plays many important roles in digestion, metabolism, and detoxification of harmful substances. One of its main digestive functions is to manufacture and secrete **bile**, a liquid that breaks down fat into droplets. This breaking down process is called *emulsification*. Our bodies need bile to process fats before they are released into the bloodstream. Once bile is produced in the liver, it travels down the **bile duct** to the gallbladder for storage. The liver is an important organ whose functions are integrated into many of the body's systems.

### *Gallbladder*

Although the liver produces and recycles bile, the **gallbladder**, which is located in a depression under the liver, stores, condenses, and delivers the bile to the small intestine, specifically the duodenum (see Figure 13-5).

### *Pancreas*

The pancreas is an elongated feather-shaped organ that lies posterior to the stomach. It has both digestive and endocrine functions. It produces digestive enzymes that aid in processing carbohydrates and fats in foods as well as secreting hormones directly into the bloodstream (see Figure 13-5).

## DISORDERS RELATED TO THE DIGESTIVE SYSTEM

Disorders of the upper GI tract may involve oral cavity infections, such as **stomatitis** (inflammation of the mucous membranes in the mouth) and **gingivitis** (inflammation of the gums). **Parotiditis** (also known as *parotitis*) is an inflammation of the parotid gland, which is the largest of the salivary glands. (See Figure 13-1 for location of the salivary gland). Other abnormal conditions such as **dental caries** (cavities) and **bruxism** (an involuntary clenching or grinding of teeth) can occur in the mouth.

The following are a few common disorders of the upper digestive tract:

1. **Dysphagia:** difficulty in swallowing
2. **Esophagitis:** inflammation of the esophagus
3. **Hiatal hernia:** stomach protrusion through the esophageal hiatus (opening) of the diaphragm into the thoracic cavity (see Figure 13-6)
4. **Gastroesophageal reflux disease (GERD):** upward flow of stomach acid into the esophagus
5. **Gastritis:** inflammation of the stomach (gastric) mucous membranes

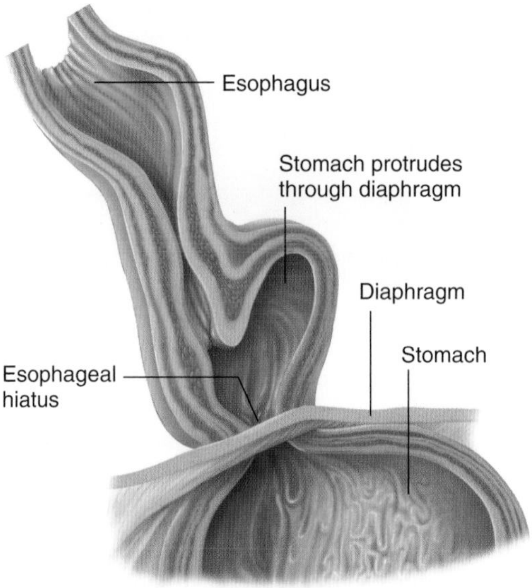


**FIGURE 13-6** Hiatal hernia.

## Quick Check

**Fill in the blanks.**

1. A small ball of masticated food is called a ______________________.

2. The stomach has two main jobs. The first is the temporary storage of food. What is the other one? ______________________

3. The three divisions of the small intestine are the ______________________, ______________________, and ______________________.

## Disorders of the Lower Gastrointestinal Tract

Disorders of the lower GI tract include obstructions, inflammation, or structural abnormalities. These conditions are listed later. A common procedure for studying the lower intestinal tract is a *barium enema* (BE), in which barium sulfate, a radiopaque dye, is injected into the rectum for X-ray imaging.

1. **Crohn's disease:** inflammation in the mucosal lining of the intestine (usually the ileum)
2. **Appendicitis:** inflammation of the appendix
3. **Peritonitis:** inflammation of the peritoneum, which is the sac that lines the abdominal cavity
4. **Diverticula:** pouches in the intestinal wall that form as increased pressure pushes the wall of the colon outward at weakened points
5. **Diverticulosis:** condition characterized by the presence of a number of diverticula
6. **Diverticulitis:** inflammation of diverticula, which fill with stagnant fecal matter and become inflamed
7. **Inguinal hernia:** protrusion of a small loop of intestine through a weak spot in the lower abdominal wall or groin

8. **Intestinal obstruction:** refers to a lack of movement of the intestinal contents through the intestine
9. **Intussusception:** a telescoping of a section of bowel inside an adjacent section
10. **Volvulus:** a twisting of the bowel



### Disorders of the Accessory Organs of the Digestive System

Many of the conditions that affect the digestive system accessory organs are obstructions caused by stones, tumors, or inflammatory processes. A few of these are described as follows:

1. **Cholelithiasis:** a condition in which calculi or stones reside in the gallbladder or bile ducts
2. **Cholecystitis:** inflammation of the gallbladder
3. **Cholangiolitis:** inflammation of a bile duct
4. **Choledocholithiasis:** obstruction of the biliary tract by gallstones
5. **Hepatitis:** inflammation of the liver
6. **Irritable bowel syndrome (IBS):** a condition characterized by abdominal pain, constipation (infrequent bowel movements with hardened feces), diarrhea, gas, and bloating
7. **Jaundice** (also called **icterus**): a symptom of hepatitis characterized by a yellowing of the skin and eyes as a result of bile accumulation
8. **Cirrhosis:** chronic liver disease characterized by inflammation and scar tissue formation; it typically results from alcoholism or hepatitis.

Additional conditions, signs, symptoms, and disorders of the digestive system include **anorexia** (loss of appetite), **bulimia** (binge eating followed by self-induced vomiting and misuse of laxatives), **eructation** (belching or burping gas), **hyperemesis** (excessive vomiting), **dyspepsia** (indigestion), and **hemorrhoids** (enlarged veins in or near the anus).

## DIAGNOSTIC TESTS, TREATMENTS, AND SURGICAL PROCEDURES

To view different parts of the GI tract, different tools are required. An **enteroscope** is an instrument for inspecting the inside of the intestine; the procedure is called an **enteroscopy**. Visual examination of the duodenum is called **duodenoscopy**. A **gastroscope** is an instrument for viewing the stomach, and the procedure is called **gastroscopy**. A **colonoscope** is a long, flexible fiber-optic endoscope used to perform a **colonoscopy** (visual examination of the colon). Endoscopic examination of the esophagus, stomach, and duodenum performed using a fiber-optic instrument is called an **esophagogastroduodenoscopy (EGD)**, whereas a radiographic contrast study using dye is called an **upper gastrointestinal series (UGIS)**.

Sometimes, a surgical procedure is necessary. The word part "ostomy," which is a word on its own meaning "mouth," is an artificial **stoma** (opening) into the GI canal. Patients with a stoma have a section of their intestines removed, so instead of waste exiting through the rectum, an artificial opening is established, and waste exits into a bag or pouch the patient wears. A **colostomy** is an opening into the colon. A **duodenostomy** is an opening into the duodenum. Notice that *-ostomy* looks very similar to *–otomy*, which is an incision (cutting), not the establishment of an opening.

## PRACTICE AND PRACTITIONERS

Apart from the specialists who treat the oral cavity and other shared organs of other systems, the specialists concerned with the digestive system are **gastroenterologists** (physicians specializing in disorders of the stomach and intestines) and **proctologists** (physicians specializing in disorders of the anus and rectum). The specialties are **gastroenterology** and **proctology**, respectively. In the hospital setting, many GI disorders are diagnosed and treated by an **internist**, a nonsurgical specialist in internal medicine.

## Abbreviation Table THE DIGESTIVE SYSTEM

| ABBREVIATION | MEANING |
|---|---|
| BE | barium enema |
| BM | bowel movement |
| EGD | esophagogastroduodenoscopy |
| GERD | gastroesophageal reflux disease |
| GI | gastrointestinal |
| HCl | hydrochloric acid |
| IBS | irritable bowel syndrome |
| LES | lower esophageal sphincter |
| NG | nasogastric |
| NPO | non per os (Latin for "nothing by mouth") |
| PO | per os (Latin for "by mouth") |
| TPN | total parenteral nutrition |
| UGIS | upper gastrointestinal series |

## Study Table THE DIGESTIVE SYSTEM

| TERM AND PRONUNCIATION | ANALYSIS | MEANING |
|---|---|---|
| **Structure and Function** | | |
| accessory organs (ak-SES-uh-ree OR-gunz) | from the Latin word *accessorius* (that which is subordinate to something else) | in the GI system: the salivary glands, liver, gallbladder, and pancreas |
| alimentary canal (al-ih-MEN-tah-ree) | from the Latin word *alimentarius* (pertaining to food) + canal | passage leading from the mouth to the anus through the pharynx, esophagus, stomach, and intestines; *digestive tract* or *GI tract* |
| appendix (uh-PEN-diks) | Latin word for "something attached" | tube-shaped sac attached into the cecum of the large intestine; *vermiform appendix* |
| bile (BILE) | from the Latin word *bilis* (fluid secreted from the liver) | yellow-brown or green liquid secreted by the liver into the duodenum to emulsify fats |
| bile duct (BILE DUKT) | from the Latin words *bilis* (fluid secreted from the liver) and *ductus* (a leading) | tube that transports bile from the liver to the gallbladder |
| bilirubin (BIHL-ee-ROO-bin) | from the Latin *bilus* (bile) and *ruber* (red) | waste produced by worn out red blood cells breaking down |

**Study Table** THE DIGESTIVE SYSTEM (*continued*)

| TERM AND PRONUNCIATION | ANALYSIS | MEANING |
|---|---|---|
| bowel movement (BM) (BOWEL MOOV-ment) | from the Latin *botellus*, a diminutive of *botulus* (sausage) | defecation |
| cardiac sphincter (KAR-dee-ak SFINGK-ter) | *cardi/o* (heart); *-ac* (adjective suffix); from the Greek word *sphingein* (to bind tight) | the ringlike muscle between the esophagus and stomach that controls food flow; LES |
| cecum (SEE-kuhm) | from the Latin word *caecus* (hidden) | a pouch connected to the junction of the small and large intestines, forming the first part of the large intestine |
| chyme (KYME) | from the Latin word *chymus* (juice produced by digestion) | the semifluid mass of partly digested food passed from the stomach into the duodenum |
| colon (KOH-luhn); also called the *large intestine* | from the Greek word *kolon* (large intestine) | the large intestine, divisible into the ascending, transverse, descending, and sigmoid colons |
| deglutition (dee-gloo-TISH-uhn) | from the Latin word *deglutire* (to swallow, overwhelm, abolish) | swallowing |
| digestive tract (dye-JES-tiv TRAKT) | from the Latin word *digero* + *-gestus* (to force apart, divide, dissolve) | passage leading from the mouth to the anus through the pharynx, esophagus, stomach, and intestines; *alimentary canal* or *GI tract* |
| duodenal (doo-OD-en-uhl) | from the Greek word *dodekadaktylon* (literally "12 fingers long"; named by Greek physician Herophilus) + *-al* (adjective suffix) | adjective form of duodenum used in the terms naming some digestive system disorders |
| duodenum (doo-OD-en-um) | from the Greek *dodekadaktylon* (12 fingers long) | segment of the small intestine connecting with the stomach |
| esophagus (ee-SOF-ah-guhs) | from the Greek *oisophagos* (gullet, literally "what carries and eats") | the part of the digestive tract between the pharynx and stomach |
| gallbladder (GAWL-blad-er) | from Old English *galla* (to shine, yellow); from Old English *bledre* (to blast, blow up, swell up) | small pear-shaped organ that stores bile |
| gastric (GAS-trik) | *gastr/o* (stomach); *-ic* (adjective suffix) | adjective form of stomach |
| gastrointestinal (GI) tract (GAS-troh-in-TES-tin-ahl TRAKT) | *gastr/o* (stomach); from Latin *intestina*, plural of *intestinus* (internal, inward, intestine) + tract | passage leading from the mouth to the anus through the pharynx, esophagus, stomach, and intestines; *alimentary canal* or *digestive tract* |

(*continued*)

**Study Table** THE DIGESTIVE SYSTEM *(continued)*

| TERM AND PRONUNCIATION | ANALYSIS | MEANING |
|---|---|---|
| ileocecal sphincter (ILL-ee-oh-see-kul SFINGK-ter) | *ile/o* (ileum); from the Latin *caecum* (blind); *-al* (adjective suffix); *sphincter* (from the Greek word *sphingein*: to bind tight) | muscular ring that separates the distal portion of the ileum (small intestine) and the beginning of the cecum (large intestine) |
| ileum (ILL-ee-uhm) | a Latin word meaning "flank," "groin" | the longest segment of the small intestine, which leads into the large intestine |
| intestine (ihn-TESS-tin) | from Latin *intestina*, plural of *intestinus* (internal, inward, intestine) | the small intestine is divisible into the duodenum, jejunum, and ileum; the large intestine comprises the cecum, colon, rectum, and anus |
| jejunum (jeh-JOO-num) | from the Latin word *jejunus* (empty, fasting, abstinent, hungry) | eight-foot-long segment of the small intestine between the duodenum and the ileum |
| liver (LIV-er) | from the Old English word *lifer* (liver) | the largest glandular organ of the body, lying beneath the diaphragm in the upper part of the gastric region, involved in many metabolic processes |
| lower esophageal sphincter (LES) (LOW-ur eh-sof-uh-JEE-ul SFINGK-ter) | from the Greek word *sphingein* (to bind tight) | the ringlike muscle between the esophagus and stomach that controls food flow; *cardiac sphincter* |
| lower GI tract (LOH-er JEE EYE TRAKT) | *gastr/o* (stomach); from Latin *intestina*, plural of *intestinus* (internal, inward, intestine) + tract | the small intestine and large intestine |
| mastication (MAS-ti-kay-shun) | from the Latin verb *masticare* (to chew) | the process of chewing food |
| oral cavity (OR-uhl KAV-i-tee) | from the Latin words *os* (mouth) and *cavus* (hollow) | the mouth |
| pancreas (PAN-kree-as) | from the Greek words *pan* (all) and *kreas* (flesh, meat) | organ of the digestive system that has both exocrine and endocrine functions; secretes enzymes that aid in digestion |
| pancreatic (pan-kree-AT-ik) | *pancreat/o* (pancreas); *-ic* (adjective suffix) | adjective for pancreas |
| peristalsis (pear-ih-STAL-sis) | from the Greek word *peristaltiko* (clasping and compressing) | wavelike muscular contractions that move food along in the digestive tract |

**Study Table** THE DIGESTIVE SYSTEM (*continued*)

| TERM AND PRONUNCIATION | ANALYSIS | MEANING |
|---|---|---|
| pharynx (FAYR ingks) | from the Greek word *pharunx* (throat) | passageway just below the nasal cavity and mouth |
| pyloric sphincter (pye-LOHR-ik SFINGK-ter) | *pylor/o* (pylorus); *-ic* (adjective suffix); sphincter (from the Greek word *sphingein*: to bind tight) | ring of muscle between the stomach and duodenum |
| rectum (REK-tuhm) | Latin word for "straight" | the terminal portion of the digestive tract |
| saliva (suh-LYE-vuh) | Latin word for "spittle" | a clear, tasteless, slightly acidic fluid secreted from the salivary glands |
| salivary glands (SAL-ih-vahr-ee GLANDZ) | from the Latin word *salivarius* (slimy, clammy) + gland from the Latin word *glans* (acorn) | collectively, the parotid, sublingual, and submandibular glands that secrete saliva |
| stoma (STOH-mah) | a Greek word meaning "mouth," "opening" | an artificial opening |
| stomach (STUM-uhk) | from the Latin word *stomachus* (throat, gullet, stomach) | digestive organ composed of four regions (cardia, fundus, body, and pylorus) |
| upper GI tract (UP-er JEE EYE TRAKT) | *gastr/o* (stomach); from Latin *intestina*, plural of *intestinus* (internal, inward, intestine) + tract | the oral cavity, pharynx, esophagus, and stomach |
| **Disorders** | | |
| anorexia (an-or-ECKS-ee-ah) | from the Greek *an* (without) + *orexis* (appetite, desire) | loss of appetite |
| appendicitis (ay-PEN-dih-SYE-tis) | from the Latin word *appendix* (something attached); *-itis* (inflammation) | inflammation of the appendix |
| ascites (uh-SYE-teez) | from the Greek word *askos* (bag) | abnormal accumulation of fluid in the peritoneal cavity |
| bruxism (BRUKS-ism) | from the Greek word *ebryxa*, root from *brykein* infinitive of the verb; *ebryxa* (to gnash the teeth) + *-ism* (condition) | involuntary grinding of the teeth that usually occurs during sleep |
| bulimia (bull-EE-mee-ah) | from the Greek word *boulemia* (hunger) | eating disorder characterized by episodes of binge eating followed by self-induced vomiting and misuse of laxatives |
| cholangiolitis (KOH-lan-jee-oh-LYE-tis) | *cholangi/o* (bile, duct); *-itis* (inflammation) | inflammation of the bile ducts |

(*continued*)

**Study Table** THE DIGESTIVE SYSTEM (*continued*)

| TERM AND PRONUNCIATION | ANALYSIS | MEANING |
|---|---|---|
| cholecystitis (KOH-lee-siss-TYE-tiss) | *cholecyst/o* (gallbladder); *-itis* (inflammation) | inflammation of the gallbladder |
| cholecystopathy (KOH-lee-siss-TOP-ah-thee) | *cholecyst/o* (gallbladder); *-pathy* (disease) | any disease of the gallbladder |
| choledocholithiasis (koh-LED-oh-koh-lith-EYE-uh-sis) | *choledoch/o* (common bile duct); *-lithiasis* (condition of having stones) | inflammation of the bile duct caused by gallstones |
| cholelithiasis (KOH-lee-lih-THYE-ah-sis) | *chol/e* (bile, gall); *-lithiasis* (condition of having stones) | formation or presence of stones in the gallbladder or bile duct |
| cirrhosis (sir-OH-sis) | from the Greek word *kirrhos* (tawny), named for the orange-yellow appearance of a diseased liver | chronic disease of the liver |
| colitis (koh-LYE-tis) | *col/o* (colon); *-itis* (inflammation) | inflammation of the colon |
| constipation (kon-stih-PAY-shun) | from the Latin word *constipare* (to press or crowd together) | decrease in the frequency of bowel movements; difficulty in passing stools; and/or hard, dry stools |
| Crohn's disease (KRONZ dih-ZEEZ) | named after American B.B. Crohn (1884–1983), one of the team that described it in 1932 | chronic inflammation of part(s) of the intestinal tract |
| dental caries (DEN-tul KAYR-eez) | *dent/i* (tooth); *-al* (adjective suffix) + *caries*, a Latin word meaning "rot," "rottenness," "corruption" | tooth decay |
| diverticulum (dye-ver-TIK-yoo-luhm); pl. diverticula (dye-ver-TIK-yoo-luh) | Latin word for "a bypath" | a pouch or sac opening from a tube, such as the gut |
| diverticulitis (dye-ver-tik-yoo-LYE-tis) | from the Latin word *diverticulum* (a bypath, side road); -*itis* (inflammation) | inflammation of a diverticulum or sac in the intestinal tract |
| diverticulosis (dye-ver-tik-yoo-LOH-sis) | *diverticulum* (bypath); *-osis* (abnormal condition) | presence of a number of diverticula of the intestine; common in middle age |
| duodenitis (doo-odd-eh-NY-tihs) | *duoden/o* (duodenum); *-itis* (inflammation) | inflammation of the duodenum |
| dyspepsia (dis-PEP-see-ah) | from the Greek word *dyspeptos* (hard to digest); *-ia* (condition of) | impairment of digestion |

**Study Table** THE DIGESTIVE SYSTEM (*continued*)

| TERM AND PRONUNCIATION | ANALYSIS | MEANING |
|---|---|---|
| dysphagia (dis-FAY-jee-ah) | *dys-* (difficulty); *phag/o* (eating, swallowing); *-ia* (condition of) | difficulty swallowing |
| enteritis (ehn-teh-RYE-tihs) | *enter/o* (intestine); *-itis* (inflammation) | inflammation of the intestine |
| enterohepatitis (EN-teh-roh- hep-ah-TI-tihs) | *enter/o* (intestine); *hepat/o* (liver); *-itis* (inflammation) | inflammation of the intestine and liver |
| enteropathy (en-tehr-OP-ah-thee) | *enter/o* (intestine); *-pathy* (disease) | any intestinal disease |
| eructation (ee-RUK-tay-shun) | from the Latin verb *eructo* (belch) | belching or burping gas up from the stomach |
| esophagitis (ih-SOF-uh-jye-tis) | *esophag/o* (esophagus); *-itis* (inflammation) | inflammation of the esophagus |
| gastric ulcers (GAS-trik UHL-serz) | *gastr/o* (stomach); *-ic* (adjective suffix) + ulcer, from the Latin *ulcus*, related to the Greek word *helkos* (wound, sore) | erosion of the gastric mucosa |
| gastritis (gas-TRY-tihs) | *gastr/o* (stomach); *-itis* (inflammation) | inflammation of the stomach |
| gastroduodenitis (GAS-troh-doo-oh-deh-NY-tihs) | *gastr/o* (stomach); *duoden/o* (duodenum); *-itis* (inflammation) | inflammation of the stomach and duodenum |
| gastroenteritis (GAS-troh-en-teh-RYE-tihs) | *gastr/o* (stomach); *enter/o* (intestine); *-itis* (inflammation) | inflammation of the stomach and intestine |
| gastroesophageal reflux disease (GAS-troh-ee-sof-a-JEE-al REE-flucks dih-ZEEZ) (GERD) | *gastr/o* (stomach); *esophag/o* (esophagus); *-al* (adjective suffix); + reflux disease | backward flow of stomach acid into the esophagus |
| gingivitis (JIN-jeh-vye-tis) | *gingiv/o* (gums); *-itis* (inflammation) | inflammation of the gums |
| hemorrhoids (HEM-oh-roydz) | from the Greek word *haimorrhoides* derived from *haima* (blood); and *rhoos* (a flowing) | enlarged veins in or near the anus that may cause pain or bleeding |
| hepatitis (hep-ah-TYE-tihs) | *hepat/o* (liver); *-itis* (inflammation) | inflammation of the liver |
| hepatogenic (heh-pah-toh-JEN-ik) | *hepat/o* (liver); *-genic* (originating) | originating in the liver |
| hepatomegaly (heh-PAH-toh-MEG-ah-lee) | *hepat/o* (liver); *-megaly* (enlargement) | enlarged liver |
| hiatal hernia (HYE-ay-tahl HER-nee-ah) | from the Latin word *hiatus* (gaping, opening); *-al* (adjective suffix) + the Latin word *hernia* (rupture) | protrusion of the stomach through the diaphragm into the thoracic cavity |

(*continued*)

**Study Table** THE DIGESTIVE SYSTEM (*continued*)

| TERM AND PRONUNCIATION | ANALYSIS | MEANING |
|---|---|---|
| hyperemesis (hy-per-EM-ih-sis) | *hyper-* (excessive); *-emesis* (vomit) | excessive vomiting |
| inguinal hernia (ING-gwi-nahl HER-nee-ah) | from the Latin word *inguinalis* (of the groin) + the Latin word *hernia* (rupture) | outpouching of intestines into the inguinal or groin region |
| intestinal obstruction (in-TES-tih-nul ob-STRUK-shun) | from the Latin words *intestinum* (gut); *-al* (adjective suffix); *obstructionem* (a barrier) | an obstruction in the intestine |
| intussusception (in-tuh-suh-SEP-shun) | from the Latin word *intus* (within); from the Latin word *suscipere* (undertake; support, accept) | one part of the intestine slipping or telescoping over another |
| irritable bowel syndrome (IBS) (IR-ih-tuh-bul BOWEL SIN-drome) | from the Latin *irritabilis* (irritate) + from the Latin *botellus*, diminutive of *botulus* (sausage) + from the Greek *sundrome*, from *sun-* (together) + *dramein* (to run) | condition characterized by abdominal pain, constipation, diarrhea, gas, and bloating |
| jaundice (JAWN-dis) or icterus (IK-tehr-us) | from Middle French word *jaunisse* (yellow) | yellowish cast to the skin, sclera (white part of the eye), and mucous membranes caused by bile deposits |
| jejunitis (jeh-joo-NYE-tihs) | *jejun/o* (jejunum); *-itis* (inflammation) | inflammation of the jejunum |
| melena (muh-LEE-nuh) | from the Greek word *melas* (black) | dark-colored, tarry stools due to the presence of blood |
| pancreatitis (PAN-kree-ah-TYE-tihs) | *pancreat/o* (pancreas); *-itis* (inflammation) | inflammation of the pancreas |
| pancreatopathy (PAN-kree-ah-TOP-ah-thee) | *pancreat/o* (pancreas); *-pathy* (disease) | any disease of the pancreas |
| parotiditis (pah-RAH-ti-DYE-tis) | parotid from the Greek words *para-* (beside) and *otos* (ear); *-itis* (inflammation) | inflammation of the parotid gland |
| peritonitis (PAYR-ih-toh-NYE-tis) | from the Greek words *peri-* (around) and *teinein* (to stretch); *-itis* (inflammation) | inflammation of the peritoneal cavity |
| polyp (PAHL-ip) | from the Latin word *polypus* (cuttlefish) | growth protruding from a stalk in the digestive tract |
| sialoadenitis (SY-ah-loh-ah-deh-NYE-tihs) | *sial/o* (saliva, salivary gland); *aden/o* (gland); *-itis* (inflammation) | inflammation of a salivary gland |

**Study Table** THE DIGESTIVE SYSTEM (*continued*)

| TERM AND PRONUNCIATION | ANALYSIS | MEANING |
|---|---|---|
| sialoangiitis (SYE-ah-loh-an-jee-EYE-tihs) | *sial/o* (saliva, salivary gland); *angi/o* (vessel); *-itis* (inflammation) | inflammation of a salivary duct |
| sialorrhea (SYE-ah-loh-REE-ah) | *sial/o* (saliva, salivary gland); *-rrhea* (discharge) | excessive production of saliva |
| sialostenosis (SYE-ah-loh-steh-NO-sihs) | *sial/o* (saliva, salivary gland); *-stenosis* (narrowed, blocked) | narrowing of a salivary duct |
| stomatitis (STOH-mah-tye-tis) | *stomat/o* (mouth); *-itis* (inflammation) | inflammation of the mucous membranes of the mouth |
| volvulus (VOL-vyuh-luhs) | from the Latin verb *volvere* "to turn, twist" | a twisting of the intestine |
| **Diagnostic Tests, Treatments, and Surgical Procedures** | | |
| antacids (ant-AS-ids) | from *anti-* (against) + acids | medications used to reduce or neutralize acidity |
| antidiarrheal (an-tee-DYE-ah-REE-al) | *anti-* (against); from the Greek *dia-* (through) + *-rrhea* (discharge); *-al* (adjective suffix) | drugs that relieve diarrhea by absorbing the excess fluid or by decreasing intestinal motility |
| antiemetic (an-tee-EE-meh-tik) | *anti-* (against); *-emesis* (vomit); *-ic* (adjective suffix) | drugs used to relieve vomiting |
| antiflatulence (an-tee-FLAT-yoo-lens) | *anti-* (against); from the Latin word *flatus* (a blowing, a breaking wind) | drugs taken to relieve gas or flatus |
| cholecystectomy (KOH-lee-siss-TEK-toh-mee) | *cholecyst/o* (gallbladder); *-ectomy* (surgical removal) | removal of the gallbladder |
| cholecystotomy (KOH-lee-siss-TOT-oh-mee) | *cholecyst/o* (gallbladder); *-tomy* (incision) | incision into the gallbladder |
| colectomy (koh-LEK-toh-mee) | *col/o* (colon); *-ectomy* (surgical removal) | removal of all or part of the colon |
| colonoscope (koh-LON-oh-skope) | *colon/o* (colon); *-scope* (instrument for viewing) | long-flexible fiber-optic endoscope used in colonoscopy |
| colonoscopy (koh-lon-OSS-koh-pee) | *colon/o* (colon); *-scopy* (viewing) | visual examination of the colon with a colonoscope |
| colopexy (KOH-loh-pehk-see) | *col/o* (colon); *-pexy* (surgical fixation) | attachment of a portion of the colon to the abdominal wall |
| colostomy (koh-LOSS-tuh-mee) | *col/o* (colon); *-stomy* (permanent opening) | surgical establishment of an opening into the colon |
| colotomy (koh-LOT-uh-mee) | *col/o* (colon); *-tomy* (incision) | incision into the colon |
| duodenectomy (doo-oh-deh-NEK-toh-mee) | *duoden/o* (duodenum); *-ectomy* (surgical removal) | removal of the duodenum |

(*continued*)

**Study Table** THE DIGESTIVE SYSTEM (*continued*)

| TERM AND PRONUNCIATION | ANALYSIS | MEANING |
|---|---|---|
| duodenoscopy (doo-oh-deh-NOS-kuh-pee) | *duoden/o* (duodenum); *-scopy* (viewing) | visual examination of the duodenum with the aid of an endoscope |
| duodenostomy (doo-oh-deh-NOS-toh-mee) | *duoden/o* (duodenum); *-stomy* (permanent opening) | surgical establishment of an opening in the duodenum |
| emetic (ee-MET-ik) | *emesis* (vomit); *-ic* (adjective suffix) | drugs that stimulate or induce vomiting; frequently used in poisoning cases |
| enteroscope (en-TEHR-oh-skope) | *enter/o* (intestine); *-scope* (instrument for viewing) | lighted instrument for visually examining the intestines |
| enteroscopy (en-tehr-OS-koh-pee) | *enter/o* (intestine); *-scopy* (viewing) | visual examination of the intestines |
| gastrectomy (gas-TREK-toh-mee) | *gastr/o* (stomach); *-ectomy* (surgical removal) | removal of part of the stomach |
| gastroscope (GAS-troh-scope) | *gastr/o* (stomach); *-scope* (instrument for viewing) | lighted instrument (endoscope) for visually examining the stomach |
| gastroscopy (gas-TROS-koh-pee) | *gastr/o* (stomach); *-scopy* (viewing) | visual examination of the stomach with a lighted instrument (endoscope) |
| H2 blockers or H2-receptor antagonists | H2 (or histamine2), a common chemical in the body, signals the stomach to make acid; H2 blockers oppose histamine's action and reduce the amount of acid the stomach produces; + blocker, a common English word | drugs that block the release of gastric acid; used to treat gastroesophageal reflux disease |
| hepatoscopy (hep-uh-TOS-kuh-pee) | *hepat/o* (liver); *-scopy* (viewing) | visual examination of the liver |
| hepatopexy (HEH-pah-to-pek-see) | *hepat/o* (liver); *-pexy* (surgical fixation) | anchoring of the liver to the abdominal wall |
| jejunectomy (jeh-joo-NEK-toh-mee) | *jejun/o* (jejunum); *-ectomy* (surgical removal) | removal of all or part of the jejunum |
| jejunoplasty (jeh-JOON-oh-plass-tee) | *jejun/o* (jejunum); *-plasty* (surgical repair) | surgical repair of the jejunum |
| jejunotomy (jeh-joo-NOT-oh-mee) | *jejun/o* (jejunum); *-tomy* (incision) | incision into the jejunum |
| nasogastric (NG) tube (nay-zoh-GAS-trik TOOB) | naso- (nose) + *gastric* (stomach) | a flexible tube passed through the nose and into the stomach to deliver nutrition or to aspirate (suction out) contents |
| pancreatotomy (PAN-kree-ah-TOT-ah-mee) | *pancreat/o* (pancreas); *-tomy* (incision) | incision into the pancreas |

**Study Table** THE DIGESTIVE SYSTEM (*continued*)

| TERM AND PRONUNCIATION | ANALYSIS | MEANING |
|---|---|---|
| sialoadenectomy (SYE-al-oh-ah-deh-NEK-tah-mee) | *sial/o* (saliva, salivary gland); *aden/o* (gland); *-ectomy* (surgical removal) | removal of a salivary gland |
| sialoadenotomy (SYE-al-oh-ah-deh-NOT-ah-mee) | *sial/o* (saliva, salivary gland); *aden/o* (gland); *-tomy* (incision) | incision of a salivary gland |
| sialography (SYE-ah-LOG-rah-fee) | *sial/o* (saliva, salivary gland); *-graphy* (the process of recording) | radiography (X-rays) of salivary glands and ducts |
| total parenteral nutrition (TPN) (TOH-tul puh-REN-ter-ul noo-TRISH-un) | from the Latin *totalis* (whole, entire); *para-* (beside) + from the Greek *enteron* (intestine); from the Latin *nutrition* (to nourish) | nutrition maintained entirely by central intravenous injection or other non-GI route |
| upper gastrointestinal series (UGIS) (UP-er gas-troh-in-TES-tin-ul seer-EEZ) | from the Middle English *up* + *-er*; *gastrointestinal* (relating to the stomach and intestines); from the Latin *sero* (to join together) | radiographic contrast study (X-rays with dye) of the esophagus, stomach, and duodenum |
| **Practice and Practitioners** | | |
| gastroenterologist (GAS-troh-en-tehr-OL-oh-jist) | *gastr/o* (stomach); *enter/o* (intestine); *-logist* (one who studies a certain field) | a specialist in the diagnosis and treatment of digestive system disorders |
| gastroenterology (GAS-troh-en-tehr-OL-oh-jee) | *gastr/o* (stomach); *enter/o* (intestine); *-logy* (the study of) | the specialty concerned with the digestive system |
| internal medicine (in-TUR-nuhl MED-uh-sin) | two common English words | specialty in the diagnosis and nonsurgical treatment of serious and/or chronic illnesses; the phrase is quite commonly used in North America (but not necessarily elsewhere); it also covers subspecialties in specific organs, such as the liver, kidneys, etc. |
| internist (IN-tur-nist) | internal (English adjective meaning "inside"); *-ist* (practitioner) | a specialist in internal medicine |
| proctologist (prok-TOL-uh-jist) | *proct/o* (anus and rectum); *-logist* (one who studies a certain field) | a specialist in the diagnosis and treatment of rectal and anal disorders |
| proctology (prok-TOL-uh-jee) | *proct/o* (anus and rectum); *-logy* (study of) | study of the rectum and anus |

(*continued*)

# END-OF-CHAPTER EXERCISES

## EXERCISE 13-1 LABELING

**Using the following list, choose the correct terms to label the diagram correctly.**

| | | |
|---|---|---|
| anus | large intestine | pharynx |
| bile duct | liver | salivary gland |
| esophagus | mouth | small intestine |
| gallbladder | pancreas | stomach |

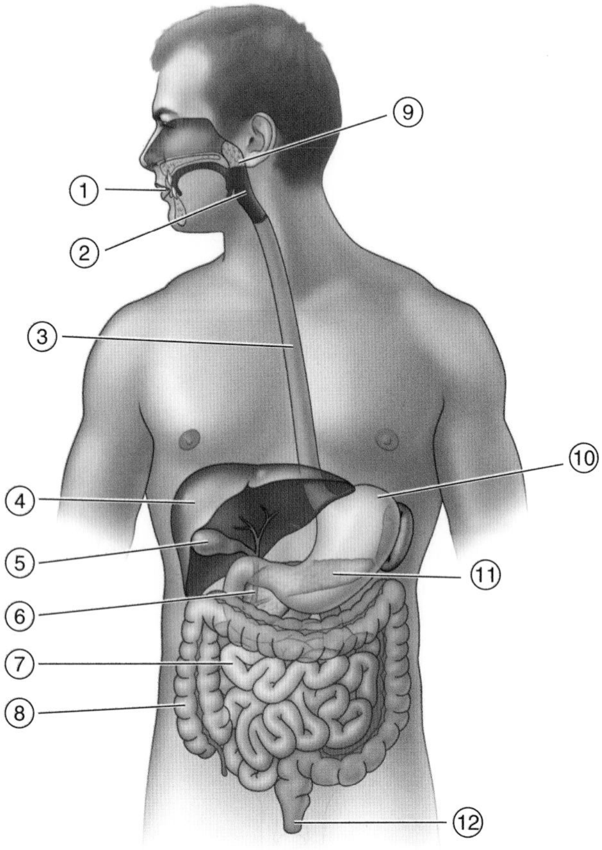


1. ______________ 5. ______________ 9. ______________

2. ______________ 6. ______________ 10. ______________

3. ______________ 7. ______________ 11. ______________

4. ______________ 8. ______________ 12. ______________

## EXERCISE 13-2 WORD PARTS

Break each of the following terms into its word parts: prefix, root, or suffix. Give the meaning of each word part and then define the term.

1. cholelithiasis

   root: ______

   suffix: ______

   suffix: ______

   definition: ______

2. enterohepatitis

   root: ______

   root: ______

   suffix: ______

   definition: ______

3. parotiditis

   prefix: ______

   root: ______

   suffix: ______

   definition: ______

4. sialorrhea

   root: ______

   suffix: ______

   definition: ______

5. colonoscopy

   root: ______

   suffix: ______

   definition: ______

6. gastroenterologist

   root: ______

   root: ______

   suffix: ______

   definition: ______

7. colectomy

   root: ______________________________

   suffix: ______________________________

   definition: ______________________________

8. jejunotomy

   root: ______________________________

   suffix: ______________________________

   definition: ______________________________

## EXERCISE 13-3 WORD BUILDING

**Use the word parts listed to build the terms defined.**

| | | | |
|---|---|---|---|
| -al | enter/o | -ia | phag/o |
| cholecyst/o | gastr/o | -ic | -pexy |
| col/o | -genic | -itis | -scope |
| duoden/o | gingiv/o | jejun/o | sial/o |
| dys- | hepat/o | -pathy | -stenosis |
| -ectomy | | | |

1. adjective form of stomach ____________________
2. any disease of the gallbladder ____________________
3. inflammation of the gums ____________________
4. narrowing of a salivary duct ____________________
5. instrument used to visually examine the intestines ____________________
6. fixation of the colon ____________________
7. removal of all or part of the jejunum ____________________
8. originating in the liver ____________________
9. difficulty swallowing ____________________
10. adjective form of duodenum ____________________

## EXERCISE 13-4  MATCHING

**Match the term with its definition.**

1. _____ buccal

2. _____ dentalgia

3. _____ esophagitis

4. _____ duodenum

5. _____ enteric

6. _____ emesis

7. _____ jaundice

8. _____ ascites

9. _____ esophagostenosis

10. _____ diarrhea

a. abnormal fluid accumulation in the abdomen

b. cheek

c. narrowing of the esophagus

d. vomiting

e. yellow

f. toothache

g. first part of small intestine

h. adjective referring to intestine(s)

i. inflammation of esophagus

j. watery discharge from the rectum; liquid stools

## EXERCISE 13-5  MULTIPLE CHOICE

**Choose the correct answer for the following multiple choice questions.**

1. Dysphagia is difficulty with _____.
   a. talking
   b. swallowing
   c. elimination
   d. digestion

2. Anorexia is _____.
   a. difficulty in digestion
   b. hyperemesis
   c. loss of appetite
   d. a small ulcer

3. Gas in the stomach or intestines is _____.
   a. gavage
   b. icterus
   c. flatus
   d. dysentery

4. Diverticulitis is an inflammation of _____.
   a. small pouches in the intestine
   b. the appendix
   c. the pharynx
   d. descending colon

5. Movement of the intestines in which contents are propelled toward the anus is termed __________.
   a. pyloroplasty
   b. volvulus
   c. peristalsis
   d. gastroenteric

6. The buccal mucosa is in the __________.
   a. nostril
   b. stomach and intestines
   c. mouth, inside the cheek
   d. greater curvature of the stomach

7. Belching is called __________.
   a. volvulus
   b. eructation
   c. gastroenteric
   d. halitosis

8. Vomiting blood is called __________.
   a. hematitis
   b. indigestion
   c. mastication
   d. hematemesis

9. Telescoping of the intestines into themselves is called __________.
   a. gastrojejunostomy
   b. intussusception
   c. volvulus
   d. sphincter

10. A colonoscopy is __________.
   a. an endoscopic study of the colon
   b. an upper endoscopy with biopsy
   c. a type of BE
   d. an endoscopic study of the small intestine

## EXERCISE 13-6 FILL IN THE BLANK

**Fill in the blank with the correct answer.**

1. The sphincter that controls flow from the ileum to the cecum is the __________.

2. The large intestine is divided into the cecum, colon, and __________.

3. Saliva is secreted by the __________.

4. The __________ is responsible for storing, condensing, and delivering bile to the small intestine.

5. A hiatal hernia is a disorder in which the ____________________ protrudes through the diaphragm.

6. Inflammation of the gallbladder is called ____________________.

7. Presence of calculi or stones in the gallbladder or bile ducts is called ____________________.

8. A drug that is used to relieve vomiting is called an ____________________.

9. The instrument used to view the stomach in a gastroscopy is a ____________________.

10. Removal of part of the stomach is called a ____________________.

## EXERCISE 13-7 ABBREVIATIONS

**Write out the term for the following abbreviations.**

1. ______________________________ PO
2. ______________________________ UGIS
3. ______________________________ TPN
4. ______________________________ BM
5. ______________________________ GI
6. ______________________________ GERD
7. ______________________________ IBS
8. ______________________________ LES

**Write the abbreviation for the following terms.**

9. ____________________ hydrochloric acid
10. ____________________ nasogastric
11. ____________________ barium enema
12. ____________________ esophagogastroduodenoscopy
13. ____________________ nothing by mouth

## EXERCISE 13-8 SPELLING

**Select the correct spelling of the medical term.**

1. The large intestine from the cecum to the rectum is also called the ____________________.
   a. colon
   b. cologne
   c. collon
   d. colin

2. The GI in GI tract stands for ____________________.
   a. gastrointestinle
   b. gastrointestinel
   c. gastrointestinal
   d. gastraentestinal

3. A loss of appetite is called ____________________.
   a. anoresia
   b. anorexia
   c. anarexia
   d. anorexsia

4. ____________________ is a chronic liver disease characterized by inflammation and degeneration.
   a. Cirosis
   b. Cirrhosis
   c. Cirrosis
   d. Cirhosis

5. A yellowish cast to the skin, scleras, and other mucous membranes caused by bile deposits is called ____________________.
   a. jandice
   b. juandice
   c. jaundise
   d. jaundice

6. A ____________________ is a surgical establishment of an opening into the colon.
   a. colostimy
   b. colostamy
   c. colostomy
   d. colostemy

7. Tarry, bloody stool is called ____________________.
   a. malena
   b. milena
   c. melena
   d. melana

8. A growth protruding from a stalk is a ____________________.
   a. polyp
   b. polip
   c. pollup
   d. pollyp

9. _____________________ is an eating disorder characterized by episodes of binge eating followed by self-induced vomiting and misuse of laxatives.
   a. Bullimia
   b. Bullemia
   c. Bulemia
   d. Bulimia

10. A _____________________ is an enlarged vein in or near the anus that may cause pain or bleeding.
    a. hemoroid
    b. hemorrhoid
    c. hemroid
    d. hemorhoid

## EXERCISE 13-9 CASE STUDY

**Reggie V., a middle-aged man, began feeling pain in his upper abdomen about a month ago. He described the pain as a burning sensation that at first disappeared after he took over-the-counter antacids. In the last 10 days or so, however, he has noticed that these measures have become less and less helpful.**

His pain is not accompanied by SOB, nausea, or chest pains, and his appetite remains normal. His BP was slightly elevated also, and he reported that on the basis of a family history of HTN, his GP had advised him to stop smoking cigarettes and restrict caffeinated drinks to one or two a day.

This patient's WBC count was normal. Endoscopy revealed a 1-cm gastric ulcer.

1. What does the abbreviation SOB stand for?

   _____________________________________________

2. What does the abbreviation BP stand for?

   _____________________________________________

3. Does the abbreviation HTN have anything to do with the first two abbreviations? Explain how each may relate to the other two.

   _____________________________________________

   _____________________________________________

4. What does WBC stand for?

   _____________________________________________

5. What word parts make up the word "endoscopy" in the case study? What does the term *endoscopy* mean?

   _____________________________________________

   _____________________________________________

6. What is a gastric ulcer?

   _____________________________________________

# The Urinary System

14

### LEARNING OUTCOMES

***Upon completion of this chapter, you should be able to:***

- Name the structures that make up the urinary system.
- Pronounce, spell, and define medical terms related to the urinary system and its disorders.
- Interpret abbreviations associated with the urinary system.

## INTRODUCTION

The **urinary system** is composed of the *kidneys*, *ureters*, *urinary bladder*, and *urethra* (see Figure 14-1A). These organs are responsible for the formation, storage, and removal of urine. These processes start with the **kidneys**, paired structures that remove wastes from the bloodstream, reclaim important electrolytes like sodium and potassium, help regulate blood pressure and fluid balance, and aid in red blood cell production. The kidneys then form **urine**, which is fluid containing water and dissolved substances. The **ureters** are tubular structures that transport urine from the kidneys to the **urinary bladder**, an organ that stores urine. The urine is then eliminated through the **urethra**, a canal leading from the urinary bladder to the exterior. This process regulates the amount of water in the body and maintains the proper balance of acids and electrolytes, which is necessary for human survival. Figure 14-1B shows the processes of urine formation, transport, storage, and elimination.

## WORD PARTS RELATED TO THE URINARY SYSTEM

Nephr/o and ren/o are both root words that mean kidney. The term *cyst* and the word part *cyst/o* mean bladder, whereas the word parts ur/o and urin/o mean urine. Table 14-1 lists word parts used in forming urinary system terms.

> What's the difference between the roots nephr/o and ren/o? Both may be used to refer to the kidneys. However, nephr/o is used in the names of most, but not all, kidney disorders and treatments. For example, nephr/o is the root in nephritis, nephralgia, nephrectomy, nephrorrhaphy, nephrotomy, and nephromegaly. In general, the term *nephrology* is also more common than renology, but the adjective renal is far more common than its counterpart, nephric. Renal is more common when naming structures, such as the renal capsule and the renal fascia.

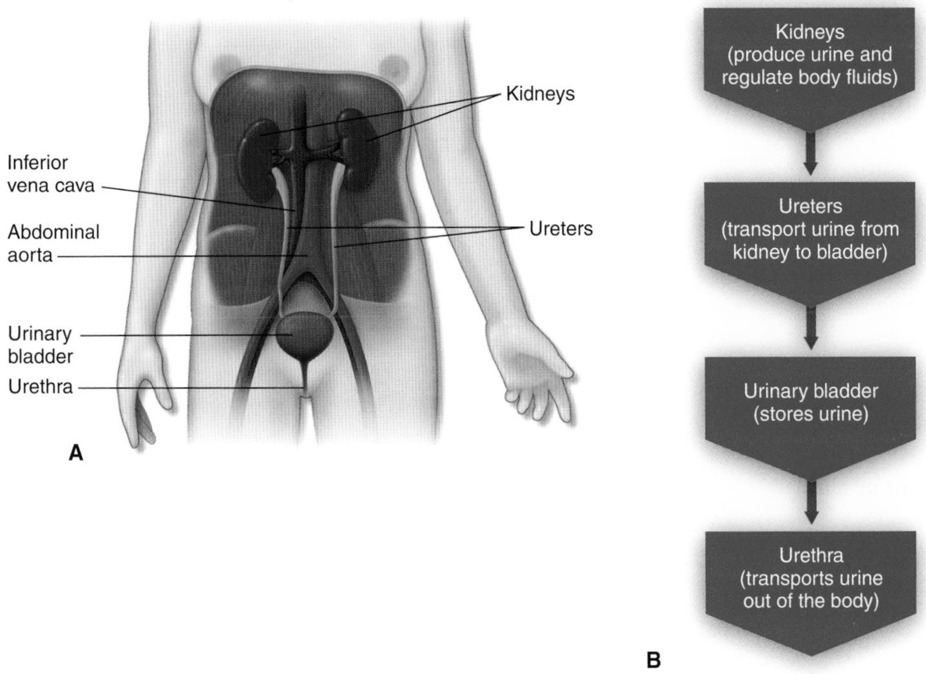


**FIGURE 14-1.** Primary organs of the urinary system. **A.** Anterior view of the kidneys, ureters, urinary bladder, and urethra (male). **B.** The process of urine formation, transport, storage, and elimination, beginning with the kidney and ending with the urethra.

## STRUCTURE AND FUNCTION

The kidneys are bean-shaped organs (hence the source for the name of the kidney bean) and are about the size of a deck of cards. They lie retroperiotoneally, which is posterior to the peritoneum in the abdominopelvic cavity, along each side of the spinal column. Each kidney is covered by a thin

**TABLE 14-1 WORD PARTS RELATED TO THE URINARY SYSTEM**

| Word Part | Meaning |
|---|---|
| cyst/o | bladder |
| glomerul/o | glomerulus |
| -iasis | condition, state |
| lith/o | stone |
| nephr/o, ren/o | kidney |
| noct/o | night |
| olig/o | few, little |
| poly- | much, many |
| py/o | pus |
| pyel/o | pelvis |
| ur/o, urin/o | urine |
| ureter/o | ureter |
| urethr/o | urethra |

## Word Parts Exercise

After studying **Table 14-1**, write the meaning of each of the word parts.

| WORD PART | MEANING |
|---|---|
| 1. ur/o, urin/o | 1. ________________ |
| 2. noct/o | 2. ________________ |
| 3. olig/o | 3. ________________ |
| 4. –iasis | 4. ________________ |
| 5. glomerul/o | 5. ________________ |
| 6. nephr/o, ren/o | 6. ________________ |
| 7. urethr/o | 7. ________________ |
| 8. lith/o | 8. ________________ |
| 9. poly- | 9. ________________ |
| 10. py/o | 10. ________________ |
| 11. pyel/o | 11. ________________ |
| 12. ureter/o | 12. ________________ |
| 13. cyst/o | 13. ________________ |



membrane called the *fibrous capsule*. A thicker layer of fatty tissue, called the **perinephric fat** or *pararenal fat body*, surrounds the fibrous capsule and thus provides protection for this vital organ. Finally, a thin layer of connective tissue, called the **renal fascia**, forms each kidney's outer covering. The two regions of the kidney are the outer **renal cortex** and the inner **renal medulla**. The **hilum** is the indented and narrowest part of the kidney, where blood vessels and nerves enter and leave. The flattened funnel-shaped expansion of the upper end of the ureter where urine collects in the kidney is called the **renal pelvis**. The cup-like structure that drains into the renal pelvis is the **calyx**. Figure 14-2 shows the anatomy of a kidney.

The kidneys form urine and remove two natural products of metabolism, **urea** and **uric acid**, along with other wastes from the blood. The kidneys also filter, reabsorb, and secrete nonwaste products back into the bloodstream.

Filtration and the urine production begin in the **nephrons**, which are the functional units of the kidneys. Each kidney has approximately 1 million nephrons, and each nephron consists of a *renal corpuscle* and the *renal tubule*. The **renal corpuscle** is a structure composed of the *glomerulus* and the *glomerular* (Bowman's) *capsule*. The **glomerulus** consists of a cluster of capillaries through which blood and wastes are filtered. The **renal tubule** consists of the *proximal convoluted tubule*, *nephron loop* (loop of Henle), and the *distal convoluted tubule* (see Figure 14-3). Fluid not returned to the bloodstream becomes urine, is collected in the *collecting duct*, and moves into the

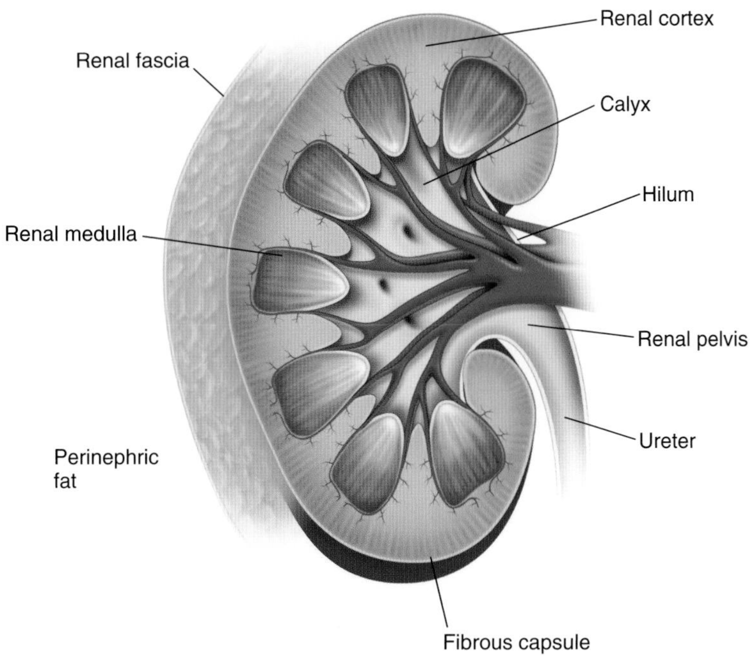


**FIGURE 14-2** Sagittal view of the kidney and internal structures.

renal pelvis before ultimately entering the ureter. The ureters carry the urine to the urinary bladder, where it is stored.

The urinary bladder stores the urine until a sufficient volume causes an increase in pressure and triggers the urge to urinate via the *micturition reflex*. The **micturition reflex** is a contraction of the

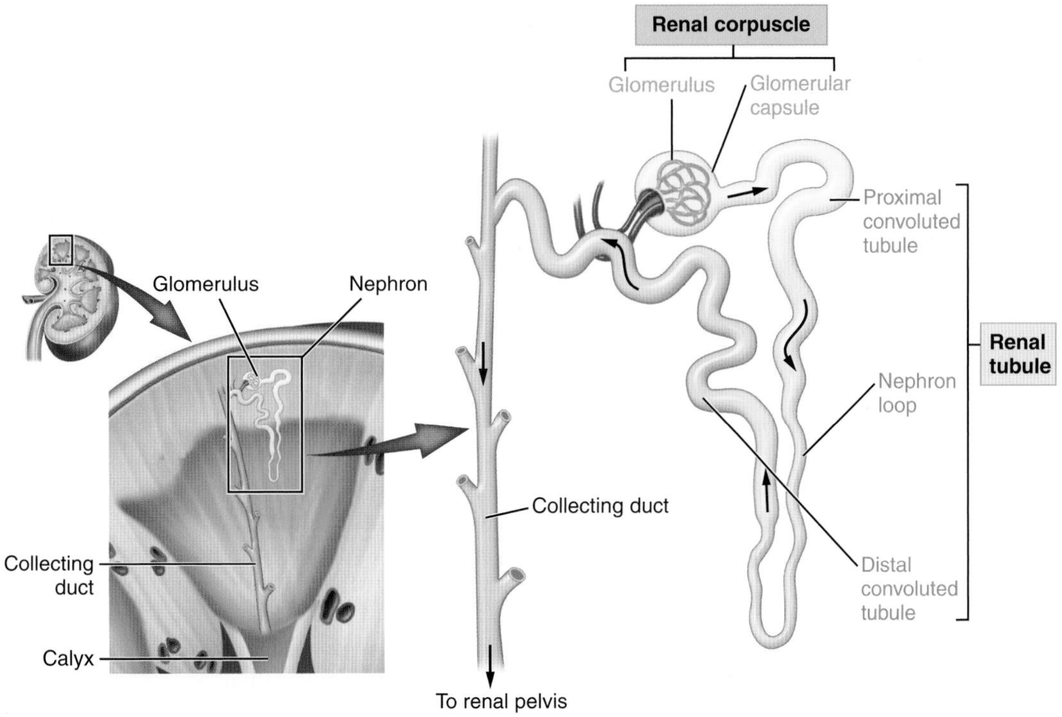


**FIGURE 14-3** Section of the kidney showing a representative nephron.

walls of the urinary bladder and relaxation of the urethral sphincter in response to the rise in urinary bladder pressure. Micturition is also called *urination*, *uresis*, or *voiding*. Urination is regulated by two sphincters, the circular muscles that surround the urethra. They are the *internal urethral sphincter*, which is located at the entrance to the urethra and is involuntarily controlled, and the *external urethral sphincter*, which is located at the distal end of the urethra and is under voluntary control.

### Quick Check

**Fill in the blanks.**

1. Name the primary organs of the urinary system. ________________, ________________, ________________ ________________
2. The indented part of the kidney, where blood vessels and nerves enter or exit, is called the ________________.
3. Name the two urethral sphincters. ________________________________



## DISORDERS RELATED TO THE URINARY SYSTEM

Disorders of the urinary system can affect any urinary structures. Some of these disorders are listed as follows:

- **Dysuria**: painful, difficult urination
- **Incontinence**: the loss of urinary control
- **Retention**: the inability to empty the bladder
- **Urinary tract infections (UTIs)**: infection of the urinary tract. Examples of UTIs include the following:
  - **Cystitis**: inflammation of the urinary bladder, usually caused by infection
  - **Glomerulonephritis**: inflammation of the glomerulus, which can involve one or both kidneys, usually caused by infection
  - **Nephritis**: inflammation of the kidney(s), usually caused by infection
  - **Pyelonephritis**: inflammation of the calyces and renal pelvis, typically due to bacterial infection
  - **Urethritis**: inflammation of the urethra, usually caused by infection
- **Renal failure** or *end-stage renal disease* (ESRD) is loss of renal function that results in kidneys ceasing urine production. It can be acute renal failure (ARF) or chronic renal failure (CRF).

## DIAGNOSTIC TESTS, TREATMENTS, AND SURGICAL PROCEDURES

The root cyst/o is used to form terms having to do with the urinary bladder. Examples include **cystalgia** (pain in the urinary bladder), **cystectomy** (excision of the urinary bladder), and **cystopexy** (surgical attachment of the urinary bladder to the abdominal wall or to other supporting structures). All of these terms come from the Greek word *kystis*, which means bladder.

A test of kidney function is the *glomerular filtration rate* (GFR). This test determines the volume of water filtered out of the blood plasma through the capillary walls into the glomerular capsule per unit of time. An X-ray or computed tomography (CT) scan of the kidneys, ureters, and bladder (KUB) after intravenous injection of a contrast dye is known as an *intravenous pyelogram* (IVP). The contrast is injected into a vein and is excreted by the kidneys to show the urinary system. Blood urea nitrogen (BUN) is a blood test that measures kidney function by assessing the level of nitrogenous waste and urea that are in the blood.

## PRACTICE AND PRACTITIONERS

A physician who specializes in the diagnosis and treatment of urinary disorders is called a **urologist**, and the specialty practice is **urology**. A physician who treats the kidney and kidney disorders is called a **nephrologist**. This area of specialty is named **nephrology**.

### Abbreviation Table THE URINARY SYSTEM

| ABBREVIATION | MEANING |
|---|---|
| ARF | acute renal failure |
| BUN | blood urea nitrogen |
| CAPD | continuous ambulatory peritoneal dialysis |
| CRF | chronic renal failure |
| CT | computed tomography |
| ESRD | end-stage renal disease |
| GFR | glomerular filtration rate |
| IVP | intravenous pyelogram |
| KUB | kidneys, ureter, and bladder |
| UA | urinalysis |
| UTI | urinary tract infection |

### Study Table THE URINARY SYSTEM

| TERM AND PRONUNCIATION | ANALYSIS | MEANING |
|---|---|---|
| **Structure and Function** | | |
| calyx (KAY-liks) | from the Greek *kalux* (cup of a flower) | cup-like structure that drains into the renal pelvis |
| electrolyte (ee-LEK-troh-lyte) | from the Greek words *electron* (able to produce static electricity by friction) and *lytos* (soluble) | an ionizable substance, such as sodium or potassium, in solution within body cells |
| glomerulus (gloh-MER-yu-luhs) | from the Latin word *glomus* (ball of yarn) | capillary network found inside each nephron |
| hilum (HY-luhm) | a Latin word meaning “a small thing,” “a trifle” | narrow part of the kidney where blood vessels and nerves enter and leave |
| kidney (KID-nee) | originally *kidenere*, perhaps a compound of Old English *cwith* (womb) + *neere* (kidney) in reference to the shape of the organ | organ that excretes urine, removes nitrogenous wastes of metabolism, reclaims electrolytes and water, and contributes to blood pressure and red blood cell production |

(continued)

**Study Table** THE URINARY SYSTEM *(continued)*

| TERM AND PRONUNCIATION | ANALYSIS | MEANING |
|---|---|---|
| micturition (mik-chuh-RISH-uhn) | from the Latin *micturio* (to desire to urinate) | urination; *uresis*; *voiding* |
| micturition reflex (mik-chuh-RISH-uhn REE-fleks) | from the Latin *micturio* (to desire to urinate) and the Latin word *reflexus* (to bend back) | contraction of the bladder walls and relaxation of the bladder and urethral sphincter in response to a rise in pressure within the bladder |
| nephron (NEFF-ron) | from the Greek word *nephros* (kidney) | tiny structure within the kidney in which the urine-production process begins |
| perinephric fat (PERH-ih-NEF-rik FAT) | *peri-* (around); *nephr-* (kidney) *-ic* (adjective suffix) | fatty tissue surrounding the renal capsule; *pararenal fat body* |
| renal capsule (REE-nul KAP-suhl) | *ren/o* (kidney); *-al* (adjective suffix); *capsula*, a Latin word meaning "a small box" | thin membrane covering each kidney, deep to the perinephric fat and renal fascia |
| renal corpuscle (REE-nul KOR-pus-el) | from the Latin word *renalis* (kidneys) + the Latin word *corpusculum* (body) | the collection of glomerular capillaries and the glomerular (Bowman's) capsule that encloses them |
| renal cortex (REE-nul KOR-teks) | from the Latin words *renalis* (kidneys) and *cortex* (bark) | outer region of the kidney |
| renal fascia (REE-nul FASH-ee-ah) | *ren/o* (kidney); *-al* (adjective suffix); *fascia*, a Latin word meaning band or sash | protective outer covering of the kidney |
| renal medulla (REE-nul me-DOO-luh) | from the Latin word *renalis* (kidneys); from the French word *medius* (middle) | inner region of the kidney |
| renal pelvis (REE-nul PEL-vis) | from the Latin words *renalis* (kidneys) and *pelvis* (basin) | a reservoir in each kidney that collects urine |
| renal tubule (REE-nul TOO-byool) | from the Latin words *renalis* (kidneys) and *tubulus* (tube) | small tubes including the proximal convoluted tubule, nephron loop (loop of Henle), and the distal convoluted tubule that convey urine from the glomeruli to the renal pelvis |
| retroperitoneal (reh-troh-pehr-ih-toh-NEE-al) | *retro-* (backward, behind); from the Greek word *periteinein* (to stretch over) | external or posterior to the peritoneum, which is a serous membrane lining the abdominopelvic cavity |
| sphincters (SFINK-tehrs) | from the Greek word *sphincter* (band, anything that binds tight) | circular muscle that surrounds a tube such as the urethra and constricts the tube when it contracts |

**Study Table** THE URINARY SYSTEM (*continued*)

| TERM AND PRONUNCIATION | ANALYSIS | MEANING |
|---|---|---|
| urea (yu-REE-ah) | from the French word *uree* (urine) | natural waste product of metabolism that is excreted in urine |
| ureters (yu-REE-tehrs; also YUR-eh-tehrs) | from the Greek word *oureter,* from *ourein* (to urinate) | two tubes that transfer urine from the kidneys to the urinary bladder |
| urethra (yu-REE-thrah) | from the Greek word *ourethra,* from *ourein* (to urinate) | tube that conducts urine away from the bladder for expulsion |
| uric acid (YUR-ik AS-id) | *ur/o* (urine); *-ic* (adjective suffix) + acid from the Latin word *acidus* (sour-tasting) | natural waste product of metabolism that is excreted in urine |
| urinary bladder (YUR-ihn-ayr-ee BLAD-dehr) | from the Greek word *ouron* (urine); Anglo-Saxon, *blaedre* (bladder) | temporary storage receptacle for urine |
| urinate (YUR-ihn-ayt) | *urin/o* (urine); *-ate* (verb suffix) | passing of urine |
| urine (YUR-ihn) | from the Greek word *ouron* (urine) | water and soluble substances excreted by the kidneys |
| void (voyd) | from Old French *voide* (empty, hollow, waste) | to urinate |
| **Disorders** | | |
| albuminuria (al-byu-mihn-YUR-ee-ah) | from the Latin *albumen* (egg white); *ur/o* (urine); *-ia* (condition) | presence of the protein, albumin, in the urine, typically a sign of kidney disease |
| anuria (an-YUR-ee-ah) | *an-* (without); *ur/o* (urine); *-ia* (condition) | failure of the kidneys to produce urine |
| calculus (KAL-kyu-luhs); plural: calculi (KAL-kyu-lye) | a Latin word meaning small pebble | a kidney stone (in the context of this body system) |
| cystalgia (sihs-TAL-jee-ah) | *cyst/o* (bladder); *-algia* (pain) | pain in the urinary bladder |
| cystitis (sihs-TYE-tihs) | *cyst/o* (bladder); *-itis* (inflammation) | inflammation of the urinary bladder |
| cystocele (SIHS-toh-seel) | *cyst/o* (bladder); *-cele* (hernia) | hernia of the urinary bladder |
| cystolith (SIS-toh-lith) | *cyst/o* (bladder); *-lith* (stone) | urinary bladder stone |
| dysuria (dihs-YUR-ee-ah) | *dys-* (difficult); *ur/o* (urine); *-ia* (condition) | difficult or painful urination |
| enuresis (en-yoo-REE-sis) | from Greek *enourein* (to urinate in) | bedwetting |
| glomerulonephritis (gloh-mer-yoo-loh-ne-FRY-tis) | *glomerul/o* (glomerulus); *nephr/o* (kidney); *-itis* (inflammation) | inflammation of the kidney glomeruli typically caused by an immune response and not an acute response to kidney infection |

(*continued*)

**Study Table** THE URINARY SYSTEM (*continued*)

| TERM AND PRONUNCIATION | ANALYSIS | MEANING |
|---|---|---|
| glycosuria (gly-kohs-YUR-ee-ah) | *glycos-* (sugar); *ur/o* (urine); *-ia* (condition) | presence of carbohydrates (sugar) in the urine; *glucosuria* |
| hematuria (hee-ma-TYOO-ree-uh) | *hemat/o* (blood); *ur/o* (urine); *-ia* (adjective suffix) | presence of blood in the urine |
| incontinence (in-KON-tih-nents) | from the Latin word *incontinentia* (inability to retain) | inability to control urination |
| nephralgia (neh-FRAL-jee-ah) | *nephr/o* (kidney); *-algia* (pain) | pain in the kidneys |
| nephritis (neh-FRY-tihs) | *nephr/o* (kidney); *-itis* (inflammation) | inflammation of the kidney |
| nephrolithiasis (NEFF-ro-lih-THY-ah-sihs) | *nephr/o* (kidney); *lith/o* (stone); *-iasis* (condition) | the presence of renal calculi |
| nephromegaly (neh-fro-MEG-ah-lee) | *nephr/o* (kidney); *-megaly* (enlargement) | enlargement of one or both kidneys; *renomegaly* |
| nephropathy (neh-FROP-ah-thee) | *nephr/o* (kidney); *-pathy* (disease) | any disease of the kidney |
| nephroptosis (neh-FROP-toh-sis) | *nephr/o* (kidney); *-ptosis* (falling downward, prolapse) | prolapse (slipping out of position) of the kidney |
| nocturia (noc-TUR-ee-ah) | *noct/o* (night); *ur/o* (urine); *-ia* (condition) | excessive urination at night |
| oliguria (oh-lih-GUR-ee-ah) | *olig/o* (little); *ur/o* (urine); *-ia* (condition) | diminished urine production |
| polyuria (pol-ee-YUR-ee-ah) | *poly-* (much, many); *ur/o* (urine); *-ia* (condition) | excessive urine production |
| pyelonephritis (pye-eh-loh-neh-FRY-tis) | *pyel/o* (pelvis); *nephr/o* (kidney); *-itis* (inflammation) | inflammation of the renal calyces and renal pelvis due to local bacteria infection |
| pyuria (pu-YOUR-ee-ah) | *py/o* (pus); *ur/o* (urine); *-ia* (condition) | pus in the urine |
| renal calculus (REE-nahl KAL-ku-luhs) | *ren/o* (kidney); *calculus,* a Latin word meaning "stone" | a kidney stone |
| renal failure (REE-nahl FAIL-yur) | *ren/o* (kidney); *-al* (adjective suffix); failure, common English word | impairment of renal function, either acute or chronic, with retention of urea, creatinine (compound produced by the metabolism of creatine), and other waste products |
| renal hypoplasia (REE-nahl HY-poh-PLAYZ-ee-ah) | *ren/o* (kidney); *hypo-* (below normal); *-plasia* (formation, development) | an underdeveloped kidney |

**Study Table** THE URINARY SYSTEM (*continued*)

| TERM AND PRONUNCIATION | ANALYSIS | MEANING |
|---|---|---|
| retention (ree-TEN-shun) | from the Latin word *retentio* (a retaining, a holding back) | the inability to empty the bladder |
| uremia (yu-REE-mee-ah) or azotemia (ays-oh-TEAM-ee-ah) | *ur/o* (urine); *-emia* (blood condition) | an excess of urea in the blood |
| ureteritis (yoo-ree-ter-EYE-tis) | *ureter/o* (ureter); *-itis* (inflammation) | inflammation of a ureter |
| urethralgia (yu-ree-THRAL-jee-ah) | *urethr/o* (urethra); *-algia* (pain) | pain in the urethra; *urethrodynia* |
| urethritis (yu-ree-THRY-tihs) | *urethr/o* (urethra); *-itis* (inflammation) | inflammation of the urethra |
| urethrostenosis (yu-REE-throh-steh-NO-sihs) | *urethr/o* (urethra); *sten/o* (narrow); *-sis* (condition) | narrowing of the urethra |
| urinary tract infection (yur-ih-NAIR-ee TRAKT in-FEK-shun) | *urin/o* (urine); *-ary* (adjective suffix); 1 tract 1 infection | microbial infection of any part of the urinary tract |
| **Diagnostic Tests, Treatments, and Surgical Procedures** | | |
| antibiotic (an-tee-BYE-ot-ik) | from *anti-* (against) + the Greek word *biotikos* (fit for life) | medicine that inhibits the growth of bacteria |
| catheter (CATH-eh-tehr) | from the Greek word *kathienai* (to let down, thrust in) | a flexible tube that enables passage of fluid from or into a body cavity |
| cystectomy (sihs-TEK-toh-mee) | *cyst/o* (bladder); *-ectomy* (excision) | excision of the urinary bladder |
| cystopexy (SIHS-toh-pek-see) | *cyst/o* (bladder); *-pexy* (fixation) | surgical attachment (fixation) of the urinary bladder to the abdominal wall or other supporting structures |
| cystoscopy (sihs-TOS-ko-pee) | *cyst/o* (bladder); *-scopy* (use of an instrument for viewing) | visual inspection of the urinary bladder by means of an instrument called a cystoscope |
| dialysis (dy-AL-ih-sihs) | a Greek word meaning "dissolution," "separation" | filtration to remove colloidal particles from a fluid; a method of artificial kidney function; types include continuous ambulatory peritoneal dialysis (CAPD) and extracorporeal dialysis |
| diuretic (dy-yu-REHT-ik) | from the Greek words *dia-* (through) and *ourein* (urine) | drug that promotes urination |
| hemodialysis (HEE-mo-dy-AL-ih-sihs) | *hemo-* (blood); *dialysis*, a Greek word meaning "dissolution," "separation" | removal of unwanted substances from the blood by passage through a semipermeable membrane; *kidney dialysis* |

(*continued*)

**Study Table** THE URINARY SYSTEM (*continued*)

| TERM AND PRONUNCIATION | ANALYSIS | MEANING |
|---|---|---|
| kidney transplant (KID-nee TRANS-plant) | originally *kidenere,* perhaps a compound of Old English *cwith* (womb) +*neere* (kidney) in reference to the shape of the organ; from the late Latin *transplantare* (something moved to a new place) | operation in which a donor kidney is placed into a recipient |
| lithotripsy (LITH-oh-trip-see) | *lith/o* (stone); *-tripsy* (crushing) | treatment in which a stone in the kidney, urethra, or urinary bladder is broken up into small particles |
| nephrectomy (neh-FREK-toh-mee) | *nephr/o* (kidney); *-ectomy* (removal) | removal of a kidney |
| nephrolithotomy (NEH-froh-lih-THOT-oh-mee) | *nephr/o* (kidney); *lith/o* (stone); *-tomy* (incision into) | incision into the kidney to remove a kidney stone |
| nephropexy (NEF-roh-pek-see) | *nephr/o* (kidney) + the Greek work *pexis* (fixation) | operative fixation of a floating or mobile kidney |
| ureteroplasty (yu-REE-tehr-oh-plass-tee) | *ureter/o* (ureter); *-plasty* (surgical repair) | surgical repair of a ureter |
| ureterorrhaphy (yu-ree-ter-OR-uh-fee) | *ureter/o* (ureter); *-rrhaphy* (surgical suturing) | suture of a ureter |
| ureteroscope (yu-REE-tehr-oh-skohp) | *ureter/o* (ureter); *-scope* (instrument for viewing) | instrument used to visually examine the ureter |
| urinalysis (UA) (yur-ih-NAL-ih-sihs) | *urin/o* (urine); *-alysis* from the English word analysis | analysis of urine by physical, chemical, and microscopic means to test for the presence of substances or disease |
| **Practice and Practitioners** | | |
| nephrologist (neh-FROL-oh-jist) | *nephr/o* (kidney); *-logist* (one who studies a special field) | a medical specialist who diagnoses and treats disorders of the kidney |
| nephrology (neh-FROL-oh-jee) | *nephr/o* (kidney); *-logy* (study of) | medical specialty dealing with the kidneys |
| urologist (yu-ROL-oh-jist) | *ur/o* (urine); *-logist* (one who studies a special field) | a medical specialist who diagnoses and treats disorders of the urinary system |
| urology (yu-ROL-oh-jee) | *ur/o* (urine); *-logy* (study of) | the medical specialty dealing with the urinary system |

# END-OF-CHAPTER EXERCISES

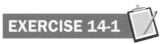

## EXERCISE 14-1 LABELING

**Using the following word list, choose the correct terms to label the diagram correctly.**

| | | |
|---|---|---|
| abdominal aorta | kidneys | urethra |
| inferior vena cava | ureters | urinary bladder |

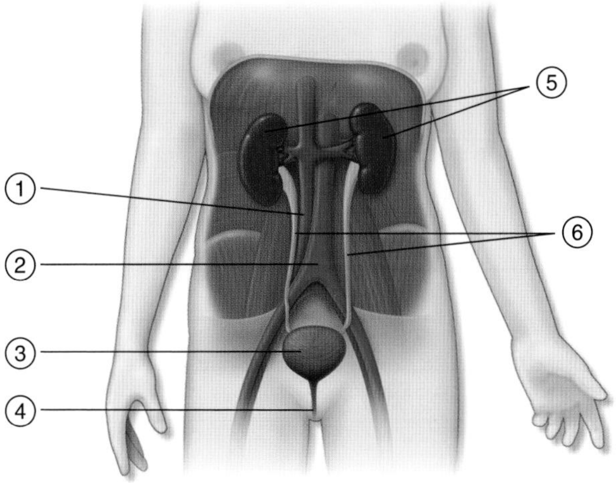


1. ____________________  3. ____________________  5. ____________________

2. ____________________  4. ____________________  6. ____________________

## EXERCISE 14-2 WORD PARTS

**Break each of the following terms into its word parts: root, prefix, or suffix. Give the meaning of each word part and then define each term.**

1. *anuria*

   prefix: ____________________

   root: ____________________

   suffix: ____________________

   definition: ____________________

2. *cystalgia*

   root: ____________________

   suffix: ____________________

   definition: ____________________

3. *nephrolithiasis*

   root: ______________________________

   root: ______________________________

   suffix: ______________________________

   definition: ______________________________

4. *hematuria*

   root: ______________________________

   root: ______________________________

   suffix: ______________________________

   definition: ______________________________

5. *glomerulonephritis*

   root: ______________________________

   root: ______________________________

   suffix: ______________________________

   definition: ______________________________

6. *nephrologist*

   root: ______________________________

   suffix: ______________________________

   definition: ______________________________

7. *urology*

   root: ______________________________

   suffix: ______________________________

   definition: ______________________________

8. *nephrectomy*

   root: ______________________________

   suffix: ______________________________

   definition: ______________________________

## EXERCISE 14-3 WORD BUILDING

**Use the word parts listed to build the terms defined.**

| | | | |
|---|---|---|---|
| albumen | urethro | -tripsy | cyst/o |
| -ur/o | -stenosis | ur/o | -ectomy |
| -ia | ur/o | -logist | -scope |
| nephro | -emia | nephr/o | urter/o |
| -aliga | lith/o | -logy | -rrhaphy |

1. presence of protein in urine ____________________
2. pain in the kidneys ____________________
3. narrowing of the urethra ____________________
4. an excess of urea in the blood ____________________
5. treatment in which a stone is broken into smaller particles ____________________
6. one who studies the urinary system ____________________
7. study of the kidney ____________________
8. excision of the bladder ____________________
9. instrument used to examine the bladder ____________________
10. suture of a ureter ____________________

## EXERCISE 14-4 MATCHING

**Match the term with its definition.**

| | | |
|---|---|---|
| 1. ________________ | nephron | a. capillary network found inside each nephron |
| 2. ________________ | urethra | b. urination |
| 3. ________________ | renal calculus | c. pain in the bladder |
| 4. ________________ | glomerulus | d. tube that conducts urine away from the bladder for excretion |
| 5. ________________ | micturition | e. an ionizable substance in solution within body cells |
| 6. ________________ | uric acid | f. narrow part of the kidney where blood vessels and nerves enter and exit |
| 7. ________________ | ureters | g. functional unit of the kidney |
| 8. ________________ | hilum | h. two tubes that transfer urine from the kidneys to the urinary bladder |
| 9. ________________ | electrolyte | i. X-ray of the ureter |
| 10. ________________ | UA | j. natural waste product of metabolism excreted in the urine |
| 11. ________________ | nephralgia | k. a kidney stone |
| 12. ________________ | nephritis | l. excision of a kidney, ureter, and at least part of the urinary bladder |
| 13. ________________ | urethrostenosis | m. inflammation of the kidney |
| 14. ________________ | nephrolithotomy | n. narrowing of the urethra |
| 15. ________________ | nephroureterocystectomy | o. any disease of the kidney |
| 16. ________________ | ureterography | p. pain in the kidneys |
| 17. ________________ | cystalgia | q. incision into the kidney to remove a calculus (kidney stone) |
| 18. ________________ | nephropathy | r. urinalysis |

## EXERCISE 14-5 MULTIPLE CHOICE

**Choose the correct answer for the following multiple choice questions.**

1. The _________________ carry the urine from the renal pelvis to the urinary bladder.
   a. urethra
   b. meatus
   c. cortex
   d. ureters

2. The inability to hold urine is called _________________.
   a. polyuria
   b. incontinence
   c. hematuria
   d. enuresis

3. Excretion of urine from the bladder is properly termed as _________________.
   a. voiding
   b. micturition
   c. urination
   d. all of the above

4. The functioning unit of the kidney is the _________________.
   a. nephron
   b. cortex of the kidney
   c. glomeruli
   d. pelvis of the kidney

5. What does anuria mean?
   a. failure to produce urine
   b. no urine from the kidney
   c. painful urination
   d. pus in the urine

6. What term means destruction of kidney tissue?
   a. nephrolithiasis
   b. neurolysis
   c. nephrolysis
   d. resection

7. What is the correct plural form of the word calculus?
   a. calcula
   b. calculuses
   c. calculi
   d. calculae

8. What is the term for surgical repair of a ureter?
   a. ureterectomy
   b. ureteroplasty
   c. ureterectasia
   d. ureterolysis

9. A hernia of the urinary bladder is called a ________________.
   a. cystitis
   b. cystocele
   c. cystalgia
   d. cystolith

10. Which of the following is NOT a correct match between a word part and its definition?
    a. cyst/o; bladder
    b. py/o; pus
    c. pyel/o; pelvis
    d. urethr/o; ureter



## EXERCISE 14-6 FILL IN THE BLANK

**Fill in the blank with the correct answer.**

1. Tom suffered from CRF. His sister donated one of her normal kidneys to him and he had a(n) ________________.
2. Cindy had a floating kidney that required surgical fixation. Her urologist performed a surgical procedure known as a(n) ________________.
3. The surgeons operated on Robert to remove a kidney stone (calculus) from his kidney. The name of this surgery is ________________.
4. Gabbi had to have one of her ureters repaired because of a stricture. This procedure is called ________________.
5. The physician had to examine Joshua's bladder for blood. They used a special instrument. This procedure is called a(n) ________________.
6. ________________ are medications that promote urination.
7. The two tubes that transfer urine from the kidneys to the urinary bladder are the ________________.
8. Natural waste products of metabolism that are excreted in urine include ________________.
9. Filtration to remove colloidal particles from a fluid is called ________________.
10. The word part *-logist* in urologist means ________________.

## EXERCISE 14-7 ABBREVIATIONS

**Write out the term for the following abbreviations.**

1. ______________________________ UTI
2. ______________________________ GFR
3. ______________________________ ESRD
4. ______________________________ BUN
5. ______________________________ CRF

**Write the abbreviation for the following terms.**

6. ____________ urinalysis
7. ____________ kidney, ureter, and bladder
8. ____________ acute renal failure
9. ____________ intravenous pyelogram
10. ____________ continuous ambulatory peritoneal dialysis

## EXERCISE 14-8 SPELLING

**Select the correct spelling of the medical term.**

1. The ____________ is a tiny structure within the kidney in which the urine production process begins.
   a. nephron
   b. nephran
   c. nephren
   d. nefron

2. An ____________ is an ionizable substance in solution.
   a. electrolyte
   b. electralyte
   c. electrolite
   d. electrelyte

3. A circular muscle that surrounds a tube and constricts the tube when it contracts is called a ____________.
   a. spincter
   b. sphincter
   c. sphicter
   d. sphinter

4. The presence of protein in the urine is ________________.
   a. albumineria
   b. albumineralia
   c. albumineuria
   d. albuminuria

5. A ________________ is a drug that promotes the excretion of urine.
   a. diretic
   b. diuritic
   c. diuretic
   d. duiretic

6. Excessive urination at night is known as ________________.
   a. nocturia
   b. nocturnia
   c. nocteria
   d. nockturia

7. A ________________ is a flexible tube that enables passage of fluid from or into a body cavity.
   a. cathater
   b. cathiter
   c. catheter
   d. cathuter

8. Difficult or painful urination is called ________________.
   a. dysurea
   b. disuria
   c. disurea
   d. dysuria

9. A treatment in which a stone in the kidney, urethra, or urinary bladder is broken up into small particles is called ________________.
   a. lithutripsy
   b. lithetripsy
   c. lithotripsy
   d. lithotripsee

10. The purpose of a ________________ is to detect and manage a wide range of disorders, which can include diabetes, kidney disease, or UTI's.
   a. urinalasis
   b. urinealysis
   c. urinlasis
   d. urinalysis

## EXERCISE 14-9 CASE STUDY

**Read the following case study. There are 11 phrases that can be reworded with a medical term that was introduced in this chapter. Determine what the term is and write your answers in the space provided.**

Heather is a 40-year-old female who saw a (1) specialist who treats disorders of the urinary system for complaints of urinary frequency, (2) painful urination, (3) blood in her urine, and low abdominal pain. She was also experiencing a low-grade fever and general fatigue. The doctor ordered a (4) laboratory reading of her urine and an (5) X-ray of her kidneys, ureters, and bladder. The laboratory results showed red blood cells in the urine, and the urine was cloudy with an odor. Tests indicated multiple (6) small, round, calcified objects in the (7) urine reservoir. Heather was diagnosed with a (8) condition of having bacteria in the urinary tract and also (9) stones in her bladder. The doctor ordered a(n) (10) drug used to kill bacteria, and he told Heather that she needed to have a (11) procedure in which a scope is inserted into the bladder to remove the stones. Heather's signs and symptoms improved, and she returned to have the procedure. Her recovery was uneventful.

1. ______________________________
2. ______________________________
3. ______________________________
4. ______________________________
5. ______________________________
6. ______________________________
7. ______________________________
8. ______________________________
9. ______________________________
10. ______________________________
11. ______________________________

15

# The Reproductive System

## LEARNING OUTCOMES

***Upon completion of this chapter, you should be able to:***

- Label diagrams of the male and female reproductive systems.
- Name the structures that make up the male and female reproductive systems.
- Understand medical terms related to pregnancy.
- Pronounce, spell, and define medical terms related to the reproductive system and its disorders.
- Interpret abbreviations associated with the reproductive system.

## INTRODUCTION

The primary function of the reproductive system is to perpetuate life. The reproductive process begins with fertilization, which occurs when sex cells called **gametes** fuse. Male gametes are known as **sperm** and female gametes are known as **oocytes**. The name for the organ that produces a gamete is **gonad**. Male gonads are *testes*, whereas female gonads are *ovaries*.

The single cell formed at **fertilization** (the fusion of a sperm with an oocyte) is called a **zygote**. A zygote contains more than a trillion molecules, despite its diameter of only 0.1 mm. These trillion or so molecules all communicate and work together forming a human organism.

## WORD PARTS RELATED TO THE REPRODUCTIVE SYSTEM

The reproductive system is the one body system where both structure and function vary greatly between the sexes. For this reason, there are very different word parts to describe the male and the female reproductive systems. Word parts that refer to the testes, prostate, sperm, and penis are only applicable to the male system, whereas word parts that refer to the breasts, vagina, ovaries, uterine tubes, and uterus apply to the female system.

Anatomists and clinicians use the singular term *testis* or the plural term *testes* to refer to the male gonad(s), but *testicle* and *testicles* are also commonly used. The Latin word for "testis" is *testis*, but the Latin word for "testicle" is *testiculus*, which is a diminutive form of *testis*. The Greek word for testicle is *orkheos*, which is where the roots orch/o, orchi/o, and orchid/o originate. The roots for sperm are spermat/o and sperm/o, which comes from the Late Latin word *sperma*, meaning seed or sperm.

There are two word roots for vagina: colp/o and vagin/o. The root colp/o comes from the Greek word *kolpos* (womb) but refers to the vagina and not the uterus. *Vagina* is actually a Latin word meaning "sheath" or "covering."

There are also three word roots for uterus: metr/o, hyster/o, and uter/o. *Uterus* is a Latin word, meaning womb. Hyster/o comes from the Greek word *hystera*, which also translates to womb. Table 15-1 shows common word parts related to the reproductive system.

TABLE 15-1 WORD PARTS RELATED TO THE REPRODUCTIVE SYSTEM

| Word Part | Meaning |
|---|---|
| amni/o | amnion |
| balan/o | glans penis |
| cervic/o | cervix, neck |
| circum/o | around |
| colp/o | vagina |
| gonad/o | gonads, sex glands |
| gynec/o | woman, female |
| hyster/o | uterus |
| lact/o | milk |
| mamm/o | breast |
| mast/o | breast |
| men/o | menses, menstruation |
| metr/o | uterus |
| nat/o | birth |
| oophor/o | ovary, egg-bearing |
| orch/o, orchi/o, orchid/o | testes |
| ovari/o | ovary, egg-bearing |
| prostat/o | prostate gland |
| salping/o | tube, uterine tube |
| sperm/o, spermat/o | sperm |
| uter/o | uterus |
| vagin/o | vagina |
| vas/o | vessel, vas deferens |
| vulv/o | vulva |

## Word Parts Exercise

After studying Table 15-1, write the meaning of each of the word parts.

| WORD PART | MEANING |
|---|---|
| 1. mast/o, mamm/o | 1. ________________ |
| 2. spermat/o, sperm/o | 2. ________________ |
| 3. salping/o | 3. ________________ |
| 4. vas/o | 4. ________________ |
| 5. circum/o | 5. ________________ |
| 6. ovari/o | 6. ________________ |
| 7. colp/o | 7. ________________ |

*(continued)*

**Word Parts Exercise** ***(continued)***

| WORD PART | MEANING |
|---|---|
| 8. prostat/o | 8. ______________________ |
| 9. amni/o | 9. ______________________ |
| 10. nat/o | 10. ______________________ |
| 11. hyster/o | 11. ______________________ |
| 12. vulv/o | 12. ______________________ |
| 13. orchid/o | 13. ______________________ |
| 14. cervic/o | 14. ______________________ |
| 15. balan/o | 15. ______________________ |
| 16. gonad/o | 16. ______________________ |
| 17. gynec/o | 17. ______________________ |
| 18. lact/o | 18. ______________________ |
| 19. men/o | 19. ______________________ |
| 20. oophor/o | 20. ______________________ |



## STRUCTURE AND FUNCTION

This section describes the male reproductive system and then the female reproductive system. Functions of the male reproductive system include synthesizing the hormone testosterone; producing, storing, and transporting sperm; and making and releasing fluid from glands that support the sperm. This male reproductive fluid is called **semen**. Main functions of the female reproductive system are producing the hormones estrogen and progesterone; propagating life by producing oocytes; transporting oocytes to sites where they can be fertilized by sperm; supporting and nurturing a developing human organism; and providing an infant's first source of nutrition and protective antibodies through breast milk. Note that in males, the urethra is part of both the urinary and reproductive systems. In females, the urethra does not play a role in reproduction but the opening to the exterior is enclosed by the **vulva**, the term for the female external genitalia.

### The Male Reproductive System

The male reproductive system is divided into internal *genitalia* (reproductive organs) and external genitalia. Internal genitalia include the testes, epididymis, ductus deferens (vas deferens), seminal glands (seminal vesicles), prostate, and bulbo-urethral glands. **Testes** are two oval-shaped gonads, located in a sac known as the *scrotum*, that produce sperm and testosterone. The **seminal glands**, also called the **seminal vesicles**, are two glands located at the base of the urinary bladder that produce seminal fluid, which becomes a component of semen. The gland that surrounds the beginning of the urethra (inferior to the bladder) that secretes a fluid that becomes part of the semen is the **prostate**.

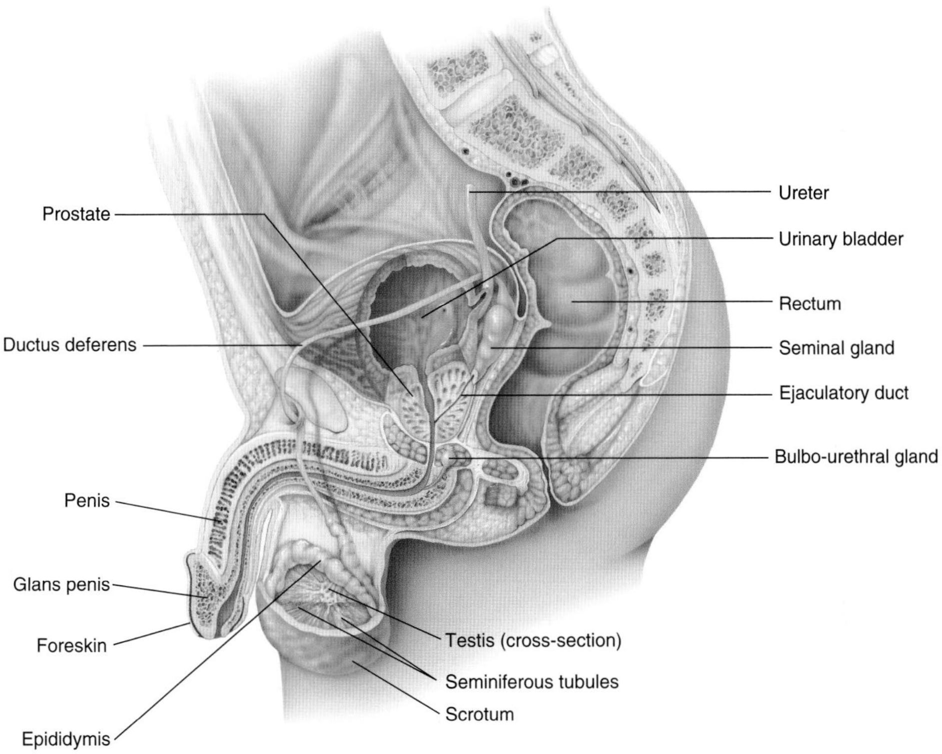


**FIGURE 15-1** A sagittal view of the male reproductive system and adjacent structures.

The **bulbo-urethral glands** (*Cowper's glands*) are two glands inferior to the prostate that secrete a sticky fluid that also becomes a component of semen. External genitalia include the penis and scrotum. The **penis** is the external male organ used in urination and sexual intercourse, whereas the **scrotum** is a pouch that is suspended on either side of and behind the penis that encloses the testes. The rounded head of the penis forms a structure called the **glans penis**. A free fold of skin covers the glans penis and is known as the **foreskin** or **prepuce**. Figure 15-1 shows the structures of the male reproductive system.

An important function of the male reproductive system is to produce sperm. The process, called **spermatogenesis**, involves stem cells dividing and differentiating into sperm. It involves cell division known as **meiosis**, which reduces the number of chromosomes from 46 to 23.

Meiosis is a type of cell division that occurs in sex cells to reduce the number of chromosomes. Mitosis is a different type of cell division that occurs in cells to produce two daughter cells that both have the same number of chromosomes as the original cell. *Meiosis* is a Greek word meaning "a lessening." Mitosis comes from the Greek word *mitos* meaning "thread" and reflects what the process of mitosis looks like when the chromosomes, which look thread-like when they bend and twist as they replicate.

Spermatogenesis begins in the *seminiferous tubules* of the testes and is initiated by the secretion of **androgens**, which are a group of hormones that have masculinizing effects. The most significant androgen is **testosterone**. After spermatogenesis is complete, the sperm migrate from the seminiferous tubules to the **epididymis**, a coil-shaped tube at the upper part of the testis where the sperm mature as they are stored. Sperm are released during the process of ejaculation, which begins with erection. When stimulated, the tissues in the penis become filled with blood, causing an *erection*. During erection, mature sperm leave the epididymis and enter the muscular tube of the **ductus deferens**, which leads to the *ejaculatory duct* that passes through the prostate. Fluid from the seminal glands is secreted into the duct. This fluid nourishes the sperm and forms much of the volume of the semen. The ductus deferens and the duct of the seminal gland unite to form the **ejaculatory duct**. The sperm and the fluid are now propelled through the ejaculatory duct toward the urethra. As the urethra passes through the prostate, milky secretions are added, forming semen. During ejaculation, the semen is expelled from the urethra at the tip of the penis. Figure 15-2 shows the pathway of sperm, beginning with production in the testes.

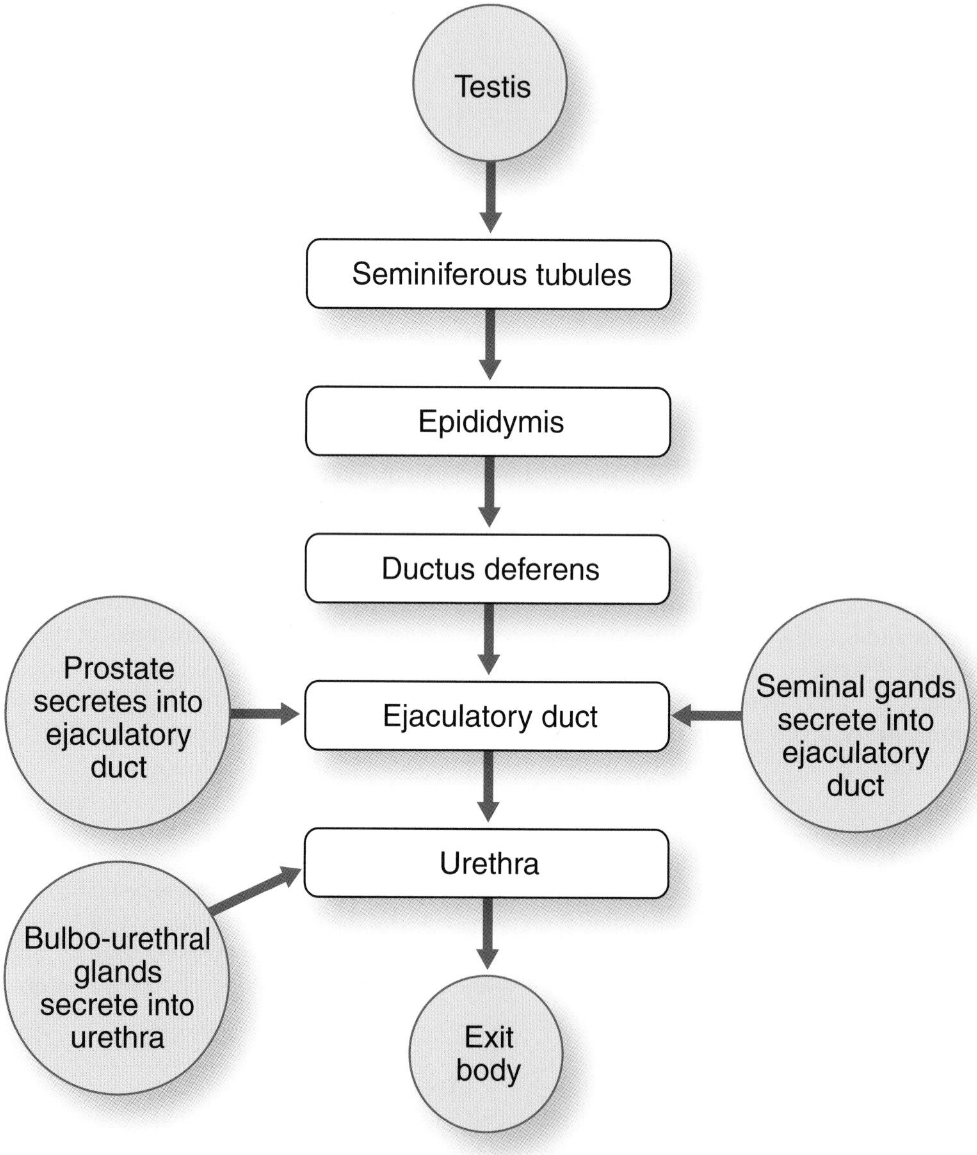


**FIGURE 15-2** Pathway of sperm. The secretions from the glands that contribute to seminal fluid are shown in circles.

## The Female Reproductive System

Like the male reproductive system, the female reproductive system is also divided into internal and external genitalia. The internal female reproductive organs are the *uterus*, two *ovaries*, two *uterine tubes*, and the *vagina*. Female external genitalia include the *clitoris*, *labium majus*, and *labium minus* (see Figure 15-3). Breasts are technically part of the integumentary system because their tissue contains modified sweat glands. We will discuss them here because breasts are the female organs of milk secretion.

The **uterus** is a pear-shaped organ that has a dome-shaped top portion called the **fundus** and a lower, narrow portion referred to as the **cervix**, which extends into the vagina. The uterus is composed of three layers of tissues: the **perimetrium**, which is the outer surrounding layer; the **myometrium**, which is the middle muscular layer; and the **endometrium**, which is the inner layer. The endometrium reacts to hormonal changes every month, and the result is **menstruation**, which involves a shedding of the endometrial lining.

Two **ovaries** lie on either side of the uterus in the pelvic cavity. The ovaries produce oocytes, the female gametes (sex cells). When an oocyte is fertilized by a sperm, it develops into an **ovum** (egg) and is capable of developing into a new individual.

The **uterine tubes** (*Fallopian tubes*) extend from the ovaries the uterus. They provide the path by which an oocyte travels from the ovary to the uterus. Fertilization takes place in the uterine tube.

The vagina is a muscular tube that extends from the cervix to the outside of the body. The vagina has the following functions:

- Allows for passage outside the body of the monthly menstrual flow of blood and tissue
- Is the organ for sexual intercourse
- Serves as the birth canal during a normal vaginal birth

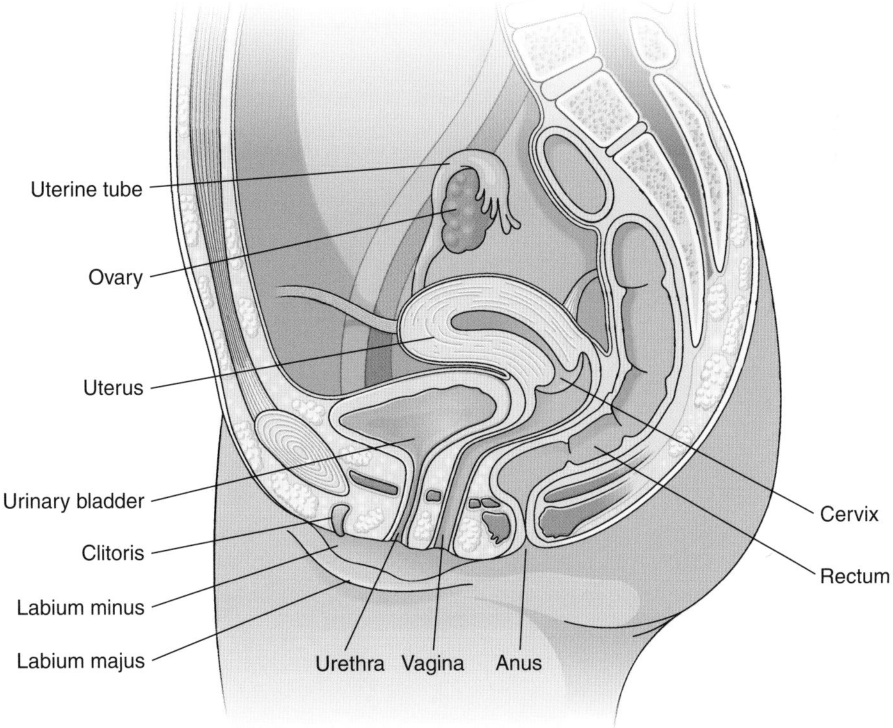


**FIGURE 15-3** The sagittal view of the female reproductive system and adjacent structures.

The external genitalia, commonly known as the **vulva**, include organs that enable sperm to enter the body, protect the internal genital organs from infectious organisms, and provide sexual pleasure. The **clitoris** is a small mass of erectile tissue that responds to sexual stimulation. *Labia* are two sets of skin folds that cover the female external genitalia and tissues. The **labium majus** (plural, *labium majora*) is one of two rounded external folds, and the **labium minus** (plural, *labium minora*) is one of two inner folds that surround the openings to the vagina and urethra (see Figure 15-3).

Breasts are protruding organs that have a *nipple* and an *areola*. The **nipple** is a projection on the breast surface through which *lactiferous* (milk) *ducts* open onto the body surface. The **areola** is the dark-pigmented area around the nipple.

Each breast contains a **mammary gland**, the modified sweat gland that produces milk. The subdivisions of the mammary gland are called *lobules* (see Figure 15-4). Breast milk provides nourishment for the newborn. **Lactation** is the term given to the production of milk.

Like the male reproductive system, the female reproductive system provides gametes for fertilization, but its function in the process continues by providing an environment for a fertilized egg to develop into to a fully formed baby.

The preparation for the process is accommodated by the **menstrual cycle** (also called the **uterine cycle**), a recurrent periodic change in the ovaries and uterus that occurs approximately every 28 days. The first time this cycle occurs in a female, around age 11 or 12, it is called **menarche**. When this monthly cycle stops occurring for the final time, around age 45 to 55, it is called **menopause**. Hormones control the menstrual cycle, which has three phases: **menstrual phase** (days 0 to 7; destruction and shedding of the endometrium), **proliferative phase** (days 7 to 14; repair and regeneration of the endometrium and preparation of the endometrial lining for implantation if fertilization occurs

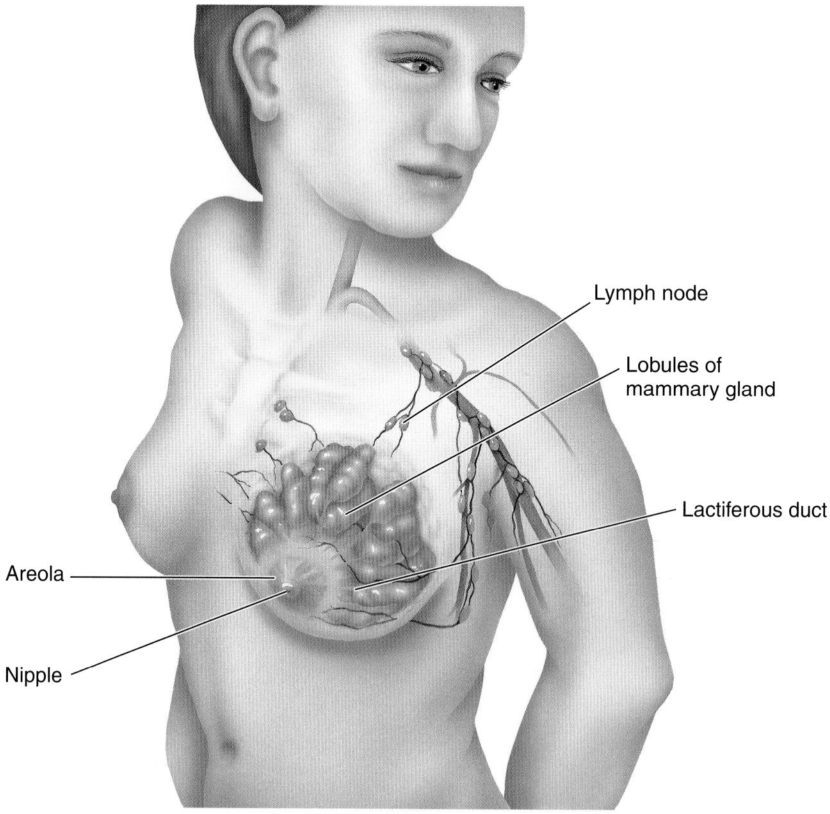


**FIGURE 15-4** Frontal view of the breasts.

after ovulation on day 14), and the **secretory phase** (days 14 to 28; secretion of hormones). If male sperm are present during **ovulation** (the release of an oocyte), the possibility of fertilization exists.

## Pregnancy

**Pregnancy**, or **gestation**, is the condition of having a developing embryo or fetus in the uterus. When a secondary oocyte is fertilized by the male sperm, it forms a *zygote*, which travels through the uterine tube and implants into the uterus. Once implanted, the zygote is called an **embryo** during the first 8 weeks of gestation. Between the end of the 8th week and birth, which under normal circumstances occurs between weeks 38 and 40, the term **fetus** is used. The fetus receives nourishment from the uterine wall through the *umbilical cord* and the *placenta*. The **umbilical cord** is the structure that contains blood vessels and connects the embryo or fetus to the placenta, whereas the **placenta** is a temporary organ implanted in the uterus formed during pregnancy. The **amnion** (*amniotic sac*) is the inner layer of the membrane that surrounds the fetus and contains *amniotic fluid*. **Amniotic fluid** encases the fetus and provides a cushion for the fetus as the mother moves (see Figure 15-5).

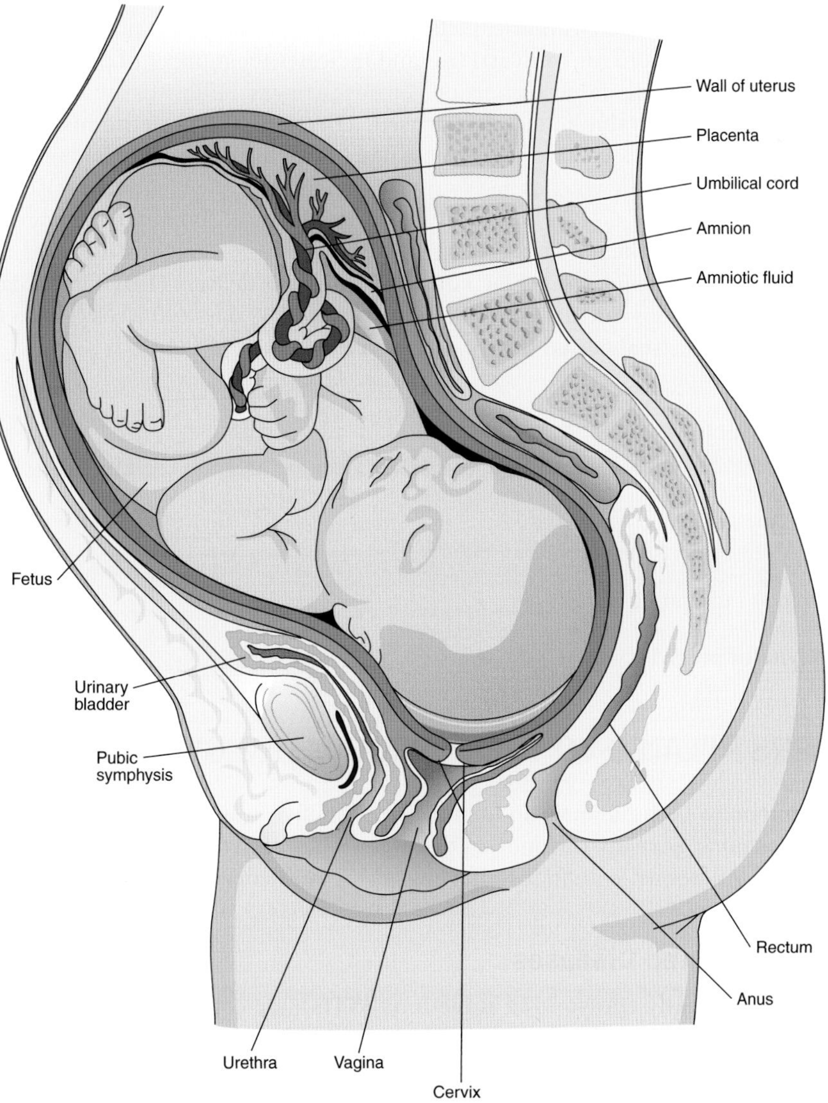


**FIGURE 15-5** A pregnant uterus with fetus.

## Terms Associated with Pregnancy

Gravida, para, and abortus are shorthand notations for a woman's pregnancy history. The term **gravida (G)**, derived from the Latin word *gravidus* (heavy), means a pregnant woman. Gravida is usually followed by a Roman numeral or Arabic numeral and indicates the number of pregnancies. For example, gravida I, GI, and G1 all refer to a woman in her first pregnancy and gravida II, GII, and G2 refer to a woman in her second pregnancy. The term can also be preceded by the Latin prefix primi- for first and secundi- for second, as in primigravida (first pregnancy) and secundigravida (second pregnancy). The number following gravida indicates the number of times a patient has been pregnant regardless of whether these pregnancies were carried to term. A current pregnancy, if any, is included in this count. The term **para (P)**, derived from the Latin word *pario* (to bring forth) refers to a woman who has given birth to one or more infants. Like gravida, it is followed by a Roman numeral or Arabic numeral or preceded by a Latin prefix. For example, para I, primipara, PI, and P1 refer to a woman who has given birth for the first time, whereas para II, secundipara, PII, and P2 refer to a woman who has given firth for a second time to one or more infants. Para indicates the number of births that occurred after 20 weeks (including viable and nonviable [i.e., stillbirths]). Pregnancies consisting of multiples, such as twins or triplets, count as one birth for the purpose of this notation. **Abortus (A)** is the Latin word for "miscarriage" and indicates the number of pregnancies that were lost for any reason, including induced abortions or miscarriages. Stillbirths are not included.

In the United States, Arabic numerals are used. Therefore, the obstetric history of a woman who has had two pregnancies (both of which resulted in live births) would be noted as G2P2. The obstetrical history of a woman who has had four pregnancies, one of which was a miscarriage before 20 weeks, would be noted as G4P3A1. That of a woman who has had one pregnancy of twins with successful outcomes would be noted as G1P1.

The *estimated date of confinement* (EDC) or *estimated date of delivery* (EDD) is the date an infant is expected to be born and is calculated by counting forward 280 days (40 weeks) from the first day of the mother's last menstrual period (LMP). It is also called the due date.

### Quick Check

**Fill in the blanks.**

1. List functions of the male reproductive system. ______________________________

2. The term for milk production is ______________________________.

3. A synonym for pregnancy is ______________________________.



## DISORDERS RELATED TO THE REPRODUCTIVE SYSTEM

Disorders common to both the male and female reproductive systems are briefly described under the following sections: sexually transmitted diseases (STDs), inflammation, structural abnormalities, and tumors. Additional conditions affecting males and females, respectively, are included at the end of this section.

## Sexually Transmitted Diseases

**STDs**, also called **sexually transmitted infections (STIs)**, are contagious diseases acquired during sexual contact. Examples include human immunodeficiency virus (HIV), herpes simplex virus (HSV), gonorrhea (GC), chlamydia, pelvic inflammatory disease (PID), syphilis, and human papillomavirus (HPV) infection.

The **HIV** attacks the immune system after it is transmitted through blood or other infected body fluids. **HSV** is a variety of infections caused by herpesvirus types 1 and 2 that produce cold sores, genital inflammation, and conjunctivitis. **GC** is a highly contagious disease caused by *Neisseria gonorrhoeae* bacteria that may also be transmitted to a child from an infected mother during birth. **Chlamydia** is another common infection spread through sexual contact and is caused by a very small parasitic bacterium from the *Chlamydia* genus. **PID**, an infection of the uterus, ovaries, and uterine tubes, can prevent fertilization. If a woman has PID and an oocyte does become fertilized, the zygote may implant outside the uterus, which is known as an **ectopic** (*ektopos* is Greek for "out of place") pregnancy. An ectopic pregnancy can be life threatening. **Syphilis** is a highly contagious disease caused by the *Treponema pallidum* bacterium. A developing fetus can contract the disease through an infected mother. **HPV** is a sexually transmitted virus that can lead to cervical cancer.

## Inflammation

Infections of the female reproductive system may result from exposure to bacteria, fungi, or viruses. Many of the conditions are marked by inflammation, the terms for which are indicated by the suffix *-itis*, which you learned in earlier chapters.

Male reproductive system inflammation conditions include **epididymitis** (inflammation of the epididymis), **prostatitis** (inflammation of the prostate), **balanitis** (inflammation of the glans penis), and **orchitis** (inflammation of a testis). Balanitis occurs in uncircumcised males who still have an intact glans penis.

Female reproductive system inflammation disorders include **mastitis** (breast inflammation), **oophoritis** (ovary inflammation), **salpingitis** (uterine tube inflammation), **cervicitis** (inflammation of the uterine cervix), and **vaginitis** (inflammation of the vagina). Salpingitis can lead to a closing of the uterine tubes, thereby causing infertility.

## Female Structural Abnormalities

In adult women, the uterus may be out of position or actually may have a bend in its body. **Anteflexion** (forward bending) is the normal position of the uterus (see Figure 15-6A). **Anteversion** (forward turning) is the normal position of the uterus in which it is angled anteriorly relative to the long axis of the vagina, so that it rests on the urinary bladder (see Figure 15-6B). **Retroflexion** (backward bending) is an abnormal tipping with the body of the uterus bent back on itself, forming an angle with the cervix (see Figure 15-6C). **Retroversion** (backward turning) is an abnormal tipping of the entire uterus backward (see Figure 15-6D). A **prolapsed uterus** involves the descent of the uterus or cervix into the vaginal canal. Two other conditions involving structural abnormalities of the female reproductive system are a **cystocele**, which is a protrusion of the urinary bladder into the anterior wall of the vagina, and a **rectocele**, which is a protrusion of the rectum into the posterior wall of the vagina.



## Tumors

Benign tumors of the uterus are called *fibroleiomyomas* or **fibroids**. Cysts, which may also be considered a benign tumor, are usually caused by hormonal disturbances.

Cancer of the endometrium is the most common type of cancer in the female reproductive system. A **hysterectomy** (removal of the uterus) is a common treatment. **Endometriosis** is a condition in which endometrial tissue grows outside the uterus, frequently forming cysts, and causing pelvic pain.

## Menstrual Cycle Disorders

Menstruation, commonly called a *period*, generally occurs once per month. However, menstrual cycle disorders are common. **Amenorrhea** is the absence of menstruation. **Dysmenorrhea** is painful menstruation. **Menorrhagia** is an increased amount and duration of blood flow. **Oligomenorrhea** is a reduced blood flow along with abnormally infrequent menstruation.

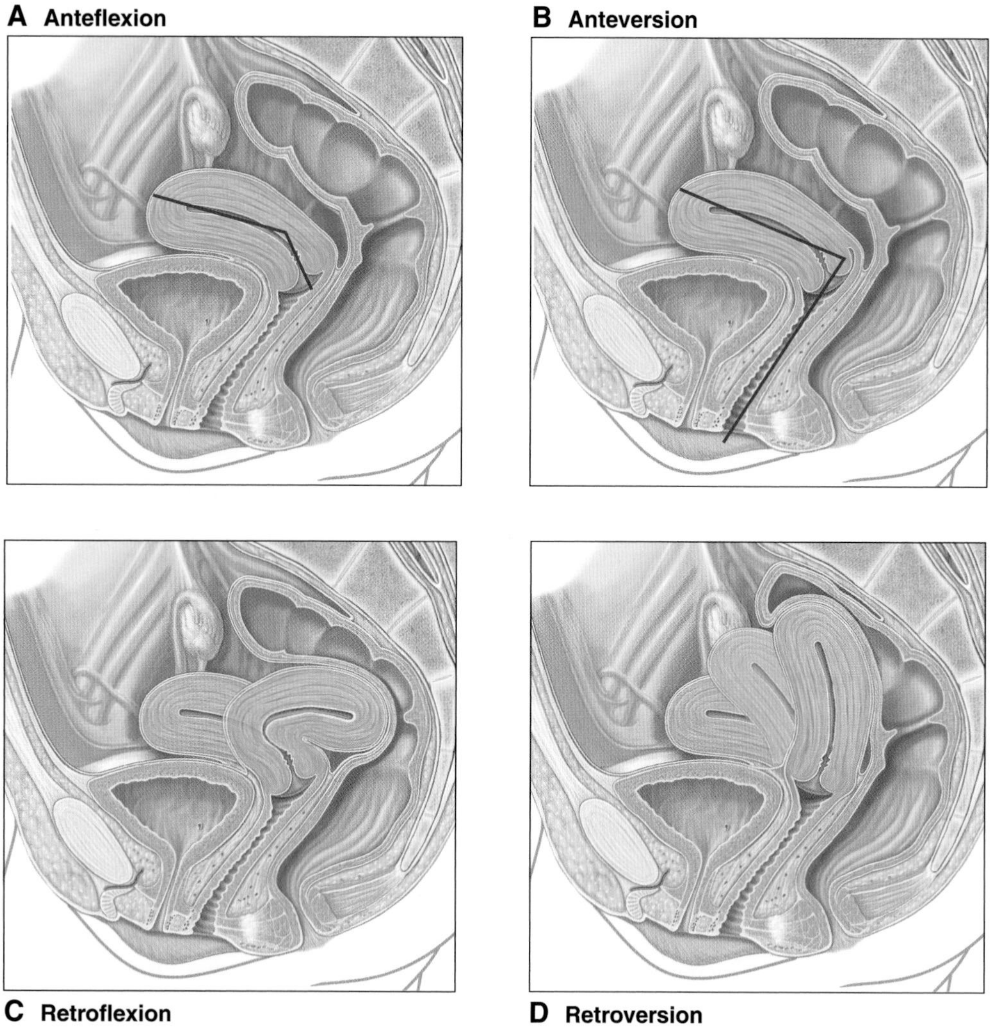


**FIGURE 15-6** Variants of uterine position within the pelvis. The pink-shaded organ is the uterus.



## Disorders that Affect Males

Any disease that affects the testes is called **orchiopathy**. This includes **azoospermia** (absence of living sperm in the semen), **oligospermia** (low sperm count), **orchialiga** (pain in the testes), **anorchism** (absence of one or both testes; may be congenital or acquired), and **cryptorchism** (failure of one or both testes to descend into the scrotum).

Other disorders that affect the male reproductive system include the following condition listed as follows:

- **Benign prostatic hyperplasia (BPH):** an enlarged, noncancerous prostate
- **Hydrocele:** fluid accumulation in the scrotum
- **Phimosis:** narrowing of the opening of the foreskin so it cannot be retracted or pulled back to expose the glans penis
- **Varicocele:** enlargement of veins in the spermatic cord (bundle of nerves and blood vessels connecting the testes to the abdominal cavity)

## DIAGNOSTIC TESTS, TREATMENTS, AND SURGICAL PROCEDURES

Some diagnostic and surgical treatments and procedures of the male reproductive system are listed as follows:

- **Circumcision:** a surgical procedure to remove the foreskin of the penis
- **Orchiectomy:** removal of one or both testes
- **Orchioplasty:** surgical repair of a testis
- **Transurethral resection of the prostate (TURP):** the removal of part or all of the prostate through the urethra
- **Varicocelectomy:** the removal of a portion of an enlarged vein to remove a varicocele
- **Vasovasostomy:** procedure to restore fertility to a vasectomized male by reconnecting the ductus (vas) deferens

Some diagnostic and surgical treatments and procedures of the female reproductive system are listed as follows:

- **Amniocentesis:** amniotic fluid is tested for fetal abnormalities; can also help determine fetal lung maturity, age, and sex of fetus (see Figure 15-7).
- **Colposcopy:** visual examination of the tissues of the cervix and vagina using a surgical instrument called a colposcope
- **Papanicolaou test (Pap smear):** scraping of the cervical tissues to diagnose cervical cancer or other conditions of the cervix and surrounding tissues
- **Dilation and curettage (D&C):** dilation (widening) of the cervix and scraping the lining of the uterus with a surgical instrument called a curette, which has a loop, ring, or scoop with sharpened edges attached to a handle
- **Cone biopsy:** surgical removal of a cone-shaped section of the cervix
- **Laparoscopy:** visual examination of the interior of the abdomen by means of a surgical instrument called a laparoscope
- **Oophorectomy:** removal of one ovary
- **Bilateral oophorectomy:** removal of both ovaries
- **Salpingo-oophorectomy:** removal of an ovary and uterine tube
- **Bilateral salpingo-oophorectomy:** removal of both ovaries and uterine tubes
- **Hysterosalpingography:** a radiographic examination of the uterus and uterine tubes
- **Hysterectomy:** surgical removal of the uterus
- **Mammography:** radiographic examination of the breast
- **Mastectomy:** removal of a breast
- **Tubal ligation:** surgical procedure that involves severing and tying the uterine tubes to prevent future conception

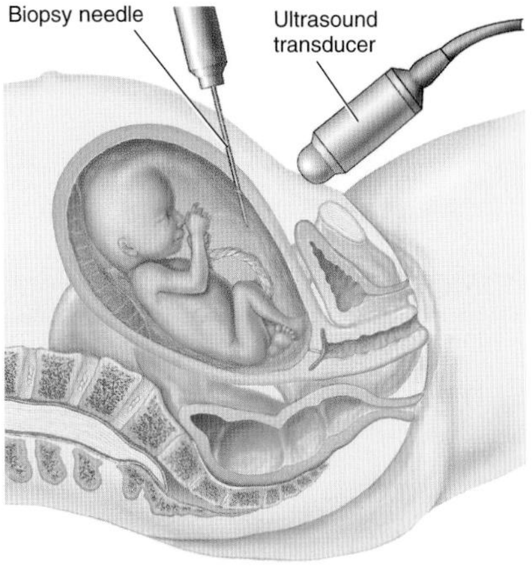

**FIGURE 15-7** Amniocentesis. A biopsy needle is inserted through the abdominal wall into the uterus, and a sample of amniotic fluid is removed from the amniotic sac using guided ultrasound.

## PRACTICE AND PRACTITIONERS

**Obstetrics (OB)** is the medical specialty concerned with the medical care of women during pregnancy and childbirth, and **obstetricians** (from *obstetrix*, the Latin word for midwife) are the specialists who provide medical care to pregnant women and deliver babies. **Gynecology (GYN)** is the study of the female reproductive system and **gynecologists** diagnose and treat disorders of the female reproductive system. **Urologists** diagnose and treat disorders of the urinary and male reproductive systems. **Neonatology** is the medical specialty dealing with newborns, and **pediatrics** is the medical specialty dealing with children. The specialists in these fields are the **neonatologist**, who specializes in newborns, and the **pediatrician**, who specializes in the diagnosis and treatment of childhood disorders.

## Abbreviation Table THE REPRODUCTIVE SYSTEM

| ABBREVIATION | MEANING |
|---|---|
| A | abortus |
| BPH | benign prostatic hyperplasia |
| CS | cesarean section |
| C-section | cesarean section |
| D&C | dilation and curettage |
| EDC | estimated date of confinement (due date) |
| EDD | estimated date of delivery (due date) |
| G | gravida |
| GC | gonorrhea |
| GYN | gynecology |
| HIV | human immunodeficiency virus |
| HPV | human papillomavirus |
| HSV | herpes simplex virus |
| LMP | last menstrual period |
| OB | obstetrics |
| P | para |
| Pap smear | papanicolaou smear |
| PID | pelvic inflammatory disease |
| STD | sexually transmitted disease |
| STI | sexually transmitted infection |
| TURP | transurethral resection of the prostate |



## Study Table THE REPRODUCTIVE SYSTEM

| TERM AND PRONUNCIATION | ANALYSIS | MEANING |
|---|---|---|
| **Structure and Function** | | |
| abortus (uh-BOR-tus) | from the Latin word *abortus* (miscarriage) | any product of a miscarriage |
| amniotic fluid (am-nee-OT-ik FLOO-id) | *amni/o* (amnion); *-ic* (suffix meaning pertaining to); fluid (from the Latin word for fluid, *fluidus*) | the fluid within the amnion (amniotic sac) that surrounds the embryo/fetus and helps to protect it from mechanical injury |
| amnion (AM-nee-on) | from the Greek word, *amnion* (membrane around the fetus) and diminutive of *amnos* (lamb) | innermost membrane enveloping the embryo/fetus in the uterus; *amniotic sac* |

**Study Table** THE REPRODUCTIVE SYSTEM (*continued*)

| TERM AND PRONUNCIATION | ANALYSIS | MEANING |
|---|---|---|
| amniotic sac (am-nee-OT-ik SAK) | *amni/o* (amnion); *-ic* (suffix meaning pertaining to); sac (from the Latin word for bag, *saccus*) | innermost membrane enveloping the embryo/fetus in the uterus; *amnion* |
| androgens (AN-droh-jenz) | from the Greek words *andros* (man) and *genein* (to produce) | hormones that stimulate the activity of accessory male sex hormones; testosterone is an androgen |
| areola (uh-REE-oh-luh) | Latin word for "small area" | circular pigmented area surrounding the nipple |
| bulbo-urethral gland (buhl-boh-yoo-REE-thruhl GLAND) | from the Latin word *bulbus* (bulb); from the Greek word *ourethra* (passage for urine) | one of two small glands along the urethra; *Cowper's gland* |
| cervix (SER-viks) | Latin word for "neck" (as in the neck of the uterus) | common term for the neck of the uterus that dips into the vagina |
| chromosome (KROH-moh-sohm) | from the Greek word *khroma* (color) and *soma* (body), so called because the structures contain a substance that stains readily with basic dyes | a gene-bearing bundle of DNA found in the nucleus of all cells |
| clitoris (KLIT-or-is) | from the Greek word *kleitoris* (small, sensitive, erectile part) | small (less than 2 cm) mass of erectile tissue in females that responds to sexual stimulation |
| embryo (EHM-bree-oh) | from the Greek word *embryon* (young animal, literally, "that which grows") | name change from *zygote* after the first cell division until the 8th week of pregnancy |
| endometrium (en-doh-MEE-tree-uhm) | endo- (within); from the Greek *metra* (uterus) | membrane forming the inner layer of the uterine wall |
| epididymis (ehp-ih-DIHD-ih-muhs) | from the Greek words *epi* (on) + *didymos* (testicle) | organ in which the male sperm become functional |
| fallopian tubes (fah-LOH-pee-ahn TOOBZ) | named after Gabriello Fallopio (1523–1562), an Italian anatomist who first described them | tubular structures between the ovaries and the uterus; *uterine tubes* |
| fertilization (fer-til-ih-ZAY-shun) | from the Latin word *fertilis* (fruitful) | the joining of the male and female gametes (in the context of the human reproductive system) |
| fetus (FEE-tuhs) | Latin word meaning "the bearing," "bringing forth," or "hatching of young" | name change from *embryo* after the 8th week of pregnancy to birth |

(*continued*)

**Study Table** THE REPRODUCTIVE SYSTEM *(continued)*

| TERM AND PRONUNCIATION | ANALYSIS | MEANING |
|---|---|---|
| fundus (FUHN-duhs) | Latin word for "bottom" | the upper rounded portion of the uterus above the openings of the uterine tubes |
| gamete (GAH-meet) | Greek word meaning "a wife"; also *gametes* (a husband), from *gamein* (to take a wife, to marry) | term given to both the sex cells; female oocyte and male sperm |
| gestation (jehs-TAY-shun) | from the Latin word *gestare* (to bear, carry, gestate) | period of development that occurs between the formation of the zygote and birth of the child; *pregnancy* |
| gonad (GOH-nad) | from the Greek word *gone* (seed, act of generation, race, family) | gamete-generating organ (ovary or testis) |
| gravida (GRAV-ih-duh) | from the Latin word *gravis* (heavy, profound, important) | a pregnant woman |
| lactation (lak-TAY-shun) | from the Latin word *lactare* (to suckle, entice, lead on, induce); derived from the Latin word *lac* (milk) | milk production |
| labium majus (LAY-bee-um MAY-jus) | from the Latin words *labium* (lip) + *magnus* (great) | part of the labia that covers and protects the female external genital organs |
| labium minus (LAY-bee-um MYE-nus) | from the Latin words *labium* (lip) + *minor* (smaller) | Inner folds of the labia that surround the openings to the vagina and urethra |
| mammary gland (MAM-uh-ree GLAND) | from the Latin word *mamma* (breast) | modified sweat gland that produces milk |
| meiosis (migh-OH-sis) | Greek word meaning "a lessening" | cell division comprising two nuclear divisions in rapid succession that results in four gametocytes |
| menarche (meh-NAR-kee) | from the Greek words *men* (month) and *arkhe* (beginning) | beginning of menstruation (menses) |
| menopause (MEN-oh-pawz) | from the Latin words *mensis* (month) and *pausis* (a cessation, a pause) | normal stopping of the monthly menstrual cycle (periods) |
| menses (MEN-seez) | plural form of the Latin word *mensis* (month) | periodic bleeding occurring at intervals of about 4 weeks in which the endometrial lining is shed; *menstruation* |

**Study Table** THE REPRODUCTIVE SYSTEM (*continued*)

| TERM AND PRONUNCIATION | ANALYSIS | MEANING |
|---|---|---|
| menstruation (men-stroo-AYE-shuhn) | from the Latin word *menstruus* (monthly); *-atio* (process) | cyclic endometrial shedding and discharge of a bloody fluid from the uterus; *menses* |
| menstrual (MEN-stroo-uhl) | from the Latin word *mensis* (month) | relating to the menses (menstruation) |
| menstrual cycle (MEN-stroo-ul SIGH-kul) | from the Latin word *mensis* (month) | part of the reproductive system process in women, comprising three phases: menstrual, proliferative, and secretory; *uterine cycle* |
| mitosis (my-TOH-sihs) | from the Greek word *mitos* (wrap, thread); *-osis* (process) | process of cell division by which one cell becomes two, both of which contain the maternal and paternal chromosomes |
| myometrium (my-oh-MEE-tree-uhm) | *myo-* (muscle); from the Greek *metra* (uterus) | the muscular wall of the uterus |
| ovary (OH-vah-ree) | from the Latin word *ovum* (egg) | small almond-shaped organ located on either side of the uterus that produces hormones and releases oocytes |
| ovulation (OV-yoo-lay-shun) | from the Latin word *ovum* (egg); *-atio* (process) | release of an oocyte from the ovary |
| ovum (OH-vuhm); plural, ova (OH-vah) | Latin word meaning "egg" | fertilized oocyte before implantation |
| para (PAR-ah) | from the Latin verb *pario* (to bring forth, produce, create) | a woman who has given birth to a viable fetus |
| penis (PEE-nihs) | from the Latin *penis* (tail) | external male sex organ used in urination and sexual intercourse that transports the male sperm into the female vagina |
| placenta (pla-SEN-tah) | Latin word meaning "cake" | a spongy organ that is attached to the fetus by the umbilical cord and that provides nourishment to the fetus |
| pregnancy (PREG-nan-see) | *pre-* (before); from the Latin word *gnascor* (to be born) | period of time when the fetus grows inside of the uterus; *gestation* |
| proliferative phase (pro-LIF-er-uh-tiv FAZE) | from the Latin words *proles* (offspring) and *ferre* (to carry, to bear) | menstrual phase (days 7–14) controlled by estrogen secreted by ovarian follicles (cell aggregation in the ovary that contains an oocyte), simultaneous with their development |

(*continued*)

**Study Table** THE REPRODUCTIVE SYSTEM *(continued)*

| TERM AND PRONUNCIATION | ANALYSIS | MEANING |
|---|---|---|
| prostate (PROS-tate) | from the Greek word *prostates*(one standing in front) | male gland that produces and stores prostatic fluid, a fluid medium that is part of semen; *prostate gland* |
| scrotum (SKROH-tum) | from the Latin word *scrotum* cognate with Old English *scrud* (garment, source of shroud) | the sac that encloses and protects the testes |
| secretory phase (se-KREE-toh-ree FAZE) | from the Latin verb *secretionem* (to separate) | menstrual phase (days 14–28) controlled by the hormone progesterone that coincides with the formation of the corpus luteum (a hormone-secreting structure that develops in the ovary after the oocyte has been released, but degenerates after a few days unless fertilization occurs) |
| semen (SEE-mehn) | a Latin word meaning "seed" | combination of sperm, their associated glandular secretions, and prostatic fluid |
| seminal gland (SEH-min-ahl GLAND) | from the Latin word *semen* (seed); -al (adjective suffix) | gland at the base of the urinary bladder that secretes a thick substance that nourishes sperm; *seminal vesicle* |
| seminal vesicle (SEH-min-ahl VES-i-kuhl) | from the Latin words *semen* (seed) and *vesica* (bladder, balloon) | gland at the base of the urinary bladder that secretes a thick substance that nourishes sperm; *seminal gland* |
| sperm (SPURM) | from the Greek words *sperma* (seed) and *zoion* (animal) | the male gamete; sperm is singular or plural |
| spermatogenesis (SPUR-mah-toh-JEHN-ih-sihs) | *spermat/o* (sperm); + *genesis* (production) | production of sperm |
| testes (TES-teez); singular: testis (TES-tihs) | from the Latin word *testiculus* dim. of *testis* (witness) (the organ being evidence of virility) | the organs that produce and store the male gametes |
| testosterone (tehs-TOSS-teh-rohn) | from the Latin word *testis* (witness); *-sterone* (steroid hormone) | the male reproductive hormone (androgen) prominent in male gamete production |
| umbilical cord (um-BILL-ih-kul KORD) | from the Latin words *umbilicus* (navel) + *chorda* (string) | connecting stalk between the embryo/fetus and the placenta that contains two arteries and one vein |

**Study Table** THE REPRODUCTIVE SYSTEM *(continued)*

| TERM AND PRONUNCIATION | ANALYSIS | MEANING |
|---|---|---|
| urethra (yu-REETH-rah) | from the Greek word *ourethra* (passage for urine) | canal leading from the bladder to the exterior; male ductwork that acts as a part of both the male urinary system and male reproductive system |
| uterine cervix (YOO-ter-in SUR-viks) | *uter/o* (uterus); *-ine* (adjective suffix) + *cervix*, Latin word for neck | the "neck" located at the lower end of the uterus |
| uterine cycle (YOO-ter-in SIGH-kul) | *uter/o* (uterus); *-ine* (adjective suffix); from the Latin word tubus (tube) | part of the reproductive system process in women, comprising three phases: menstrual, proliferative, and secretory; *menstrual cycle* |
| uterine tubes (YOO-ter-in TOOBZ) | *uter/o* (uterus); *-ine* (adjective suffix); from the Latin word *tubus* (tube) | tubular structures between the ovaries and the uterus; *fallopian tubes* |
| uterus (YOO-ter-us) | Latin word meaning "womb" or "belly" | reproductive organ in which the fertilized oocyte is implanted and in which the embryo/fetus develops |
| vagina (vuh-JYE-nuh) | Latin word for sheath | the female genital canal extending between the cervix of the uterus and the exterior |
| vas deferens (vas DEHF-eh rehnz) | from the Latin words *vas* (vessel) and *deferens* (carrying down) | duct leading out of the epididymis; *ductus deferens* |
| vulva (VUL-vuh) | from the Latin word *vulva* (wrapper or covering) | female external genital organs |
| zygote (ZY-goht) | from the Greek word *zygotos* (yoked) | single cell formed at fertilization from the union of the oocyte with the sperm |
| **Disorders** | | |
| amenorrhea (ah-MEN-oh-REE-ah) | *a-* (without); *men/o* (menses); *-rrhea* (flowing, discharge) | absence of menstruation |
| anorchism (an-OR-kizm) | *an-* (without); *orch/o* (testes); *-ism* (condition) | congenital absence of one or both testes |
| anteflexion (an-tee-FLEX-shun) | *ante-* (something positioned in front of); from the Latin word *flectere* (to bend) | forward bend of the uterus |
| anteversion (an-tee-VER-shun) | *ante-* (something positioned in front of); from the Latin word *versio* (turning) | turning forward of the entire uterus |

*(continued)*

**Study Table** THE REPRODUCTIVE SYSTEM (*continued*)

| TERM AND PRONUNCIATION | ANALYSIS | MEANING |
|---|---|---|
| azoospermia (ay-ZOH-oh-SPER-mee-ah) | *a-* (without); from the Greek word *azoos* (lifeless); *sperm/o* (sperm) | absence of living sperm in the semen |
| balanitis (bal-ah-NIGH-tis) | *balan/o* (glans penis); *-itis* (inflammation) | inflammation of the glans penis |
| benign prostatic hyperplasia (BPH) (bee-NINE pros-TAT-ik high-per-PLAY-zhee-uh) | benign (common English word) + *prostat/o* (prostate) + *-ic* (adjective suffix); *hyper-* (above normal); *-plasia* (development, growth) | an enlarged, noncancerous prostate; *prostatomegaly* |
| cervicitis (sur-vih-SY-tihs); also trachelitis (trak-ih-LY-tihs) | *cervic/o* (cervix); *-itis* (inflammation) | inflammation of the uterine cervix |
| cryptorchidism (kript-OR-kid-iz-um) | from the Greek word *kryptos* (hidden); *orch/o* (testes); *-ism* (condition) | undescended testes or when one or both testes fail to descend into the scrotum; *cryptorchism* |
| cystocele (SIS-toh-seel) | *cyst/o* (bladder); *-cele* (hernia) | protrusion of the bladder into the anterior wall of the vagina |
| dysmenorrhea (dis-MEN-oh-REE-ah) | *dys-* (bad, difficult); *men/o* (menses); *-rrhea* (flowing, discharge) | painful menstruation |
| ectopic (ek-TOP-ik) | from the Greek word ektopos (away from a place, distant) | out of place; a pregnancy occurring elsewhere than in the uterus |
| endometriosis (EN-doh-MEE-tree-OH-sis) | from the Greek words *endon* (within) and *metra* (womb) + *-osis* (condition) | presence of endometrial tissue outside the uterus |
| epididymitis (ep-ih-did-ih-MY-tis) | from the Greek words *epi* (on) and *didymos* (testicle); *-itis* (inflammation) | inflammation of the epididymis |
| fibroids (FIGH-broidz) | from the Latin word *fibra* (a fiber, filament); -oid (resembling) | benign neoplasm derived from smooth muscle occurring in the uterus; *fibroleiomyoma* |
| gonorrhea (GC) (gon-oh-REE-ah) | from the Greek *gonos* (offspring); *-rrhea* (discharge, flowing) | highly contagious sexually transmitted disease caused by bacteria |
| herpes simplex virus (HSV) (HUR-peez SIM-pleks VYE-rus) | *herpes* (Latin for a spreading skin eruption); *simplex* (Latin for simple); *virus* (Latin for poison) | infections caused by herpesvirus types 1 and 2; symptoms include groups of vesicles and lesions on the genitalia |
| human immunodeficiency virus (HIV) (HYOO-mun IM-yoo-noh-dee-fish-en-see VYE-rus) | *immunis* (Latin for exempt); *deficientem* (Latin for deficient); *virus* (Latin for poison) | virus that attacks the immune system; can be sexually transmitted |

15 | Reproductive System

**Study Table** THE REPRODUCTIVE SYSTEM (*continued*)

| TERM AND PRONUNCIATION | ANALYSIS | MEANING |
|---|---|---|
| human papillomavirus (HPV) (HYOO-mun pap-ih-LOH-muh VYE-rus) | *papilla* (Latin for nipple; *-oma* (tumor); *virus* (Latin for poison) | most common sexually transmitted disease; causes certain types of genital warts |
| hydrocele (HIGH-droh-seel) | *hydro-* (water); *-cele* (hernia) | hernia filled with fluid in the testes |
| hysteralgia (HIHS-teh-RAL-jee-ah); also hysterodynia (HIHS-teh-roh-DIHN-ee-ah) | *hyster/o* (womb, uterus); *-algia/-dynia* (pain) | pain in the uterus |
| hysteropathy (hiss-ter-ROP-ah-thee) | *hyster/o* (womb, uterus); *-pathy* (disease) | any disease of the uterus |
| mastitis (mast-EYE-tis) | *mast/o* (breast); *-itis* (inflammation) | inflammation of the breast |
| menorrhagia (MEN-oh-RAY-jee-ah) | *men/o* (menses); *-rrhagia* (rapid flow of blood) | increased amount and duration of menstrual flow |
| oligomenorrhea (oh-LIG-oh-MEN-oh-REE-ah) | *olig/o* (having little); *men/o* (menses); *-rrhea* (discharge, flowing) | markedly reduced menstrual flow along with abnormally infrequent menstruation |
| oligospermia (oh-LIG-oh-SPER-mee-ah) | *olig/o* (having little); *-sperm/o* (sperm); *-ia* (condition) | low sperm count |
| oophoritis (oh-of-or-EYE-tis) | *oophor/o* (ovary); *-itis* (inflammation) | inflammation of an ovary; *ovaritis* |
| orchialgia (or-kee-AL-jee-ah) | *orchi/o* (testes); *-algia* (pain) | pain in the testes |
| orchitis (or-KIGH-tis) | *orchi/o* (testes); *-itis* (inflammation) | inflammation of a testis |
| ovarialgia (oh-vahr-ee-AL-jee-ah) | *ovari/o* (ovary); *-algia* (pain) | pain in an ovary |
| ovaritis (ohv-ah-RY-tihs) | *ovari/o* (ovary); *-itis* (inflammation) | inflammation of an ovary; *oophoritis* |
| pelvic inflammatory disease (PID) (PEL-vik in-FLAM-uh-tawr-ee dih-ZEEZ) | common English words | acute or chronic suppurative inflammation of female pelvic structures (endometrium, uterine tubes, pelvic peritoneum) due to infection by *Neisseria gonorrhoeae*, *Chlamydia trachomatis*, or other organisms |
| phimosis (fi-MOH-sis) | from the Greek word *phimoo* (to muzzle); *-osis* (condition) | narrowing of the opening of the foreskin so it cannot be retracted or pulled back to expose the glans penis |
| prolapsed uterus (proh-LAPSED YOO-ter-uhs) | common English word; *uterus* is a Latin word meaning "womb" | descent of the uterus or cervix into the vagina |

(*continued*)

**Study Table** THE REPRODUCTIVE SYSTEM (*continued*)

| TERM AND PRONUNCIATION | ANALYSIS | MEANING |
|---|---|---|
| prostatitis (PROS-tah-TYE-tis) | *prostat/o* (prostate); + *itis* (inflammation) | inflammation of the prostate |
| rectocele (REK-toh-seel) | *rect/o* (rectum); *-cele* (hernia) | protrusion of the rectum into the posterior wall of the vagina |
| retroflexion (re-troh-FLEX-shun) | *retro-* (backward) + flexion, from the Latin word *flectere* (to bend) | abnormal tipping with the body of the uterus bent back on itself |
| retroversion (re-troh-VER-shun) | *retro-* (backward); from the Latin word *versio* (to turn) | an abnormal tipping of the entire uterus backward |
| salpingitis (sal-pin-JY-tis) | *salping/o* (tube, uterine tube); *-itis* (inflammation) | inflammation of the uterine tube |
| sexually transmitted disease (STD) (SEK-shoo-uh-lee trans-MIT-ted dih-ZEEZ) | common English words | diseases that are transmitted through sexual intercourse or sexual contact (HIV, syphilis, chlamydia); STI |
| syphilis (SIF-ih-lis) | from a poem *Syphilis sive Morbus Gallicus* by Fracastorius, *Syphilus* being a shepherd and principal character | a highly contagious STD that is caused by a bacterium |
| vaginitis (VAJ-ih-NIGH-tis) | *vagin/o* (vagina); *-itis* (inflammation) | inflammation of the vaginal tissues that may be infectious or due to several other causes |
| varicocele (VAR-ih-ko-seel) | *varic/o* (varix, varicose, varicosity); *-cele* (hernia) | a varicose vein of the testes |
| **Diagnostic Tests, Treatments, and Surgical Procedures** | | |
| amniocentesis (am-nee-oh-sen-TEE-sihs) | *amni/o* (amnion); *-centesis* (surgical puncture for aspiration) | extraction and diagnostic examination of amniotic fluid from the amniotic sac |
| bilateral oophorectomy (bye-LAT-er-ul oh-of-oh-REK-tuh-mee) | *bi-* (two); lateral (side); *oophor/o* (ovary); *-ectomy* (excision) | removal of both ovaries |
| bilateral salpingo-oophorectomy (bye-LAT-er-ul sal-ping-oh-oh-of-oh-REK-tuh-mee | *bi-* (two); lateral (side); *salping/o* (tube, fallopian tube); *oophor/o* (ovary); + *ectomy* (excision) | removal of both sets of ovaries and uterine tubes |
| cervicectomy (surv-ih-SEK-toh-mee) | *cervic/o* (cervix); + *ectomy* (excision); | excision of the uterine cervix; *trachelectomy* |
| cervicoplasty (SURV-ih-ko-plass-tee) | *cervic/o* (cervix); + *plasty* (surgical repair) | surgical repair of the uterine cervix |
| cervicotomy (surv-ih-KOT-oh-mee) | *cervic/o* (cervix); + *-tomy* (incision into); | incision into the uterine cervix |

**Study Table** THE REPRODUCTIVE SYSTEM (*continued*)

| TERM AND PRONUNCIATION | ANALYSIS | MEANING |
|---|---|---|
| cesarean section (CS or C-section) (seh-SAYR-ee-ahn SEK-shuhn); other spellings are caesarean and caesarian | etymology uncertain | surgical operation through the abdominal wall and uterus for delivery of the baby |
| circumcision (SER-kum SIZH-un) | *circum/o* (around); from the Latin word *caedo* (cut) | a surgical procedure to remove the foreskin of the penis |
| colposcope (kol-POH-skope) | *colp/o* (vagina); *-scope* (instrument used to view) | endoscopic instrument used to magnify and examine the tissues of the vagina and cervix |
| colposcopy (kol-POSS-koh-pee) | *colp/o* (vagina); *-scopy* (use of an instrument for viewing) | using an endoscopic instrument to examine the vagina and cervix |
| dilation and curettage (D&C) (dye-LAY-shun and KYOO-ruh-tahzh) | from the Latin word *dilatare* (to make wider, enlarge); from the French word *curette* (scoop) | dilation of the cervix and curettage, which involves scraping of the lining of the uterus |
| hysterectomy (his-ter-EK-tuh-mee) | *hyster/o* (uterus); *-ectomy* (excision) | surgical removal of the uterus |
| hysteropexy (his-ter-oh-PEK-see) | *hyster/o* (uterus); *-pexy* (fixation) | surgical fixation of the uterus |
| hysteroplasty (his-ter-oh-PLAS-tee) | *hyster/o* (uterus); *-plasty* (surgical repair) | surgical repair of the uterus |
| hysterosalpingography (HISS-ter-roh-sal-ping-goh-gruh-fee) | *hyster/o* (uterus); *salping/o* (tube, fallopian tube); *-graphy* (process of recording) | radiography of the uterus and uterine tubes |
| hysterotomy (his-ter-OT-oh-mee) | *hyster/o* (uterus); *-tomy* (incision into) | incision of the uterus |
| laparoscopy (lap-uh-ROS-kuh-pee) | *lapar/o* (of or pertaining to the abdominal wall, flank); *-scopy* (use of an instrument for viewing) | direct visualization of the interior of the abdomen with the use of a laparoscope |
| mammography (mah-MOG-ruh-fee) | *mamm/o* (breast); *-graphy* (process of recording) | examination of the breast by means of an imaging technique, such as radiography |
| mastectomy (mas-TEK-toh-mee) | *mast/o* (breast); *-ectomy* (excision) | removal of a breast |
| oophorectomy (OH-of-oh-rek-tuh-mee) | *oophor/o* (ovary); *-ectomy* (excision) | excision of an ovary; *ovariectomy* |
| oophoroplasty (oh-of-or-oh PLAS-tee) | *oophor/o* (ovary); *-plasty* (surgical repair) | surgical repair of an ovary |

(*continued*)

**Study Table** THE REPRODUCTIVE SYSTEM (*continued*)

| TERM AND PRONUNCIATION | ANALYSIS | MEANING |
|---|---|---|
| oophorotomy (oh-of-or-OT-uh-mee) | *oophor/o* (ovary); *-tomy* (incision into) | incision into an ovary |
| orchiectomy (or-kee-EK-toh-mee) | *orchi/o* (testes); *-ectomy* (excision) | removal of one or both testes; *orchechtomy*; *orchidectomy* |
| orchioplasty (OR-kee-oh-plass-tee) | *orchi/o* (testes); *-plasty* (surgical repair) | surgical repair of a testis |
| orchiotomy (or-kee-OT-ah-mee) | *orchi/o* (testes); *-tomy* (incision into) | incision into a testis |
| ovariectomy (oh-vahr-ee-EK-toh-mee) | *ovari/o* (ovary); *-ectomy* (excision) | excision of one or both ovaries |
| ovariotomy (oh-vahr-ee-OT-oh-mee) | *ovari/o* (ovary); *-tomy* (incision into) | incision of an ovary |
| Pap smear (Papanicolaou) (pap smeer) | named after George Papanicolaou, who developed the technique | exfoliative biopsy or a scraping of the cervix to diagnose conditions of the cervix and surrounding tissues |
| salpingo-oophorectomy (sahl-ping-goh oh-uh-fuh-REK-tuh-mee) | *salping/o* (tube, uterine tube); *oophor/o* (ovary); *-ectomy* (excision) | removal of an ovary and uterine tube |
| transurethral resection of the prostate (TURP) (TRANS-yoo-ree-thrul ree-SEK-shun of the PROS-tate) | from the Latin *trans* (across); from the Greek word *ourethra* (urethra); re- (again) from the Latin *secare* (to cut) | the removal of part or all of the prostate through the urethra |
| tubal ligation (TOO-ball lie-GAY-shun) | tube; *-al* (adjective suffix); ligation, from the Latin word *ligare* (to bind) | surgical procedure performed for female sterilization where each fallopian tube is tied off or "ligated" to prevent the oocyte from reaching the uterus |
| uteropexy (yoo-ter-oh-PEK-see) | *uter/o* (uterus); *-pexy* (fixation) | surgical fixation of the uterus; *hysteropexy* |
| uteroplasty (yoo-ter-oh-PLAS-tee) | *uter/o* (uterus); *-plasty* (surgical repair) | surgical repair of the uterus; *hysteroplasty* |
| uterotomy (yoo-ter-OT-uh-mee) | *uter/o* (uterus); *-tomy* (incision into) | incision of the uterus; *hysterotomy* |
| varicocelectomy (VAIR-ih-koh-seh-LEK-tuh-mee) | *varic/o* (varix, varicose, varicosity); *-cele* (hernia); *-ectomy* (excision) | the removal of a portion of an enlarged vein to remove a varicocele |
| vasovasostomy (vay-soh-vay-ZOS-toh-mee) | *vas/o* (vessel, vas deferens); *-stomy* (creation of an opening) | procedure to restore fertility to a vasectomized male; reconnect the ductus (vas) deferens |

**Study Table** THE REPRODUCTIVE SYSTEM (*continued*)

| TERM AND PRONUNCIATION | ANALYSIS | MEANING |
|---|---|---|
| **Practice and Practitioners** | | |
| gynecologist (guy-neh-KOL-oh-jist) | *gynec/o* (woman, female); *-logist* (one who studies a certain field) | a specialist of the female reproductive system |
| gynecology (guy-neh-KOL-oh-jee) | *gynec/o* (woman, female); *-logy* (study of) | the study of the female reproductive system |
| neonatology (NEE-oh-nay-TOL-oh-jee) | *neo-* (new); *nat/o* (birth); *-logy* (study of) | the medical specialty dealing with newborns |
| neonatologist (NEE-oh-nay-TOL-oh-jist) | *neo-* (new); *nat/o* (birth); *-logist* (one who studies a certain field) | the medical specialist dealing with newborns |
| obstetrician (OB-steh-trish-uhn) | from the Latin word *obstetricis* (midwife), derived from the Latin word *obstare* (to stand opposite to) | a physician who specializes in the medical care of women during pregnancy and childbirth |
| obstetrics (OB) (ob-STET-riks) | from the Latin word *obstetricis* (midwife), derived from the Latin word *obstare* (to stand opposite to) | medical specialty concerned with the medical care of women during pregnancy and childbirth |
| pediatrician (pee-dee-a-TRISH-an) | from the Greek *paid-*, stem of *pais* (child); *-iatr/o* (pertaining to medicine) | medical specialist of children |
| pediatrics (pee-dee-AT-riks) | from the Greek *paid-*, stem of *pais* (child); *-iatr/o* (pertaining to medicine) | medical specialty dealing with children |
| urologist (yoo-ROL-uh-jist) | *uro-* (urinary) + *logos* (study) | medical specialists who diagnose and treat disorders of the urinary and male reproductive systems |

## END-OF-CHAPTER EXERCISES

### EXERCISE 15-1 LABELING

**Using the following list, choose the correct terms to label the diagrams correctly.**

Label the figure of the male reproductive system.

| | | |
|---|---|---|
| ductus deferens or vas deferens | glans penis | scrotum |
| epididymis | penis | seminal gland |
| foreskin | prostate | testis |

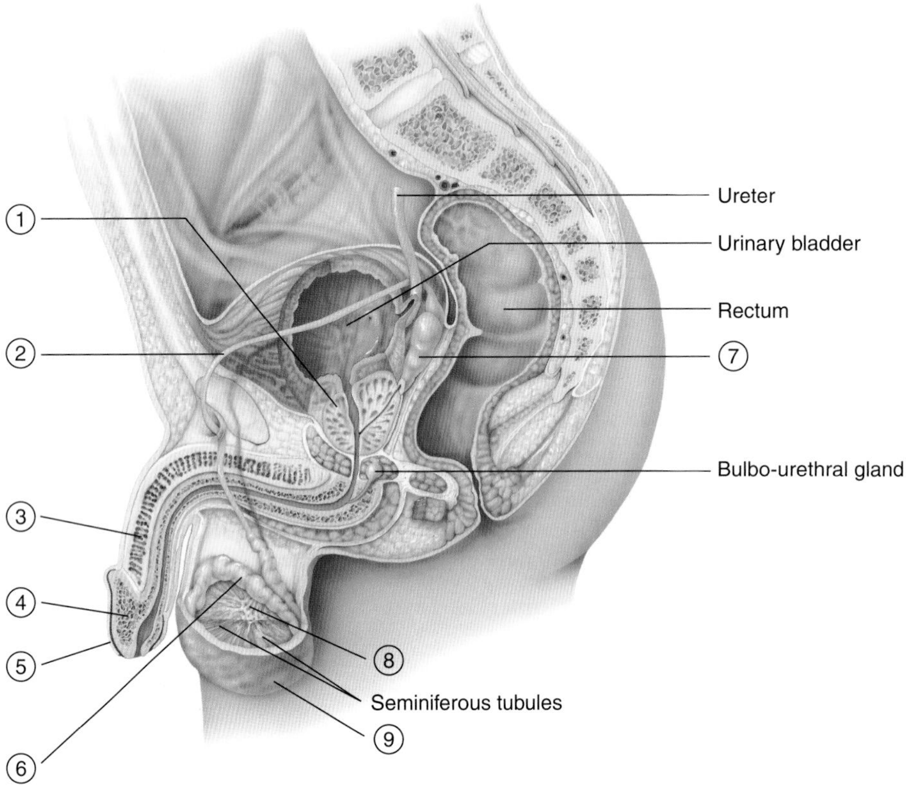


1. ______________________ 4. ______________________ 7. ______________________

2. ______________________ 5. ______________________ 8. ______________________

3. ______________________ 6. ______________________ 9. ______________________

Label the figure of the female reproductive system.

| | | |
|---|---|---|
| anus | labium minus | urinary bladder |
| cervix | ovary | uterine tube |
| clitoris | rectum | uterus |
| labium majus | urethra | vagina |

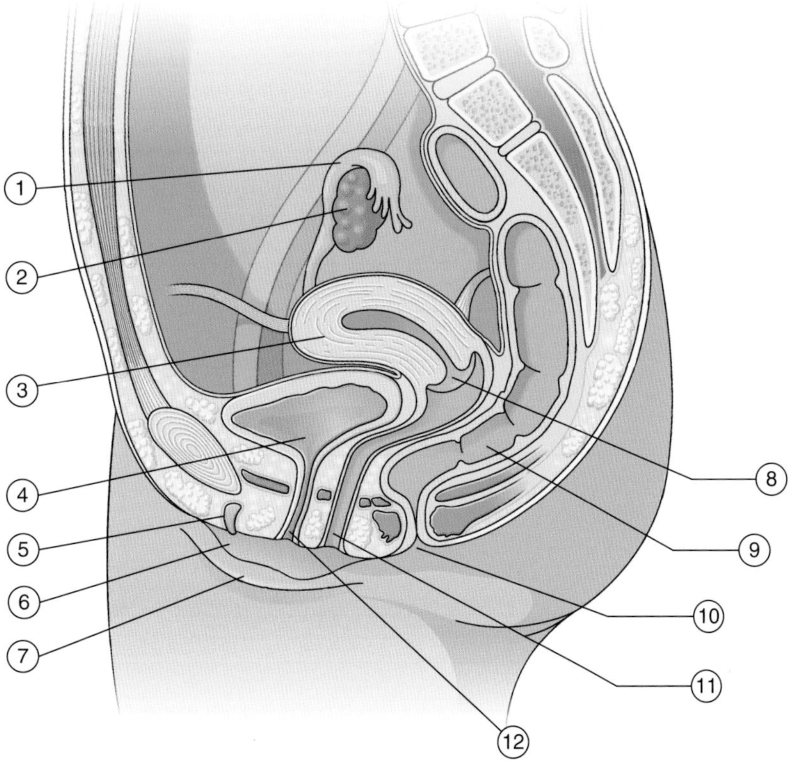


1. ____________________
2. ____________________
3. ____________________
4. ____________________
5. ____________________
6. ____________________
7. ____________________
8. ____________________
9. ____________________
10. ____________________
11. ____________________
12. ____________________

## EXERCISE 15-2 WORD PARTS

**Break each of the following terms into its word parts: prefix, root, or suffix. Give the meaning of each word part and then define the term.**

1. *amenorrhea*

   prefix: ______

   root: ______

   suffix: ______

   definition: ______

2. *azoospermia*

   prefix: ______

   prefix: ______

   root: ______

   suffix: ______

   definition: ______

3. *dysmenorrhea*

   prefix: ______

   root: ______

   suffix: ______

   definition: ______

4. *menorrhagia*

   root: ______

   suffix: ______

   definition: ______

5. *prostatitis*

   root: ______

   suffix: ______

   definition: ______

6. *hysterotomy*

   root: ______

   suffix: ______

   definition: ______

7. *mastectomy*

   root: ____________________

   suffix: ____________________

   definition: ____________________

8. *neonatology*

   prefix: ____________________

   root: ____________________

   suffix: ____________________

   definition: ____________________

## EXERCISE 15-3 WORD BUILDING

**Use the word parts listed to build the terms defined.**

| | | | |
|---|---|---|---|
| -algia | -graphy | -logist | -pexy |
| amni/o | gynec/o | mamm/o | -pathy |
| -cele | hyster/o | mast/o | -scopy |
| -centesis | -itis | oophor/o | -tomy |
| cyst/o | lapar/o | orchi/o | uter/o |

1. protrusion of the bladder into the anterior wall of the vagina ____________________
2. pain in the uterus ____________________
3. inflammation of the breast ____________________
4. any disease of the testes ____________________
5. extraction and diagnostic examination of amniotic fluid from the amniotic sac ____________________
6. examination of the breast by means of an imaging technique, such as radiography ____________________
7. direct visualization of the interior of the abdomen with the use of a laparoscope ____________________
8. incision into an ovary ____________________
9. surgical fixation of the uterus ____________________
10. specialist of the female reproductive system ____________________

## EXERCISE 15-4 MATCHING

**Match the term with its definition.**

| | | |
|---|---|---|
| 1. ________________ | vas deferens | a. combination of sperm and associated liquids that nourish the sperm |
| 2. ________________ | prostate | b. pain in the ovary |
| 3. ________________ | spermatogenesis | c. organs that produce and store male gametes |
| 4. ________________ | epididymis | d. duct leading out of the epididymis |
| 5. ________________ | semen | e. production of sperm |
| 6. ________________ | orchialgia | f. inflammation of an ovary |
| 7. ________________ | testes | g. pain in the testes |
| 8. ________________ | hysterectomy and bilateral oophorectomy | h. release of the female gamete from the ovary |
| 9. ________________ | ovarialgia | i. organ in which the male sperm become functional; lies on top of the testes |
| 10. ________________ | hysteropexy | j. excision of the uterine cervix |
| 11. ________________ | period of gestation | k. surgical fixation of the uterus |
| 12. ________________ | oophoritis | l. the female gamete |
| 13. ________________ | ovulation | m. surgical removal of the uterus and right and left ovaries |
| 14. ________________ | oocyte | n. time lapse between zygote formation and birth |
| 15. ________________ | cervicectomy | o. gland that surrounds the urethra; secretes alkaline fluid that assists in sperm motility |

## EXERCISE 15-5 MULTIPLE CHOICE

**Choose the correct answer for the following multiple choice questions.**

1. The surgical removal of testes is called ____________________.
   a. orchiectomy
   b. vasectomy
   c. circumcision
   d. cauterization

2. A prolapsed uterus means that the uterus is ____________________.
   a. bent backward on itself
   b. descended down into the vagina
   c. tipped forward
   d. tipped backward

3. Menarche is ____________________.
   a. the beginning of menstruation
   b. the end of menopause
   c. part of the first trimester
   d. another name for gestation

4. Cryptorchidism is ____________________.
   a. underdeveloped testes
   b. small ovaries
   c. ruptured ovaries
   d. undescended testes

5. Removal of fluid from the area around the fetus to analyze it is called ____________________.
   a. cervicentesis
   b. amniocentesis
   c. intrauterine analysis
   d. uterocentesis

6. The surgical procedure that removes the prostate is called a ____________________.
   a. vasectomy
   b. prostatectomy
   c. vasoligation
   d. circumcision

7. A Papanicolaou test is done to detect ____________________.
   a. fibroids
   b. metritis
   c. cancer of the cervix
   d. ovarian cancer

8. A difficult or painful monthly blood flow is termed __________.
   a. dysmenorrhea
   b. menorrhea
   c. dysmetrorrhagia
   d. menometrorrhagia

9. A colposcope is used to visualize the __________.
   a. testis
   b. epididymis
   c. breast
   d. vagina

## EXERCISE 15-6 FILL IN THE BLANK

**Fill in the blank with the correct answer.**

1. A male gamete is also called a __________.
2. A female gamete is also called an __________
3. Spermatogenesis is initiated by the secretion of the androgen __________.
4. The male glands located at the base of the urinary bladder that produce a fluid that nourishes the sperm are the __________.
5. The inner layer of the uterus is the __________.
6. A fertilized egg is call an __________ during the first 8 weeks of gestation.
7. A fertilized egg that implants outside the uterus is called an __________ pregnancy.
8. A Pap smear uses tissue from the __________.
9. The plural of ovum is __________.
10. The plural of ovary is __________.

## EXERCISE 15-7 ABBREVIATIONS

**Write out the term for the following abbreviations.**

1. BPH ______________________
2. G ______________________
3. HIV ______________________
4. EDD ______________________
5. CS ______________________
6. OB ______________________
7. EDC ______________________
8. STD ______________________
9. GYN ______________________
10. PID ______________________
11. HSV ______________________

**Write the abbreviation for the following terms.**

12. abortus ______________
13. sexually transmitted infection ______________
14. transurethral resection of the prostate ______________
15. gonorrhea ______________
16. last menstrual period ______________
17. dilation and curettage ______________
18. para ______________
19. human papillomavirus ______________

## EXERCISE 15-8 SPELLING

**Select the correct spelling of the medical term.**

1. The Latin word for neck is ____________________, which is a common term for a structure found in the uterus.
   a. cirvix
   b. cervics
   c. cerviks
   d. cervix

2. The term for a female oocyte and a male sperm is ____________________.
   a. gameat
   b. gameet
   c. gamete
   d. gemete

3. The beginning of menses is called ____________________.
   a. menarche
   b. menarch
   c. menerch
   d. mennarche

4. The plural of testis is ____________________.
   a. testeas
   b. testes
   c. testies
   d. testees

5. A gene-bearing bundle of DNA found in the nucleus of all cells is a ____________________.
   a. cromosome
   b. chromasome
   c. chromosome
   d. chromosone

6. The absence of menstruation is called ____________________.
   a. amenorrhea
   b. amenorhea
   c. amenorea
   d. amenoria

7. A low sperm count is known as ____________________.
   a. oligaspermia
   b. oligospermia
   c. oligospermea
   d. oliguspermiea

8. The STD caused by the bacterium *Treponema pallidum* is ____________________.
   a. sipilis
   b. siphilis
   c. siphylis
   d. syphilis

9. A ____________________ is a practitioner who specializes in the female reproductive system.
   a. gynacologist
   b. gynecologist
   c. gynicologist
   d. gynocologist

10. The extraction and diagnostic examination of amniotic fluid from the amniotic sac is called ____________________.
    a. amiocentesis
    b. aminocentesis
    c. amniocentesis
    d. amnoicentesis

## EXERCISE 15-9 CASE STUDY

**A 27-year-old gravida II, para I woman without significant medical history. Blood work was normal before delivery of a stillborn 1-pound, 11-ounce infant during week 21. Although ultrasound studies during week 14 and amniocentesis during week 15 were unremarkable, intrauterine fetal demise had occurred during week 18.**

1. What does gravida II para I mean? ____________________________________________

   ____________________________________________

2. What is amniocentesis? ____________________________________________

   ____________________________________________

3. Using your knowledge of word parts, define intrauterine ____________________________________________

   ____________________________________________

# APPENDIX A Answers

## CHAPTER 1

### Quick Check

prefix = intra-
root = cran/i
suffix = -al

### EXERCISE 1-1 DEFINING TERMS

1. cardiology
2. gerontology
3. hematology
4. dermatology
5. neurology
6. psychology

### EXERCISE 1-2 ANALYZING TERMS

| TERM | ROOT | SUFFIX | DEFINITION |
|---|---|---|---|
| 1. neuropathy | neuro | -pathy | disease of the nerves |
| 2. psychology | psycho | -logy | the study and science of mental processes and behavior |
| 3. pathogenic | patho | -genic | causing disease |
| 4. neuralgia | neur | -algia | pain in one or more nerves |
| 5. systemic | system | -ic | relating to a body system or systems |
| 6. psychiatrist | psych iatr | -ist | a medical doctor who specializes in the diagnosis and treatment of mental and emotional disorders |
| 7. pediatrician | ped iatr | -ician | a physician who deals with the care and treatment of babies and children |
| 8. iatrogenic | iatro | -genic | refers to ailments caused by a doctor or other medical personnel |
| 9. cardialgia | cardi | -algia | pain in the heart (or stomach) |
| 10. neuritis | neur | -itis | inflammation of a nerve or nerves |

### EXERCISE 1-3 FILL IN THE BLANK

1. around
2. study of
3. skin
4. roots, suffix
5. logos, word
6. inflammation, tendon
7. before
8. Pain, -dynia
9. -itis
10. psychology

# CHAPTER 2

## Quick Check

| | | |
|---|---|---|
| 1. anti- | definition: not | refers to: negation |
| 2. hyper- | definition: above | refers to: position |
| 3. tachy- | definition: rapid | refers to: speed |

### EXERCISE 2-1 ADDING PREFIXES OF TIME OR SPEED

1. anteroom; outer room that leads into another room
2. neoclassic; new classic work
3. postglacial; following the glacial period
4. predominant; important
5. tachometer; instrument used to compute speed based on travel time or distance based on speed

### EXERCISE 2-2 ADDING PREFIXES OF DIRECTION

1. abnormal; adjective meaning "away from normal"
2. adjoining; adjective meaning "next to"
3. concentric; having the same center
4. contralateral; the other side
5. diagram; illustration that gives an overall view
6. sympathetic; sharing emotions with another person
7. synthesis; assembling parts into a whole

### EXERCISE 2-3 ADDING PREFIXES OF POSITION

1. eccentric; outside the center; unusual
2. ectomorph; slightly built person
3. enslave; to make a slave of
4. endocardial; adjective meaning "inside the heart"
5. epidemic; great number of occurrences of a particular disease
6. exchange; give something in return for another
7. exosphere; the far reaches of the atmosphere
8. extraterrestrial; beyond the earth
9. hypersensitive; highly sensitive
10. hypothesis; a possible explanation underlying the facts
11. infrastructure; the internal framework of a system or organization
12. intercollegiate; participation involving at least two colleges
13. intramural; inside the walls; often applied to sports teams within a school
14. mesosphere; the middle part of the earth's atmosphere
15. metaphysics; beyond physics
16. panorama; a wide expansive view of everything
17. paralegal; a trained assistant to a lawyer

### EXERCISE 2-4 ADDING PREFIXES OF SIZE OR NUMBER

1. biannual; occurring twice a year
2. hemisphere; half of a sphere
3. macrocosm; the universe
4. microscope; a device for viewing objects invisible to the human eye
5. monorail; a railway system on which the vehicle travels on one rail
6. oligarchy; rule by a small group of people
7. quadrilateral; having four sides
8. semiannual; twice a year
9. triangle; three-sided geometric shape
10. unicycle; a vehicle having one wheel

## EXERCISE 2-5 COMBINING ROOTS AND SUFFIXES THAT DENOTE MEDICAL CONDITIONS

1. card/i/o
   a. cardiocele; herniation of the heart
   b. cardiodynia; heart pain
   c. cardiectasia; dilation of the heart
   d. carditis; inflammation of the heart
   e. cardiomalacia; softening of the heart
   f. cardiomegaly; enlargement of the heart
   g. cardioptosis; drooping of the heart
   h. cardioplegia; paralysis of the heart
   i. cardiorrhexis; rupture of the heart wall
   j. cardiospasm; spasm of the heart
2. dermat/o
   a. dermatitis; inflammation of the skin
   b. dermatoma; tumor of the skin
   c. dermatomegaly; enlargement of the skin
   d. dermatosis; abnormal condition of the skin
3. hem/o, hemat/o
   a. hemolysis; destruction of the blood cells
   b. hematogenesis; produced by the blood
   c. hematoma; localized mass of blood
   d. hematosis; abnormal condition of the blood
4. neur/o
   a. neuralgia; nerve pain
   b. neurectasis; dilation of a nerve
   c. neuritis; inflammation of a nerve
   d. neuroma; tumor of a nerve
5. oste/o
   a. osteodynia; bone pain
   b. osteoma; bone tumor
   c. osteomalacia; softening of the bone
   d. osteopenia; reduction of bone density
   e. osteoporosis; porous bone, condition resulting in decreased bone mass
   f. osteitis; inflammation of the bone
6. psych/o
   a. psychosis; severe mental and behavioral disorder

## EXERCISE 2-6 COMBINING ROOTS AND SUFFIXES THAT DENOTE DIAGNOSTIC TERMS, TEST INFORMATION, OR SURGICAL PROCEDURES

1. card/i/o
   a. cardiogenic; originating in the heart
   b. cardiogram; graphic record of the heart
   c. cardiograph; machine that produces a cardiogram
   d. cardiography; process of electrically measuring heart function
   e. cardiopathy; heart disease
   f. cardiorrhaphy; suture of the wall of the heart
2. dermat/o
   a. dermatoplasty; surgical repair of the skin
3. hemat/o
   a. hematogenesis; originating with or in the blood
   b. hematometry; examination of blood
4. neur/o
   a. neurectomy; removal of a nerve or part of a nerve
   b. neurogenic; adjectival form of *neurogenesis; originating in the nervous system*
   c. neurogenesis; originating in the nervous system
5. oste/o
   a. osteorrhaphy; suturing broken bone together
   b. osteoplasty; surgical repair of the bone
   c. osteogenesis; formation of bone
   d. ostectomy; excision of bone
   e. osteotomy; cutting of bone
6. path/o
   a. pathogen; a disease-causing agent
   b. pathogenic; adjectival form of *pathogen; disease causing*
   c. pathogenesis; development of a disease
7. psych/o
   a. psychogenic; adjectival form of *psychogenesis; of mental origin*
   b. psychogenesis; mental development
   c. psychometry; mental testing
   d. psychopathy; mental illness or disorder

## EXERCISE 2-7 COMBINING ROOTS AND SUFFIXES ASSOCIATED WITH A MEDICAL SPECIALIST OR SPECIALTY

1. card/i/o
   a. cardiology; medical specialty that diagnoses and treats heart diseases
   b. cardiologist; heart specialist
2. derm/o, dermat/o
   a. dermatology; medical specialty that diagnoses and treats skin disorders
   b. dermatologist; skin specialist
3. ger/o/nt/o
   a. geriatrics; medical specialty that diagnoses and treats the aged
   b. gerontology; the study of the process and results of aging
   c. gerontologist; specialist in gerontology

4. hem/o, hemat/o
   a. hematology; medical specialty that diagnoses and treats blood disorders
   b. hematologist; a specialist who treats blood disorders
5. neur/o
   a. neurology; medical specialty that diagnoses and treats the nervous system
   b. neurologist; specialist who treats the nervous system
6. oste/o
   a. osteology; medical specialty that diagnoses and treats disorders of the skeletal system
   b. osteologist; a bone specialist
7. path/o
   a. pathology; study of disease
   b. pathologist; a medical specialist who studies pathology
8. psych/o
   a. psychology; study of the mind
   b. psychiatry; the medical specialty that diagnoses and treats mind disorders
   c. psychiatrist; a medical specialist in psychiatry

## EXERCISE 2-8 COMBINING ROOTS AND SUFFIXES THAT DENOTE ADJECTIVES

1. card/i/o
   a. cardiac; refers to the heart
2. hem/o, hemat/o
   a. hemotoxic; destructive of red blood cells
3. derm/o, dermat/o
   a. dermal; adjective denoting skin
   b. dermatic; adjective denoting skin
4. ger/o, geront/o
   a. geriatric; adjective meaning "pertaining to the elderly or aging"
   b. gerontal; adjective meaning "old-age related"
5. neur/o
   a. neural; adjective meaning "related to the nervous system"
   b. neurotic; adjective meaning "pertaining to neurosis"
6. spin/o
   a. spinal; adjective referring to spinal column
   b. spinous; adjective meaning "having spines"
7. oste/o
   a. osteal; adjective meaning "bone"
   b. osteoid; adjective meaning "resembling bone"

## EXERCISE 2-9 MATCHING SUFFIXES WITH MEANINGS

1. g
2. i
3. b
4. m
5. j
6. d
7. c
8. h
9. f
10. e
11. a
12. o
13. n
14. k
15. l

## EXERCISE 2-10 FILL IN THE BLANK

1. -algia, -dynia
2. angiectasis
3. adjective
4. suture of a blood vessel
5. -graphy
6. tumor of the blood vessel
7. surgical repair
8. dermatologist
9. old patients
10. gerontology is the study of old age; geriatrics is the branch of medicine dealing with the care of older people
11. ad-
12. ante-
13. abnormally slow heartbeat
14. beyond
15. hyper-
16. medicine to prevent coagulation (clotting)
17. three
18. the instrument will make objects visible that are too small to be seen with the unaided eye
19. endocarditis; inflammation of the inside of the heart
20. tachypnea is rapid breathing; dyspnea is difficulty or painful breathing

# CHAPTER 3

## Word Parts Exercise

1. across
2. back
3. near
4. cartilage
5. front, anterior
6. muscle
7. superior
8. neck
9. groin
10. spinal cord

## Quick Check

1. distal: proximal
2. inferior: superior
3. anterior: posterior
4. dorsal: ventral

## EXERCISE 3-1 MATCHING

### A. Planes of the Body

1. c
2. b
3. a

### B. Directional Terms

1. f
2. g
3. h
4. j
5. i
6. e
7. a
8. d
9. c
10. b

## EXERCISE 3-2 FILL IN THE BLANK

1. distal
2. proximal
3. anterior, ventral
4. medial
5. superior
6. lateral
7. posterior, dorsal
8. inferior

## EXERCISE 3-3 WORD BUILDING

1. hypo-, -ic; hypogastric
2. -al; dorsal
3. -itis; chondritis
4. trans-, -ic; transthoracic
5. -itis; neuritis
6. epi-, -al; epicardial

## EXERCISE 3-4 SHORT ANSWER

1. lateral
2. toward the back
3. proximal
4. anterior or forward
5. ventral

## EXERCISE 3-5 TRUE OR FALSE

1. False
2. True
3. False
4. True
5. True
6. False
7. True
8. False
9. False
10. True

# CHAPTER 4

## Word Parts Exercise

1. skin
2. fungus
3. cell
4. sweat
5. red
6. dry
7. to carry
8. below
9. sebum (oil; fat)
10. upon
11. white
12. blue
13. dry, scaly (fishlike)
14. skin
15. horny tissue or cells
16. skin
17. nail
18. black
19. hair
20. hardening
21. yellow

## Quick Check

| Suffix | Term |
|---|---|
| -ous | subcutaneous |
| -cyte | melanocyte |
| -aceous | sebaceous |

## EXERCISE 4-1 LABELING THE SKIN

1. hair
2. epidermis
3. dermis
4. hypodermis (subcutaneous) layer
5. nerve
6. artery
7. vein
8. adipose tissue
9. sudoriferous (sweat) gland
10. hair follicle
11. arrector pili muscle
12. sebaceous (oil) gland
13. pore (opening of sweat gland)

## EXERCISE 4-2 WORD PARTS

1. avascular
   prefix: a-, without;
   root: vascular, small vessels;
   definition: without blood vessels
2. epidermis
   prefix: epi-, upon;
   root: dermis, skin;
   definition: outer layer of the skin
3. melanocyte
   root: melano;
   suffix: -cyte, cell;
   definition: cell that produces melanin
4. scabicide
   root: scabies, infection caused by mites;
   suffix:-icide, destruction;
   definition: agent lethal to mites
5. dermatomycosis
   root: dermato, skin;
   root: myc, fungus;
   suffix: -osis, abnormal condition;
   definition: fungal infection of the skin
6. onychectomy
   root: onych, nail;
   suffix: -ectomy, excision;
   definition: surgical removal of a nail
7. ecchymosis
   prefix: ec-, out;
   root: chymos, juice;
   suffix: -osis, abnormal condition;
   definition: a purple patch more than 3 mm in diameter caused by blood under the skin
8. antiseptic
   prefix: anti-, against;
   root: septic, poison;
   definition: agent that inhibits the growth of infectious agents

**EXERCISE 4-3** WORD BUILDING

1. dermatoplasty
2. hemangioma
3. dermatitis
4. subcutaneous
5. onchotomy
6. dermatology
7. onchyomalacia
8. paronchia
9. ichthyosis
10. hyperhidrosis

**EXERCISE 4-4** MATCHING

1. d
2. e
3. i
4. f
5. b
6. c
7. g
8. j
9. h
10. a
11. l
12. k

**EXERCISE 4-5** MULTIPLE CHOICE

1. b
2. b
3. b
4. d
5. b
6. c
7. b
8. b
9. d
10. d
11. d
12. b
13. b
14. a
15. c

**EXERCISE 4-6** FILL IN THE BLANK

1. keloid
2. fissure
3. Cyanosis
4. scleroderma
5. alopecia
6. albinism
7. vitiligo
8. Urticaria
9. biopsy
10. polyp

**EXERCISE 4-7** ABBREVIATIONS

1. body surface area
2. incision and drainage
3. SLE
4. UV

**EXERCISE 4-8** SPELLING

1. d.
2. d
3. c
4. a
5. d
6. c
7. b
8. d
9. a
10. a

**EXERCISE 4-9** CASE STUDY

1. antibiotic; medication used to kill bacteria or treat an infection
2. impetigo; contagious superficial skin infection that presents with vesicles
3. dermatologist; medical specialist who diagnoses and treats disorders of the skin
4. dermatitis; inflammation of the skin
5. erythematous; redness of the skin
6. pustules; small elevated areas of skin that contains pus
7. edema; swelling in the tissues
8. antipruritic medication; medication used to reduce or stop itching
9. pruritus; itching
10. One reason the dermatologist may have been asking about pets is that allergies to pets may cause some of the signs and symptoms of an allergic reaction. Another possible reason to ask about children and pets is that they can carry diseases that are uncommon in adult populations, but more common in children and animals.

# CHAPTER 5

## Word Parts Exercise

1. swayback, curve
2. joined (yoked) together
3. wrist
4. foot, child
5. bone
6. bones of fingers and toes
7. pain
8. cranium
9. joined together
10. inflammation
11. muscle
12. to visually examine
13. movement
14. correct, straight
15. femur, thighbone
16. softening
17. surgical repair
18. joint
19. pelvis
20. growth
21. arm
22. finger, toe
23. rib
24. bone marrow
25. electricity
26. thorax, chest
27. humerus, upper arm bone
28. porous
29. stiff, fused, closed
30. vertebrae
31. written record of
32. movement
33. both sides
34. calcaneus, heel bone
35. hump
36. neck
37. study of
38. cartilage
39. lower back
40. removal of, excision of
41. tumor

## Quick Check

1. osteocytes
2. synovial
3. mandible

## EXERCISE 5-1 LABELING: SKELETON

1. cranium
2. facial bones
3. mandible
4. sternum
5. costal cartilage
6. vertebral column
7. ilium
8. pubis
9. sacrum
10. calcaneus
11. metatarsals
12. phalanges
13. tarsal bones
14. tibia
15. fibula
16. patella
17. femur
18. clavicle
19. scapula
20. humerus
21. ribs
22. radius
23. ulna
24. carpal bones
25. metacarpals
26. phalanges

## EXERCISE 5-2 FIGURE LABELING: LONG BONE

1. proximal epiphysis
2. diaphysis
3. distal epiphysis
4. spongy bone
5. epiphyseal plate
6. periosteum
7. compact bone
8. medullary cavity
9. endosteum

## EXERCISE 5-3 WORD PARTS

1. osteorraphy
   root: oste/o = bone
   suffix: -rrhaphy = surgical suturing
   definition: suturing together the fragments of a broken bone
2. arthrocentesis
   root: arthr/o = joint
   suffix: -centesis = surgical puncture for aspiration
   definition: aspiration of fluid from a joint by needle puncture
3. brachialgia
   root: brachi/o = arm
   suffix: -algia (pain)
   definition: pain in the arm
4. osteochondritis
   root: oste/o = bone
   root: chondr/o = cartilage
   suffix: -itis = inflammation
   definition: inflammation of bone and its overlying cartilage
5. carpectomy
   root: carp/o = wrist
   suffix: -ectomy = surgical removal
   definition: excision of a portion or all of the wrist
6. chondrosarcoma
   root: chondr/o = cartilage
   root: sarc/o = flesh
   suffix: -oma = tumor
   definition: malignant tumor derived from cartilage
7. dactylomegaly
   root: dactyl/o = finger, toe
   suffix: - megaly = enlargement
   definition: enlargement of one or more fingers or toes

## EXERCISE 5-4 WORD BUILDING

1. osteomyelitis
2. arthroscopy
3. chondromalacia
4. arthrogram
5. arthralgia
6. kinesiology
7. chondroplasty
8. intercostal
9. osteitis
10. osteosarcoma
11. arthroplasty
12. myelogram
13. chondritis
14. osteoporosis
15. costalgia

## EXERCISE 5-5 MATCHING

1. e
2. d
3. b
4. c
5. a
6. f
7. g

## EXERCISE 5-6 MULTIPLE CHOICE

1. d
2. a
3. d
4. a
5. c
6. b
7. c
8. d
9. a
10. a
11. d
12. b
13. a
14. a
15. b

**EXERCISE 5-7** FILL IN THE BLANK

1. arthritis
2. arthrocentesis
3. orthopedic surgeon
4. compound
5. medullary
6. ligament
7. herniated disc

**EXERCISE 5-8** ABBREVIATIONS

1. anterior cruciate ligament
2. computed tomography
3. cervical vertebra 1
4. total knee arthroplasty
5. lumbar vertebra 5
6. rheumatoid arthritis
7. nonsteroidal anti-inflammatory drug
8. magnetic resonance imaging
9. THR
10. Fx
11. Tx
12. ROM
13. T12
14. TKR
15. MRI

**EXERCISE 5-9** SPELLING

1. a
2. b
3. b
4. d
5. c
6. d
7. a
8. c
9. a
10. b

**EXERCISE 5-10** CASE STUDY

1. a physician who treats and diagnoses skeletal disorders
2. ROM = range of motion; unable to flex or move her wrist much
3. a wrist bone was broken in several places
4. hip bone, which is formed by the fusion of the ilium, ischium, and pubis, was broken and pressed into another part of the bone
5. realignment
6. a treatment using elastics or pulley and weights

# CHAPTER 6

## Word Parts Exercise

1. ligament
2. tendon
3. tone
4. paralysis
5. muscle
6. movement
7. partial or incomplete paralysis
8. strength
9. muscle
10. four
11. 11. fibrous membrane
12. fiber
13. half
14. alongside, near

## Quick Check

**Muscle Tissue**

| **Type** | **Location** |
|---|---|
| 1. skeletal | voluntary, striated muscle tissue found throughout the body attached to bones |
| 2. smooth | involuntary muscle tissue lining blood vessels, hollow organs, and respiratory passageways |
| 3. cardiac | involuntary, striated muscle tissue making up the heart wall |

## EXERCISE 6-1 WORD PARTS

1. fibromyalgia
   root: fibro, fiber;
   root: my/o, muscle;
   suffix: -algia, pain;
   definition: a chronic disorder characterized by widespread aching and stiffness of muscles and soft tissues
2. periostitis
   prefix: peri-, around;
   root: osteo, bone;
   suffix: -itis, inflammation;
   definition: inflammation of the periosteum or the covering that surrounds the bone
3. tendinoplasty
   root: tendo, tendon;
   suffix: -plasty, restoring function to a part;
   definition: surgical procedure to restore function to the tendon
4. myology
   root: my/o, muscle;
   suffix: -ology, study of;
   definition: study of muscles
5. electromyography
   root: electro, electricity;
   root: myo, muscle;
   suffix: -graphy, process of writing;
   definition: diagnostic technique that records the strength of muscle contractions by means of electrical stimulation
6. epicondylitis
   prefix: epi-, around;
   root: condyl, rounded end surface of bone;
   suffix: -itis, inflammation;
   definition: inflammation of the tissues around the elbow
7. hemiplegia
   prefix: hemi-, half;
   root: plegia, paralysis;
   definition: total paralysis of one side of the body
8. paralysis
   prefix: para-, not normal;
   suffix: -lysis, loosening;
   definition: loss of sensation and voluntary muscle movements caused by an injury or disease

## EXERCISE 6-2 WORD BUILDING

1. tenotomy
2. neurologist
3. paraplegia
4. myocele
5. hemiparesis
6. fasciitis
7. kinesialgia
8. fibromyalgia
9. myopathy; musculopathy
10. myositis

## EXERCISE 6-3 MATCHING

1. d
2. i
3. f
4. b
5. c
6. e
7. a
8. g
9. k
10. h
11. l
12. j

## EXERCISE 6-4 MULTIPLE CHOICE

1. c
2. c
3. b
4. d
5. a
6. a
7. c
8. a
9. d
10. a

**EXERCISE 6-5** FILL IN THE BLANK

1. Epicondylitis
2. ligament
3. plantar flexion
4. Asthenia
5. myocele
6. Plantar fasciitis
7. electromyography (EMG)
8. tendinoplasty
9. Myology
10. myalgia

**EXERCISE 6-6** ABBREVIATIONS

1. muscular dystrophy
2. rest, ice, compression, elevation
3. cumulative trauma disorder
4. myasthenia gravis
5. EMG
6. ALS
7. IM
8. Fx
9. MD

**EXERCISE 6-7** SPELLING

1. c
2. a
3. b
4. d
5. d
6. c
7. c
8. b
9. a
10. a

**EXERCISE 6-8** CASE STUDY

1. flexion (closing the angle of a joint); extension (opening the angle of a joint); rotation (turning a body part on its own axis); abduction (movement away from midline)
2. inflammation of a tendon
3. range of motion is the amount of movement that is possible at the joint
4. nonsteroidal anti-inflammatory drug

# CHAPTER 7

## Word Parts Exercise

1. slight paralysis
2. outer layer or covering
3. referring to the mind
4. paralysis
5. memory
6. physician; to treat
7. fear
8. brain
9. the cerebrum; also, the brain in general
10. water
11. a membrane
12. ganglia (*ganglion*, singular)
13. suffix meaning "morbid attraction to" or "impulse toward"
14. in connection with the nervous system, refers to the spinal cord and medulla oblongata
15. nerve, nerve tissue
16. spider
17. to split
18. head
19. mind
20. resembling
21. the cerebellum
22. spine
23. speech
24. glue

## Quick Check

1. brain and spinal cord
2. homeostasis
3. brainstem

**EXERCISE 7-1**

1. dendrites
2. nucleus
3. cell body
4. myelin
5. axon

## EXERCISE 7-2 WORD PARTS

1. psychosis
   root: psycho, of or pertaining to the mind;
   suffix: -sis, condition of;
   definition: a serious disorder involving a marked distortion of, or sharp break from, reality
2. electroencephalography
   root: electro, electic;
   root: encephalo, brain;
   suffix: -graphy, process of recording;
   definition: record of the electrical potential of the brain
3. astrocytoma
   root: astro, star;
   root: cyt, cell;
   suffix: -oma, tumor;
   definition: star-shaped tumor that usually develops in the cerebrum
4. cerebrovascular
   root: cerebro, brain;
   root: vascul;
   suffix: -ar, adjective suffix;
   definition: of or relating to the brain and its blood vessels
5. encephalitis
   root: encephal, of or pertaining to the brain;
   suffix: -itis, inflammation;
   definition: inflammation of the brain
6. epidural
   prefix: epi-, above;
   root: dura, relating to the dura mater;
   suffix: -al, adjective suffix;
   definition: on or around the dura mater
7. psychiatrist
   root: psych, of or pertaining to the mind;
   root: iatr, of or pertaining to medicine or a physician;
   suffix: -ist, one who specializes in;
   definition: a medical doctor who specializes in the diagnosis and treatment of psychological disorders
8. meningioma
   root: mening, membrane;
   suffix: -oma, tumor;
   definition: benign tumor of the meninges

## EXERCISE 7-3 WORD BUILDING

1. encephalitis
2. glioma
3. hemiparesis
4. lobotomy
5. neuroglia
6. parasympathetic
7. paranoia
8. neuroplasty
9. diencephalon
10. paresthesia

## EXERCISE 7-4 MATCHING

1. k
2. f
3. c
4. n
5. h
6. j
7. e
8. b
9. m
10. g
11. d
12. a
13. l
14. i

## EXERCISE 7-5 MULTIPLE CHOICE

1. d
2. c
3. a
4. b
5. a
6. b
7. c
8. c
9. d
10. c
11. b
12. d
13. b
14. b
15. d

### EXERCISE 7-6 FILL IN THE BLANK

1. hyperesthesia
2. poliomyelitis
3. dementia
4. multiple sclerosis
5. myelomeningocele
6. cerebral thrombosis
7. Ataxia
8. epilepsy
9. Syncope
10. neuralgia

### EXERCISE 7-7 ABBREVIATIONS

1. intracranial pressure
2. cerebral spinal fluid
3. lumbar puncture
4. electroencephalography
5. multiple sclerosis
6. obsessive-compulsive disorder
7. Parkinson's disease
8. peripheral nervous system
9. cerebrovascular accident
10. dopamine
11. PTSD
12. PNS
13. CVA
14. MRI
15. TIA

### EXERCISE 7-8 SPELLING

1. a
2. c
3. c
4. d
5. a
6. b
7. d
8. b
9. c
10. a

### EXERCISE 7-9 CASE STUDY

1. transient ischemic attack; sometimes called a ministroke
2. cerebrovascular accident
3. dys- means "difficult"; -phasia means "speak"
4. partial or incomplete paralysis
5. hemiparesis means "partially paralyzed on half the body"; hemiplegia means "complete paralysis on half the body"
6. hemi- means "half"; -plegia means "paralysis"

# CHAPTER 8

## Word Parts Exercise

1. retina
2. hard, cornea
3. tear, lacrimal apparatus
4. light, eye, vision
5. eye
6. denoting the pigmented middle eye layer
7. two, double
8. tears, lacrimal sac or lacrimal duct
9. iris
10. eye
11. lens
12. old age
13. eyelid
14. conjunctiva (plural: conjunctivae)
15. pupil
16. horny
17. relating to the sclera; hard

### Quick Check

1. fibrous, vascular, inner
2. choroid
3. pupil

## Word Parts Exercise

1. sound
2. ear
3. hearing
4. tympanic membrane (eardrum)
5. eardrum
6. ear
7. stapes
8. ear

### Quick Check

1. malleus, incus, and stapes
2. conductive hearing loss, sensorineural hearing loss, presbycusis, and anacusis
3. cochlea

## EXERCISE 8-1 LABELING

1. conjunctiva
2. cornea
3. iris
4. pupil
5. lens
6. anterior chamber (containing aqueous humor)
7. posterior chamber (containing vitreous humor)
8. sclera
9. choroid
10. retina
11. optic nerve

## EXERCISE 8-2 WORD PARTS

1. extraocular
   prefix: extra-, outside;
   root: ocul, eye;
   suffix: -ar, adjective suffix;
   definition: situated outside the eye
2. xerophthalmia
   root: xero, dry;
   root: ophthalm, eye;
   suffix: -ia, condition;
   definition: dry eyes
3. scleroiritis
   root: sclera, sclera;
   root: ir/o, iris;
   suffix: -itis, inflammation;
   definition: inflammation of the sclera and iris
4. blepharoconjunctivitis
   root: blephar, eyelid;
   root: conjunctiv, mucous membrane covering the anterior surface of the eyeball and inner eyelid;
   suffix: -itis, inflammation;
   definition: inflammation of the palpebral conjectiva, the inner lining of the eyelids
5. audiometry
   root: audio, hearing;
   suffix: -metry, process of measuring;
   definition: measuring hearing with an audiometer
6. otosclerosis
   root: oto, ear;
   root: sclero, hardening;
   suffix: -osis, abnormal condition;
   definition: formation of spongy bone in the inner ear producing hearing loss
7. mastoidectomy
   root: mastoid, mastoid process;
   suffix: -ectomy, excision;
   definition: surgical removal of the mastoid process
8. otorhinolaryngologist
   root: oto, ear;
   root: rhino, nose;
   root: laryngo, throat;
   suffix: -logist, one who studies a certain field;
   definition: physician who specializes in the diagnosis and treatment of ear, nose, and throat disorders

**EXERCISE 8-3** WORD BUILDING

1. dacryolith
2. phacolysis
3. dacryocystotomy
4. retinopexy
5. iridomalacia
6. tympanocentesis
7. otodynia
8. myringotomy
9. otorrhea
10. otitis

**EXERCISE 8-4** MATCHING: THE EYE

1. j
2. g
3. e
4. d
5. h
6. a
7. f
8. i
9. c
10. b

**EXERCISE 8-5** MATCHING: THE EAR

1. c
2. g
3. d
4. i
5. b
6. j
7. e
8. a
9. h
10. f

**EXERCISE 8-6** MULTIPLE CHOICE

1. b
2. a
3. d
4. c
5. a
6. d
7. b
8. c
9. a
10. d

**EXERCISE 8-7** FILL IN THE BLANK

1. cataract
2. presbycusis
3. diplopia
4. vertigo
5. Tinnitus
6. auricle
7. hordeolum
8. Otalgia
9. astigmatism
10. keratitis
11. cochlea
12. semicircular
13. auditory tube
14. Blepharoptosis
15. conductive

**EXERCISE 8-8** ABBREVIATIONS

1. right ear
2. otitis media
3. right eye
4. left ear
5. both eyes
6. left eye
7. laser-assisted in situ keratomileusis
8. AU
9. EOM
10. AD
11. IOP
12. OS
13. O.D.

**EXERCISE 8-9** SPELLING

1. a
2. c
3. b
4. b
5. d
6. d
7. a
8. b
9. c
10. a

### EXERCISE 8-10 CASE STUDY

1. middle ear infection or inflammation
2. incision into the tympanic membrane
3. earwax
4. passageway leading inward from the auricle to the tympanic membrane (eardrum)

# CHAPTER 9

## Word Parts Exercise

1. secreting internally
2. pituitary gland
3. adrenal glands
4. suffix used in the formation of names of chemical substances
5. suffix meaning nourishment or stimulation
6. tumor
7. pancreas
8. extremities
9. gland
10. thyroid gland
11. enlargement
12. sugar, glucose, glycogen
13. to separate or secrete
14. parathyroid gland
15. calcium

## Quick Check

1. hypophysis
2. suprarenal gland
3. Endocrine

### EXERCISE 9-1 LABELING

1. pineal gland
2. thyroid
3. adrenal glands
4. testes
5. pituitary gland
6. parathyroid glands
7. thymus
8. pancreas
9. ovaries

### EXERCISE 9-2 WORD PARTS

1. adenogenous
   root: aden/o (gland)
   suffix: -genous (originating)
   definition: originating in a gland

2. epinephrine
   prefix: epi- (upon)
   root: nephr/o (kidney)
   suffix: -ine (chemical substance)
   definition: hormone secreted from the adrenal medulla, which is the central region of the adrenal gland located on the superior border of each kidney

3. suprarenal
   prefix: supra- (above)
   root: ren/o (kidney)
   suffix: -al (pertaining to)
   definition: above the kidney

4. adrenomegaly
   root: adren/o (adrenal gland)
   suffix: -megaly (enlargement)
   definition: enlargement of the adrenal gland

5. hyperglycemia
   prefix: hyper- (above normal)
   root: glyc/o (glucose; sugar)
   suffix: -ia (condition)
   definition: excessive glucose (sugar) in the blood

6. adenotomy
   root: aden/o (gland)
   suffix: -tomy (cutting operation)
   definition: incision of a gland

7. thyroparathyroidectomy
   root: thryr/o (thyroid gland)
   root: parathyr/o (parathyroid gland)
   suffix: -ectomy (excision)
   definition: excision of the thyroid and parathyroid glands
8. endocrinology
   root: endocrin/o (endocrine)
   suffix: -ology (study of)
   definition: medical specialty of the endocrine system

**EXERCISE 9-3** WORD BUILDING

1. adrenomegaly
2. adrenalectomy
3. adrenopathy
4. hypothyroidism
5. throiditis
6. throidotomy
7. thyromegaly
8. pancreatoma
9. pancreatitis
10. pancreatogenic

**EXERCISE 9-4** MATCHING

1. d
2. k
3. g
4. i
5. a
6. e
7. f
8. m
9. j
10. b
11. c
12. l
13. h

**EXERCISE 9-5** MULTIPLE CHOICE

1. a
2. b
3. b
4. c
5. b
6. a
7. d
8. a
9. d

**EXERCISE 9-6** FILL IN THE BLANK

1. thyromegaly
2. diabetes mellitus
3. hyperglycemia
4. polyuria
5. glycosuria
6. glucagon
7. acromegaly
8. Homeostasis

**EXERCISE 9-7** ABBREVIATIONS

1. glucose tolerance test
2. parathyroid hormone
3. thyroxine or tetraiodothyronine
4. fasting blood sugar
5. antidiuretic hormone
6. hemogloboin $A_{1c}$
7. growth hormone
8. parathyroid hormone
9. ACTH
10. FSH
11. DM
12. CT
13. MSH
14. $T_3$
15. PRL
16. TSH
17. LH

### EXERCISE 9-8 SPELLING

1. d
2. c
3. b
4. a
5. a
6. c
7. d
8. b
9. b
10. d

### EXERCISE 9-9 CASE STUDY

1. difficulty speaking
2. goiter, thyromegaly
3. thyroid stimulating hormone

## CHAPTER 10

### Word Parts Exercise

1. ven/o or phlebo
2. cardi/o
3. angi/o or vas/o
4. endo-
5. tachy-
6. thromb/o
7. peri-
8. ather/o
9. atri/o
10. -gram
11. -emia
12. my/o
13. -stenosis
14. hem/o, hemat/o
15. arteri/o
16. phleb/o or ven/o
17. valv/o, valvul/o
18. aort/o
19. brady-
20. varic/o
21. coron/o
22. -ectasis
23. vas/o or angi/o
24. electr/o
25. ventricul/o
26. isch

### Quick Check

1. arterioles
2. Veins
3. red blood cell

### EXERCISE 10-1 LABELING

1. superior and inferior vena cava
2. right atrium
3. right AV (tricuspid) valve
4. right ventricle
5. pulmonary valve
6. pulmonary arteries
7. pulmonary veins
8. left atrium
9. left AV (mitral) valve
10. left ventricle
11. aortic valve
12. aorta

### EXERCISE 10-2 WORD PARTS

1. erythrocyte
   root: erythr/o (red)
   suffix: -cyte (cell)
   definition: red blood cell
2. atherosclerosis
   root: ather/o (fatty)
   root: scler/o (hardening)
   suffix: -osis (abnormal condition)
   definition: hardening and narrowing of the arteries

3. cardiomyopathy
   root: cardi/o (heart)
   root: my/o (muscle)
   suffix: -pathy (disease)
   definition: disease of the heart muscle
4. endocarditis
   prefix: endo- (within)
   root: cardi/o (heart)
   suffix: -itis (inflammation)
   definition: inflammation of the endocardium
5. thrombocytopenia
   root: thromb/o (blood clot)
   root: cyt/o (cell)
   suffix: -penia (deficiency)
   definition: abnormal decrease in the number of thrombocytes
6. angiogram
   root: angi/o (blood vessel)
   suffix: -gram (record or picture)
   definition: printed record of a blood vessel
7. hematology
   root: hemat/o (blood)
   suffix: -logy (study of)
   definition: medical specialty dealing with blood
8. pericardiotomy
   prefix: peri- (surrounding)
   root: cardi/o (heart)
   suffix: -tomy (cutting operation)
   definition: incision into the pericardium

**EXERCISE 10-3** WORD BUILDING

1. cardiogenic
2. atriotomy
3. erythrocyte
4. hemophilia
5. vasospasm
6. thrombectomy
7. vasodilation
8. cardiomegaly
9. arteriostenosis
10. atheroma
11. leukocyte
12. valvectomy
13. cardiac
14. hemolysis, erythrolysis
15. interventricular
16. anemia
17. myocardium
18. atherectomy
19. arrhythmia

**EXERCISE 10-4** MATCHING

1. g
2. i
3. b
4. a
5. f
6. h
7. j
8. c
9. e
10. d

**EXERCISE 10-5** MULTIPLE CHOICE

1. b
2. a
3. b
4. b
5. a
6. a
7. b
8. d
9. d
10. d

**EXERCISE 10-6** FILL IN THE BLANK

1. hypotension
2. tachycardia
3. hematologist
4. pulmonary
5. O, AB
6. cardiology
7. phlebotomy
8. hyperlipidemia
9. bicuspid
10. superior vena cava, inferior vena cava

### EXERCISE 10-7 ABBREVIATIONS

1. blood pressure
2. atrial fibrillation
3. low-density lipoprotein
4. shortness of breath
5. white blood cell
6. atrioventricular
7. coronary artery disease
8. congestive heart failure
9. heart rate
10. hemoglobin
11. myocardial infarction
12. transient ischemic attack
13. Hb
14. A-fib
15. RBC
16. SA
17. CHF
18. ECG or EKG
19. CABG
20. HTN
21. DIC
22. HDL
23. PTCA

### EXERCISE 10-8 SPELLING

1. b
2. a
3. c
4. d
5. a
6. b
7. d
8. b
9. c
10. a

### EXERCISE 10-9 CASE STUDY

1. pain in the chest due to ischemia
2. shortness of breath
3. high blood pressure
4. electrocardiogram; record of the heart's electrical activity
5. aspirin—anticoagulant effect; antiarrhythmics—decrease abnormal atrial heart beats; diuretics—decrease fluid volume by increasing urination; vasodilators—increase diameter of blood vessels to decrease blood pressure and increase blood flow
6. myocardial infarction or heart attack; lack of blood supply (infarction) to the heart muscle; my/o means "muscle" and cardi/o means "heart"
7. irregular atrial contractions; frequently a rapid irregular rhythm

# CHAPTER 11

### Word Parts Exercise

1. immune system
2. ingest or engulf
3. protection
4. enlargement
5. tonsil
6. spleen
7. without
8. lymph nodes
9. lymph vessels
10. lymph or lymphatic system
11. thymus
12. resembling
13. disease

### Quick Check

1. fluid; fats
2. tonsils, lymph nodes, thymus, spleen, appendix, lymphoid nodules of the small intestine (Peyer's patches)
3. antigen

### EXERCISE 11-1 LABELING

1. cervical lymph nodes
2. axillary lymph nodes
3. thymus
4. mediastinal lymph nodes
5. spleen
6. superficial lymphatics of lower limb

**EXERCISE 11-2** WORD PARTS

1. lymphocyte
   root: lymph/o (lymph)
   suffix: -cyte (cell)
   definition: white blood cell in the lymphatic system
2. phagocytosis
   root: phag/o (ingest or engulf)
   root: cyt/o (cell)
   suffix: -osis (condition of)
   definition: process carried out by white blood cells to ingest and digest solid substances
3. anaphylaxis
   prefix: ana- (without)
   root: phylaxis (protection)
   definition: life-threatening reaction to a foreign substance
4. hemolysis
   root: hem/o (blood)
   suffix: -lysis (destruction)
   definition: destruction of red blood cells
5. lymphoma
   root: lymph/o (lymph)
   suffix: -oma (tumor)
   definition: tumor of lymph tissue
6. splenectomy
   root: splen/o (spleen)
   suffix: -ectomy (excision)
   definition: excision (removal) of the spleen
7. thymectomy
   root: thym/o (thymus)
   suffix: -ectomy (excision)
   definition: excision (removal) of the thymus
8. immunology
   root: immun/o (immune system)
   suffix: -logy (study of)
   definition: study of the immune system

**EXERCISE 11-3** WORD BUILDING

1. lymphadenitis
2. lymphoma
3. thymomegaly
4. lymphangitis
5. lymphadenopathy
6. immunologist
7. lymphography
8. phagocytosis

**EXERCISE 11-4** MATCHING

1. e
2. f
3. g
4. i
5. a
6. j
7. b
8. d
9. h
10. c

**EXERCISE 11-5** MULTIPLE CHOICE

1. b
2. c
3. c
4. a
5. d
6. b
7. c
8. b
9. c
10. d

**EXERCISE 11-6** FILL IN THE BLANK

1. lymphocytes
2. maintain fluid balance
3. lymph nodes
4. Innate
5. tonsils
6. lymphedema
7. splenectomy
8. allergist
9. thymus
10. immunodeficiency

**EXERCISE 11-7** ABBREVIATIONS

1. systemic lupus erythematosus
2. rheumatoid arthritis
3. Epstein–Barr virus
4. AIDS
5. HIV

**EXERCISE 11-8** SPELLING

1. a
2. c
3. c
4. a
5. d
6. b
7. d
8. c
9. b
10. a

**EXERCISE 11-9** CASE STUDY

1. disease of the lymph nodes
2. splenomegaly
3. an infectious disease caused by the Epstein–Barr virus

# CHAPTER 12

## Word Parts Exercise

1. voice
2. trachea
3. thorax, chest
4. bronchus
5. breathing
6. larynx
7. sinus cavity
8. rib, side, pleura
9. lungs, air
10. nose
11. oxygen
12. pharynx
13. diaphragm
14. lung
15. mouth, opening

## Quick Check

1. larynx
2. trachea
3. pharynx

**EXERCISE 12-1** LABELING

1. paranasal sinuses
2. lungs
3. trachea
4. bronchi
5. alveoli

**EXERCISE 12-2** WORD PARTS

1. nasopharynx
   root: nas/o (nose)
   root: pharyng/o (pharynx)
   definition: upper portion of the pharynx
2. pulmonary
   root: pulmon/o (lung)
   suffix: -ary (related to)
   definition: adjective meaning related to the lungs
3. dysphonia
   prefix: dys- (painful)
   root: phon/o (sound)
   suffix: -ia (condition)
   definition: condition of painful speech
4. hemoptysis
   root: hem/o (blood)
   suffix: -ptysis (spitting)
   definition: spitting or coughing up blood

5. laryngostenosis
   root: laryng/o (larynx)
   root: sten/o (narrowing)
   suffix: -osis (abnormal condition)
   definition: condition of a narrowing of the larynx
6. antipyretic
   prefix: anti- (against)
   root: pyretos (fever)
   suffix: -ic (adjective)
   definition: drug used to reduce fever
7. rhinoplasty
   root: rhin/o (nose)
   suffix: -plasty (surgical repair)
   definition: surgical repair of the nose
8. otolaryngologist
   root: ot/o (ear)
   root: laryng/o (larynx)
   suffix: -logist (one who studies)
   definition: physician who specializes in ear, nose, and throat diseases

**EXERCISE 12-3** WORD BUILDING

1. bronchitis
2. bronchiectasis
3. laryngitis
4. sinusitis
5. epiglottitis
6. tachypnea
7. bradypnea
8. dyspnea
9. orthopnea

**EXERCISE 12-4** MATCHING

1. e
2. d
3. c
4. f
5. a
6. g
7. b
8. j
9. k
10. l
11. r
12. n
13. o
14. h
15. m
16. q
17. i
18. p

**EXERCISE 12-5** MULTIPLE CHOICE

1. c
2. c
3. b
4. d
5. b
6. b
7. c
8. b
9. b
10. c

**EXERCISE 12-6** FILL IN THE BLANK

1. hemoptysis
2. bradypnea
3. pneumocentesis
4. inflammation of the pleura (membrane that surrounds the lungs and lines the walls of the thoracic cavity)
5. pleura
6. orthopnea
7. bronchiectasis
8. rhinorrhea
9. Cheyne–Stokes respirations

### EXERCISE 12-7 ABBREVIATIONS

1. chronic obstructive pulmonary disease
2. arterial blood gas
3. total lung capacity
4. cystic fibrosis
5. tonsillectomy and adenoidectomy
6. upper respiratory infection
7. TB
8. $O_2$
9. $CO_2$
10. PFT
11. RV
12. SOB

### EXERCISE 12-8 SPELLING

1. d
2. b
3. c
4. a
5. a
6. b
7. d
8. c
9. b
10. a

### EXERCISE 12-9 CASE STUDY

1. a
2. b

## CHAPTER 13

### Word Parts Exercise

1. eat or swallow
2. common bile duct
3. mouth
4. sigmoid colon
5. abdomen
6. intestine
7. abdomen
8. rectum
9. stone
10. salivary glands
11. liver
12. pylorus
13. bile, gall
14. bile duct
15. esophagus
16. vomit
17. instrument used for viewing
18. tongue
19. jejunum
20. stomach
21. lip
22. ileum
23. pancreas
24. cheek
25. gallbladder
26. digestion
27. colon
28. teeth
29. eating, swallowing
30. duodenum
31. anus and rectum
32. gums
33. visual examination
34. nutrition

### Quick Check

1. bolus
2. The stomach also secretes acid and enzymes to help break down proteins, fats, and carbohydrates.
3. duodenum, jejunum, ileum

### EXERCISE 13-1 LABELING

1. mouth
2. pharynx
3. esophagus
4. liver
5. gallbladder
6. bile duct
7. small intestine
8. large intestine
9. salivary gland
10. stomach
11. pancreas
12. anus

## EXERCISE 13-2 WORD PARTS

1. cholelithiasis
   root: chol/e (bile, gall)
   suffix: -lith (stone)
   suffix: -iasis (condition of)
   definition: formation or presence of stones in the gallbladder or common bile duct
2. enterohepatitis
   root: enter/o (intestine)
   root: hepat/o (liver)
   suffix: -itis (inflammation)
   definition: inflammation of the intestine and liver
3. parotiditis
   prefix: para- (beside)
   root: ot/o (ear)
   suffix: -itis (inflammation)
   definition: inflammation of the parotid salivary gland
4. sialorrhea
   root: sial/o (saliva, salivary gland)
   suffix: -rrhea (discharge)
   definition: excessive production of saliva
5. colonoscopy
   root: colon/o (colon)
   suffix: -scopy (viewing)
   definition: visual examination of the colon
6. gastroenterologist
   root: gastr/o (stomach)
   root: enter/o (intestine)
   suffix: -logist (one who studies)
   definition: a specialist in the diagnosis and treatment of digestive system disorders
7. colectomy
   root: col/o (colon)
   suffix: -ectomy (surgical removal)
   definition: excision of all or part of the colon
8. jejunotomy
   root: jejun/o (jejunum)
   suffix: -tomy (incision)
   definition: incision into the jejunum

## EXERCISE 13-3 WORD BUILDING

1. gastric
2. cholecystopathy
3. gingivitis
4. sialostenosis
5. enteroscope
6. colopexy
7. jejunectomy
8. hepatogenic
9. dysphagia
10. duodenal

## EXERCISE 13-4 MATCHING

1. b
2. f
3. i
4. g
5. h
6. d
7. e
8. a
9. c
10. j

## EXERCISE 13-5 MULTIPLE CHOICE

1. b
2. c
3. c
4. a
5. c
6. c
7. b
8. d
9. b
10. a

### EXERCISE 13-6 FILL IN THE BLANK

1. ileocecal sphincter
2. anus
3. salivary glands
4. gallbladder
5. stomach
6. cholecystitis
7. cholelithiasis
8. antiemetic
9. gastroscope
10. gastrectomy

### EXERCISE 13-7 ABBREVIATIONS

1. per os or nothing by mouth
2. upper gastrointestinal series
3. total parenteral nutrition
4. bowel movement
5. gastrointestinal
6. gastroesophageal reflux disease
7. irritable bowel syndrome
8. lower esophageal sphincter
9. HCl
10. NG
11. BE
12. EGD
13. NPO

### EXERCISE 13-8 SPELLING

1. a
2. c
3. b
4. b
5. d
6. c
7. c
8. a
9. d
10. b

### EXERCISE 13-9 CASE STUDY

1. shortness of breath
2. blood pressure
3. HTN stands for hypertension, which is high blood pressure. Hypertension and shortness of breath may accompany each other. Smoking and excessive caffeine intake may be related to both conditions.
4. white blood cell
5. Endo- means within; -scopy means "look" or "see". Endoscopy may be defined as looking inside, by means of an instrument called an endoscope.
6. A gastric ulcer is a sore on the lining (mucous membrane) of the stomach.

## CHAPTER 14

### Word Parts Exercise

1. urine
2. night
3. little, few
4. condition, state
5. glomerulus
6. kidney
7. urethra
8. stone
9. much, many
10. pus
11. pelvis
12. ureter
13. bladder

### Quick Check

1. kidneys, ureters, urinary bladder, and urethra
2. hilum
3. internal urethral sphincter and external urethral sphincter

### EXERCISE 14-1 LABELING

1. inferior vena cava
2. abdominal aorta
3. urinary bladder
4. urethra
5. kidneys
6. ureters

## EXERCISE 14-2 WORD PARTS

1. anuria
   prefix: an-, without
   root: ur/o, urine
   suffix: -ia, condition
   definition: absence of urine formation

2. cystalgia
   root: cyst/o, bladder
   suffix: -algia, pain
   definition: pain in the bladder

3. nephrolithiasis
   root: nephr/o, kidney
   root: lith/o, stone
   suffix: -iasis, condition
   definition: presence of a kidney stone

4. hematuria
   root: hemat/o, blood
   root: ur/o, urine
   suffix: -ia, condition
   definition: blood in the urine

5. glomerulonephritis
   root: glomerul/o, glomerulus
   root: nephr/o, kidney
   suffix: -itis, inflammation
   definition: renal disease characterized by inflammation of the glomeruli

6. nephrologist
   root: nephr/o, kidney
   suffix: -logist, one who studies
   definition: a specialist who treats kidney disorders

7. urology
   root: ur/o, urine
   suffix: -logy, study of
   definition: study of the urinary system

8. nephrectomy
   root: nephr/o, kidney
   suffix: -ectomy, removal
   definition: removal of a kidney

## EXERCISE 14-3 WORD BUILDING

1. albuminuria
2. nephralgia
3. urethrostenosis
4. uremia
5. lithotripsy
6. urologist
7. nephrology
8. cystectomy
9. cystoscope
10. ureterorrhaphy

## EXERCISE 14-4 MATCHING

1. g
2. d
3. k
4. a
5. b
6. j
7. h
8. f
9. e
10. r
11. p
12. m
13. n
14. q
15. l
16. i
17. c
18. o

## EXERCISE 14-5 MULTIPLE CHOICE

1. d
2. b
3. d
4. a
5. a
6. c
7. c
8. b
9. b
10. d

**EXERCISE 14-6** FILL IN THE BLANK

1. kidney transplant
2. nephropexy
3. nephrolithotomy
4. ureteroplasty
5. cystoscopy
6. Diuretics
7. ureters
8. urea and uric acid
9. dialysis
10. one who studies

**EXERCISE 14-7** ABBREVIATIONS

1. urinary tract infection
2. glomerular filtration rate
3. end-stage renal disease
4. blood urea nitrogen
5. chronic renal failure
6. UA
7. KUB
8. ARF
9. IVP
10. CAPD

**EXERCISE 14-8** SPELLING

1. a
2. a
3. b
4. d
5. c
6. a
7. c
8. d
9. c
10. d

**EXERCISE 14-9** CASE STUDY

1. urologist
2. dysuria
3. hematuria
4. urinalysis
5. KUB
6. calculi
7. urinary bladder
8. UTI
9. calculi
10. antibiotic
11. cystoscopy

# CHAPTER 15

## Word Parts Exercise

1. breast
2. sperm
3. uterine tube
4. vessel, vas deferens
5. around
6. ovary, egg-bearing
7. vagina
8. prostate gland
9. amnion
10. birth
11. uterus
12. vulva
13. testes
14. cervix, neck
15. glans penis
16. gonads, sex glands
17. woman, female
18. milk
19. menses, menstruation
20. ovary, egg-bearing

### Quick Check

1. synthesizing testosterone, producing and storing sperm, and making and releasing fluid from glands that support the sperm
2. lactation
3. gestation

## EXERCISE 15-1 LABELING

### Male reproductive system

1. prostate
2. ductus deferens or vas deferens
3. penis
4. glans penis
5. foreskin
6. epididymis
7. seminal gland
8. testis
9. scrotum

### Female reproductive system

1. uterine tube
2. ovary
3. uterus
4. urinary bladder
5. clitoris
6. labium minus
7. laium majus
8. cervix
9. rectum
10. anus
11. vagina
12. urethra

## EXERCISE 15-2 WORD PARTS

1. amenorrhea
   prefix: a- (without)
   root: men/o (menses)
   suffix: -rrhea (flowing, discharge)
   definition: absence of menstruation
2. azoospermia
   prefix: a- (without)
   prefix: zoo- (animal, living being)
   root: sperm/o (sperm)
   suffix: -ia (condition of)
   definition: absence of sperm in the semen
3. dysmenorrhea
   prefix: dys- (bad, difficult)
   root: men/o (menses)
   suffix: -rrhea (flowing, discharge)
   definition: painful menstruation
4. menorrhagia
   root: men/o (menses)
   suffix: -rrhagia (rapid flow of blood)
   definition: increased amount and duration of flow
5. prostatitis
   root: prostat/o (prostate)
   suffix: -itis (inflammation)
   definition: inflammation of the prostate
6. hysterotomy
   root: hyster/o (uterus)
   suffix: -tomy (incision into)
   definition: incision of the uterus
7. mastectomy
   root: mast/o (breast)
   suffix: -ectomy (excision)
   definition: removal of a breast
8. neonatology
   prefix: neo- (new)
   root: nat/o (birth)
   suffix: -logy (study of)
   definition: medical specialty dealing with newborns

## EXERCISE 15-3 WORD BUILDING

1. cystocele
2. hysteralgia
3. mastitis
4. orchiopathy
5. amniocentesis
6. mammography
7. laparoscopy
8. oophorotomy
9. uteropexy
10. gynecologist

### EXERCISE 15-4 MATCHING

1. d
2. o
3. e
4. i
5. a
6. g
7. c
8. m
9. b
10. k
11. n
12. f
13. h
14. l
15. j

### EXERCISE 15-5 MULTIPLE CHOICE

1. a
2. b
3. a
4. d
5. b
6. b
7. c
8. a
9. d

### EXERCISE 15-6 FILL IN THE BLANK

1. sperm
2. oocyte
3. testosterone
4. seminal glands or seminal vesicles
5. endometrium
6. embryo
7. ectopic
8. cervix
9. ova
10. ovaries

### EXERCISE 15-7 ABBREVIATIONS

1. benign prostatic hyperplasia
2. gravida
3. human immunodeficiency virus
4. estimated date of delivery
5. cesarean section
6. obstetrics
7. estimated date of confinement
8. sexually transmitted disease
9. gynecology
10. pelvic inflammatory disease
11. herpes simplex virus
12. A
13. STI
14. TURP
15. GC
16. LMP
17. D&C
18. P
19. HPV

### EXERCISE 15-8 SPELLING

1. d
2. c
3. a
4. b
5. c
6. a
7. b
8. d
9. b
10. c

### EXERCISE 15-9 CASE STUDY

1. Gravida II means that she has had two pregnancies. Para I means that she has had one birth after 20 weeks.
2. An amniocentesis is a transabdominal puncture of the amniotic sac to remove amniotic fluid for testing.
3. Intrauterine means within the uterus.

APPENDIX B

# Glossary of Word Parts with Meanings

| Word Part | Meaning |
|---|---|
| ab- | away from, outside of, beyond |
| abdomin/o | abdomen |
| -ac | converts a root or noun to an adjective |
| acous/o, acus/o, acoust/o | hearing |
| acr/o | extremities |
| ad- | toward, near to |
| aden/o | gland |
| adeno- | glandlike |
| adren/o | adrenal glands |
| adrenal/o | adrenal glands |
| adip/o | fat |
| -al | adjective suffix |
| albin/o | white |
| -algia | pain |
| aliment/o | nutrition |
| amni/o | amnion |
| -amphi | both sides |
| a-, an- | not; without |
| -an | converts a root or noun to an adjective |
| -aneous | converts a root or noun to an adjective |
| angi/o | blood vessel |
| ankyl/o | stiff, fused, closed |
| ante- | before |
| anter/o | front, anterior |
| anti- | against, opposed |
| aort/o | aorta |
| -ar | converts a root or noun to an adjective |
| arachn/o | spider |
| arter/i/o | artery |
| ather/o | fatty |
| arthr/o | joint |
| aspir/o | breathe in |

| Word Part | Meaning |
|---|---|
| atri/o | atrium |
| -ary | converts a root or noun to an adjective |
| audi/o | sound |
| aur/o | ear |
| auricul/o | ear |
| balan/o | glans penis |
| bi- | two |
| blephar/o | eyelid |
| brachi/o | arm |
| brady- | slow |
| bronch/o, bronchi/o | bronchus |
| bucc/o | cheek |
| calcane/o | calcaneus, heel bone |
| calc/i | calcium |
| card/i/o | heart |
| carp/o | wrist |
| -cele | protrusion, hernia |
| -centesis | surgical puncture |
| cephal/o | head |
| cerebell/o | cerebellum |
| cerebr/o | cerebrum; brain |
| cerv/o, cervic/o | neck, cervix |
| cheil/o | lip |
| chol/e, chol/o | bile, gall |
| cholangi/o | bile duct |
| cholecyst/o | gallbladder |
| choledoch/o | common bile duct |
| chondr/o | cartilage |
| circum/o | around |
| cirrh/o | yellow |
| col/o, colon/o | colon |
| colp/o | vagina |
| con- | with |
| conjunctiv/o | conjunctiva (*conjunctivae*, plural) |
| contra- | against |

| Word Part | Meaning |
|---|---|
| **corne/o** | horny |
| **coron/o** | crown; encircling, such as in the coronary blood vessels encircling the heart |
| **cortic/o** | outer layer or covering |
| **cost/o** | rib |
| **crani/o** | cranium, skull |
| **crin/o** | to separate or secrete |
| **cutane/o** | skin |
| **cyan/o** | blue |
| **cyst/o** | bladder |
| **-cyte, cyt/o** | cell |
| **dacry/o** | tears, lacrimal sac, or lacrimal duct |
| **dactyl/o** | finger, toe |
| **de-** | without, not |
| **dent/i, dent/o** | teeth |
| **derm/o, dermat/o** | skin |
| **-desis** | surgical binding |
| **di-, dipl-** | two, twice |
| **dipl/o** | two, double |
| **dia-** | across, through |
| **dis-** | remove |
| **diverticul/o** | diverticulum |
| **dors/o** | back |
| **duoden/o** | duodenum |
| **-dynia** | pain |
| **dys-** | painful, bad, difficult |
| **-eal** | converts a root or noun to an adjective |
| **ec-, ecto-** | outside |
| **-ectomy** | surgical removal |
| **-ectasis, -ectasia** | expansion or dilation |
| **-edema** | excessive fluid |
| **electr/o** | electricity |
| **-emesis** | vomiting |
| **-emia** | blood |
| **en-** | inside |
| **enchephal/o** | brain |
| **endo-** | within, inner |
| **endocrin/o** | secreting internally |
| **enter/o** | intestine |
| **-eous** | converts a root or noun to an adjective |
| **epi-** | upon, following, or subsequent to |
| **erythr/o** | red |

| Word Part | Meaning |
|---|---|
| **esophag/o** | esophagus |
| **ex-, exo-** | outside |
| **extra-** | beyond |
| **fasci/o** | fibrous membrane |
| **femur/o** | femur, thighbone |
| **fer/o** | to carry |
| **fibr/o** | fiber |
| **gangli/o** | ganglia (*ganglion*, singular) |
| **ganglion/o** | ganglia (*ganglion*, singular) |
| **gastr/o** | stomach |
| **-gen, -genesisa** | origin, cause, formation |
| **-gen, -genic, -genesis** | origin, producing |
| **gen/o** | origin, cause, formation |
| **ger/o/onto** | old age |
| **gingiv/o** | gums |
| **gli/o** | glue |
| **glomerul/o** | glomerulus |
| **gloss/o** | tongue |
| **gluc/o** | sugar, glucose, glycogen |
| **glyc/o** | sugar, glucose, glycogen |
| **gonad/o** | gonads, sex glands |
| **-gram** | a recording, usually by an instrument |
| **-graph** | the instrument for making a recording |
| **-graphy** | act of graphic or pictorial recording |
| **gynec/o** | woman, female |
| **hem/a/to** | blood |
| **hemi-** | half |
| **hem/o** | blood |
| **hemat/o** | blood |
| **hepat/o** | liver |
| **humer/o** | humerus, upper arm bone |
| **hydr/o** | water |
| **hyper-** | above, beyond normal |
| **hypo-** | low, below, below normal |
| **hypophys/o** | pituitary gland |
| **hyster/o** | uterus |
| **-iac** | converts a root or noun to an adjective |
| **-ian** | specialist |
| **-iasis** | a condition or state |
| **-iatric** | converts a root or noun to an adjective |
| **-iatrics** | medical specialty |
| **iatr/o** | physician |
| **-iatry** | medical specialty |

| Word Part | Meaning |
|---|---|
| -ic | adjective suffix denoting of: converts a root or noun to an adjective |
| -ical | converts a root or noun to an adjective |
| ichthy/o | dry, scaly |
| -ics | medical specialty |
| ile/o | ileum |
| immun/o | immune system |
| -ine | suffix used in the formation of names of chemical substances |
| infra- | inside or below |
| inguin/o | groin |
| inter- | between |
| intra- | inside, within |
| irid/o | iris |
| -ism | a condition of; a process; or a state of |
| -ist | specialist in a field of study |
| -itis | inflammation |
| jaund/o | yellow |
| jejun/o | jejunum |
| kerat/o | the cornea; horny tissue or cells |
| kine-, kinesi/o | movement |
| -kinesia | movement |
| kyph/o | hump |
| lacrim/o | tear, lacrimal apparatus |
| lact/o | milk |
| lapar/o | abdomen |
| laryng/o | larynx |
| ligament/o | ligament |
| -lith | stone, calculus, calcification |
| lob/o | lobe |
| -logy | study of |
| lord/o | swayback, curve |
| lumb/o | lower back |
| lymph/o | lymph or lymphatic system |
| lymphaden/o | lymph nodes |
| lymphangia/o | lymph vessels |
| lymphat/o | lymph or lymphatic system |
| -lysis | disintegration, breaking down |
| macro- | big |
| -malacia | softening |
| mamm/o | breast |
| -mania | morbid attraction or impulse toward |

| Word Part | Meaning |
|---|---|
| mast/o | breast |
| -megaly | enlargement |
| melan/o | black |
| meningi/o | membrane |
| men/o | menses, menstruation |
| ment/o | referring to the mind |
| meso- | middle |
| meta- | beyond |
| -meter | device for measuring |
| metr/o | uterus |
| -metry | act of measuring |
| micro- | small |
| -mnesia | memory |
| mono- | one |
| muscul/o | muscle |
| myc/o | fungus |
| my/o | muscle |
| myel/o | spinal cord and medulla oblongata; bone marrow |
| myring/o | tympanic membrane (eardrum) |
| nas/o | nose |
| natal | birth; born |
| nat/o | birth |
| neo- | new |
| nephr/o, ren/o | kidney |
| neur/o | nerve, nerve tissue |
| noct/o | night |
| ocul/o | eye |
| -oid | resembling or like: converts a root or noun to an adjective |
| olig-, oligo- | little, few |
| -oma | tumor |
| onych/o | nail |
| oophor/o | ovary, egg-bearing |
| ophthalm/o | eye |
| -opia | vision |
| -opsy | examination |
| opt/o | light, eye, vision |
| orch/o, orchi/o, orchid/o | testes |
| or/o | mouth, opening |
| -orth/o | correct, straight |
| -osis | abnormal condition |
| oste/o | bone |

| Word Part | Meaning |
|---|---|
| **-otic** | converts a root or noun to an adjective |
| **ot/o** | ear |
| **-ous** | converts a root or noun to an adjective |
| **ovari/o** | ovary, egg-bearing |
| **-oxia** | oxygen |
| **pan-** | all or everywhere |
| **panceat/o** | pancreas |
| **para-** | alongside, near |
| **parathyr/o** | parathyroid gland |
| **parathyroid/o** | parathyroid gland |
| **-paresis** | partial or incomplete paralysis |
| **path/o** | disease |
| **-pathy** | disease |
| **ped/ia** | child |
| **ped/o** | foot, child |
| **pelv/o** | pelvis |
| **-penia** | reduction of size or quantity |
| **-pepsia** | digestion |
| **peri-** | around, surrounding |
| **-pexy** | surgical fixation |
| **phac/o** | lens |
| **phag/o** | eating, swallowing |
| **-phagia** | eat or swallow |
| **phalang/o** | bones of fingers and toes |
| **pharyng/o** | pharynx |
| **-phasia** | speech |
| **phleb/o** | vein |
| **-phobia** | fear |
| **-phonia** | voice |
| **phren/o** | diaphragm |
| **-phylaxis** | protection |
| **-physis** | growth |
| **pil/o** | hair |
| **-plasia** | abnormal formation |
| **-plasty** | surgical repair |
| **-plegia** | paralysis |
| **pleur/o** | rib, side, pleura |
| **-pnea** | breathing |
| **pneumo-, pneumon/o** | lungs, air |
| **-poesis** | producing |
| **poly-** | many |
| **-porosis** | porous condition |
| **post-** | after |
| **poster/o** | posterior, back |
| **pre-** | before |
| **presby/o** | old age |

| Word Part | Meaning |
|---|---|
| **proct/o** | anus and rectum |
| **prostat/o** | prostate gland |
| **proxim/o** | near |
| **-ptosis** | downward displacement |
| **psych/o** | mind |
| **pulmon/o** | lung |
| **pupil/o** | pupil |
| **pyel/o** | pelvis |
| **pylor/o** | pylorus |
| **py/o** | pus |
| **quadri-** | four |
| **rect/o** | rectum |
| **retin/o** | retina |
| **retro-** | backward, behind |
| **rhin/o** | nose |
| **-rrhage** | flowing forth |
| **-rrhapy** | suture |
| **-rrhea** | discharge |
| **-rrhexis** | rupture |
| **salping/o** | tube, uterine tube |
| **schiz/o** | to split |
| **scler/o** | hard; relating to the sclera |
| **-sclerosis** | hardness |
| **-scope** | viewing; an instrument used for viewing |
| **-scopy** | act of viewing, to visually examine |
| **seb/o** | sebum |
| **semi-** | half, partial |
| **sial/o** | salivary glands |
| **sigmoid/o** | sigmoid colon |
| **sinus/o** | sinus cavity |
| **skelet/o** | skeleton |
| **-spasm** | muscular contraction |
| **sperm/o, spermat/o** | sperm |
| **spin/o** | spine |
| **splen/o** | spleen |
| **spondyl/o** | vertebrae |
| **staped/o** | stapes (smallest ear bone) |
| **-stasis** | level; unchanging |
| **-stenosis** | a narrowing |
| **sthen/o** | strength |
| **stomat/o** | mouth |
| **-stomy** | artificial or surgical opening |
| **sub-** | below |
| **sudor-** | sweat |
| **super/o** | superior |
| **sym-** | with |
| **syn-** | with, joined together |

| Word Part | Meaning |
|---|---|
| **tachy-** | rapid |
| **tend/o, tendin/o** | tendon |
| **tetra-** | four |
| **thorac/o, thorac/i, thoracic/o** | thorax, chest |
| **thromb/o** | clot |
| **thym/o** | thymus |
| **thyr/o** | thyroid gland |
| **thyroid/o** | thyroid gland |
| **-tic** | converts a root or noun to an adjective |
| **-tome** | instrument for cutting |
| **-tomy** | incision |
| **ton/o** | tone |
| **tonsill/o** | tonsil |
| **trache/o** | trachea |
| **trans-** | across |
| **tri-** | three |
| **-tripsy** | crushing |
| **-tropin** | suffix meaning nourishment or stimulation |
| **tympan/o** | eardrum |
| **-ular** | converts a root or noun to an adjective |
| **uni-** | one |
| **ur/o, urin/o** | urine |
| **ureter/o** | ureter |
| **urethr/o** | urethra |
| **uter/o** | uterus |
| **uve/o** | denoting the pigmented middle eye layer |
| **vagin/o** | vagina |
| **valv/o** | valve |
| **varic/o** | dilated |
| **vas/o** | vessel, vas deferens |
| **ven/o** | vein |
| **ventricul/o** | ventricle |
| **vertebr/o** | vertebrae |
| **vulv/o** | vulva |
| **xanth/o** | yellow |
| **xer/o** | dry |
| **zygo-** | joined (yoked) together |

APPENDIX C

# Glossary of Abbreviations

| Abbreviation | Meaning |
|---|---|
| A | abortus |
| ABG | arterial blood gas |
| ACL | anterior cruciate ligament |
| ACTH | aderenocorticotropic hormone |
| AD | Alzheimer's disease |
| AD | right ear |
| ADH | antidiuretic hormone |
| A-fib | atrial fibrillation |
| AIDS | acquired immunodeficiency syndrome |
| ALS | amyotrophic lateral sclerosis |
| ARF | acute renal failure |
| AS | left ear |
| AU | both ears |
| AV | atrioventricular |
| BE | barium enema |
| BM | bowel movement |
| BP | blood pressure |
| BPH | benign prostatic hyperplasia |
| BSA | body surface area |
| BUN | blood urea nitrogen |
| C (C1–C7) | cervical |
| CABG | coronary artery bypass graft |
| CAD | coronary artery disease |
| CAPD | continuous ambulatory peritoneal dialysis |
| CCU | cardiac care unit |
| CF | cystic fibrosis |
| CHF | congestive heart failure |
| CNS | central nervous system |
| c/o | complains of |
| $CO_2$ | carbon dioxide |
| COPD | chronic obstructive pulmonary disease |
| CRF | chronic renal failure |
| CS | cesarean section |
| C-section | cesarean section |
| CSF | cerebrospinal fluid |
| CT | calcitonin |
| CT | computer tomography |
| CVA | cerebrovascular accident |
| CXA | chest X-ray |
| D&C | dilation and curettage |
| DIC | disseminated intravascular coagulation |
| DM | diabetes mellitus |
| EBV | Epstein–Barr virus |
| ECG | electrocardiogram, electrocardiograph, electrocardiography, or cardiogram |
| ECT | electroconvulsive therapy |
| EDC | estimated date of confinement (due date) |
| EDD | estimated date of delivery (due date) |
| EEG | electroencephalography |
| EGD | esophagogastroduodenoscopy |
| EKG | electrocardiogram, electrocardiograph, electrocardiography, or cardiogram |
| EMG | electromyography |
| EOM | extra-ocular movement |
| ERV | expiratory reserve volume |
| ESRD | end-stage renal disease |
| F | Fahrenheit |
| FBS | fasting blood sugar |
| FSH | follicle-stimulating hormone |
| Fx | fracture |
| G | gravida |
| GC | gonorrhea |
| GERD | gastroesophageal reflux disease |
| GFR | glomerular filtration rate |
| GH | growth hormone |

| Abbreviation | Meaning |
|---|---|
| GI | gastrointestinal |
| GTT | glucose tolerance test |
| GYN | gynecology |
| Hb | hemoglobin (protein in the blood that carries oxygen) |
| $HbA_{1c}$ | hemoglobin $A_{1c}$ (glycosylated hemoglobin) |
| HCl | hydrochloric acid |
| HDL | high-density lipoprotein |
| HIV | human immunodeficiency virus |
| HPV | human papillomavirus |
| HR | heart rate |
| HSV | herpes simplex virus |
| HTN | hypertension |
| IBS | irritable bowel syndrome |
| ICP | intracranial pressure |
| ICU | intensive care unit |
| IM | intramuscular |
| IOP | intra-ocular pressure |
| IRV | inspiratory reserve volume |
| IVP | intravenous pyelogram |
| I&D | incision and drainage |
| KUB | kidneys, ureter, and bladder |
| L (L1–L5) | lumbar |
| LASIK | laser-assister in situ keratomileusis |
| LES | lower esophageal sphincter |
| LDL | low-density lipoprotein |
| LH | luteinizing hormone |
| LLQ | left lower quadrant (of abdomen) |
| LMP | last menstrual period |
| LP | lumbar puncture |
| LUQ | left upper quadrant (of abdomen) |
| MD | muscular dystrophy |
| MG | myasthenia gravis |
| MI | myocardial infarction |
| MRI | magnetic resonance imaging |
| MS | multiple sclerosis |
| MSH | melanocyte-stimulating hormone |
| NG | nasogastric |
| NPO | nothing by mouth |
| NSAID | nonsteroidal anti-inflammatory drug |
| $O_2$ | oxygen |
| OB | obstetrics |

| Abbreviation | Meaning |
|---|---|
| OCD | obsessive-compulsive disorder |
| OD | right eye |
| O.D. | doctor of optometry |
| OM | otitis media |
| OS | left eye |
| OU | both eyes |
| P | para |
| P | pulse |
| Pap smear | Papanicolaou smear |
| PID | pelvic inflammatory disease |
| PD | Parkinson's disease |
| PFT | pulmonary function test |
| PNS | peripheral nervous system |
| PO | per os or by mouth |
| PRL | prolactin |
| PT | physical therapy |
| PTCA | percutaneous transluminal coronary angioplasty |
| PTH | parathyroid hormone |
| PTSD | posttraumatic stress disorder |
| R | respiration |
| RA | rheumatoid arthritis |
| RBC | red blood cell |
| $Rh^+$, $Rh^-$ | symbol for Rh blood group; Rh positive, Rh negative |
| RICE | rest, ice, compression, elevation |
| RLQ | right lower quadrant (of abdomen) |
| ROM | range of motion |
| RUQ | right upper quadrant (of abdomen) |
| RV | residual volume (as measured with test equipment) |
| S | sacral |
| SA | sinoatrial |
| SLE | systemic lupus erythematosus |
| SOB | shortness of breath |
| STD | sexually transmitted disease |
| STI | sexually transmitted infection |
| T | temperature |
| T (T1–T12) | thoracic |
| $T_3$ | triiodothyronine |
| $T_4$ | thyroxine tetraiodothyronine |
| T and A | tonsillectomy and adenoidectomy |
| TB | tuberculosis |

| Abbreviation | Meaning |
|---|---|
| THR | total hip replacement |
| TIA | transient ischemic attack |
| TKA | total knee arthroplasty |
| TKR | total knee replacement |
| TLC | total lung capacity |
| TPN | total parenteral nutrition |
| TURP | transurethral resection of the prostate |
| UA | urinalysis |
| UGIS | upper gastrointestinal series |
| URI | upper respiratory infection |
| UTI | urinary tract infection |
| UV | ultraviolet |
| VC | vital capacity |
| WBC | white blood cell |

# APPENDIX D

# Error-Prone Abbreviations, Symbols, and Dose Designations

This list is a comprehensive list assembled from the Institute for Safe Medication Practices (ISMP), a nonprofit organization whose mission is to educate consumers and the healthcare community about safe medication practices.

The abbreviations, symbols, and dose designations found in this table have been reported to ISMP through the ISMP National Medication Errors Reporting Program (ISMP MERP) as being frequently misinterpreted and involved in harmful medication errors. They should NEVER be used when communicating medical information. This includes internal communications, telephone/verbal prescriptions, computer-generated labels, labels for drug storage bins, medication administration records, as well as pharmacy and prescriber computer order entry screens.

| ABBREVIATIONS | INTENDED MEANING | MISINTERPRETATION | CORRECTION |
|---|---|---|---|
| µg | Microgram | Mistaken as "mg" | Use "mcg" |
| AD, AS, AU | Right ear, left ear, each ear | Mistaken as OD, OS, OU (right eye, left eye, each eye) | Use "right ear," "left ear," or "each ear" |
| OD, OS, OU | Right eye, left eye, each eye | Mistaken as AD, AS, AU (right ear, left ear, each ear) | Use "right eye," "left eye," or "each eye" |
| BT | Bedtime | Mistaken as "BID" (twice daily) | Use "bedtime" |
| cc | Cubic centimeters | Mistaken as "u" (units) | Use "mL" |
| D/C | Discharge or discontinue | Premature discontinuation of medications if D/ C (intended to mean "discharge") has been misinterpreted as "discontinued" when followed by a list of discharge medications | Use "discharge" and "discontinue" |
| IJ | Injection | Mistaken as "IV" or "intrajugular" | Use "injection" |
| IN | Intranasal | Mistaken as "IM" or "IV" | Use "intranasal" or "NAS" |

| ABBREVIATIONS | INTENDED MEANING | MISINTERPRETATION | CORRECTION |
|---|---|---|---|
| HS<br>hs | Half-strength<br>At bedtime, hours of sleep | Mistaken as bedtime<br>Mistaken as half-strength | Use "half-strength" or "bedtime" |
| IU** | International unit | Mistaken as IV (intravenous) or 10 (ten) | Use "units" |
| o.d. or OD | Once daily | Mistaken as "right eye" (OD-oculus dexter), leading to oral liquid medications administered in the eye | Use "daily" |
| OJ | Orange juice | Mistaken as OD or OS (right or left eye); drugs meant to be diluted in orange juice may be given in the eye | Use "orange juice" |
| Per os | By mouth, orally | The "os" can be mistaken as "left eye" (OS-oculus sinister) | Use "PO," "by mouth," or "orally" |
| q.d. or QD** | Every day | Mistaken as q.i.d., especially if the period after the "q" or the tail of the "q" is misunderstood as an "i" | Use "daily" |
| qhs | Nightly at bedtime | Mistaken as "qhr" or every hour | Use "nightly" |
| qn | Nightly or at bedtime | Mistaken as "qh" (every hour) | Use "nightly" or "at bedtime" |
| q.o.d. or QOD** | Every other day | Mistaken as "q.d." (daily) or "q.i.d. (four times daily) if the "o" is poorly written | Use "every other day" |
| q1d | Daily | Mistaken as q.i.d. (four times daily) | Use "daily" |
| q6PM, etc. | Every evening at 6 PM | Mistaken as every 6 hours | Use "daily at 6 PM" or "6 PM daily" |
| SC, SQ, sub q | Subcutaneous | SC mistaken as SL (sublingual); SQ mistaken as "5 every;" the "q" in "sub q" has been mistaken as "every" (e.g., a heparin dose ordered "sub q 2 hours before surgery" misunderstood as every 2 hours before surgery) | Use "subcut" or "subcutaneously" |

| ABBREVIATIONS | INTENDED MEANING | MISINTERPRETATION | CORRECTION |
|---|---|---|---|
| ss | Sliding scale (insulin) or ½ (apothecary) | Mistaken as "55" | Spell out "sliding scale;" use "one-half" or "½" |
| SSRI | Sliding scale regular insulin | Mistaken as selective-serotonin reuptake inhibitor | Spell out "sliding scale (insulin)" |
| SSI | Sliding scale insulin | Mistaken as Strong Solution of Iodine (Lugol's) | |
| i/d | One daily | Mistaken as "tid" | Use "1 daily" |
| TIW or tiw | 3 times a week | Mistaken as "3 times a day" or "twice in a week" | Use "3 times weekly" |
| U or u** | Unit | Mistaken as the number 0 or 4, causing a 10-fold overdose or greater (e.g., 4U seen as "40" or 4u seen as "44"); mistaken as "cc" so dose given in volume instead of units (e.g., 4u seen as 4cc) | Use "unit" |
| UD | As directed ("ut dictum") | Mistaken as unit dose (e.g., diltiazem 125 mg IV infusion "UD" misin- terpreted as meaning to give the entire infusion as a unit [bolus] dose) | Use "as directed" |
| **DOSE DESIGNATIONS AND OTHER INFORMATION** | **INTENDED MEANING** | **MISINTERPRETATION** | **CORRECTION** |
| Trailing zero after decimal point (e.g., 1.0 mg)** | 1 mg | Mistaken as 10 mg if the decimal point is not seen | Do not use trailing zeros for doses expressed in whole numbers |
| "Naked" decimal point (e.g., .5 mg)** | 0.5 mg | Mistaken as 5 mg if the decimal point is not seen | Use zero before a decimal point when the dose is less than a whole unit |
| Abbreviations such as mg. or mL. with a period following the abbreviation | mg<br>mL | The period is unnecessary and could be mistaken as the number 1 if written poorly | Use mg, mL, etc. without a terminal period |

| DOSE DESIGNATIONS AND OTHER INFORMATION | INTENDED MEANING | MISINTERPRETATION | CORRECTION |
|---|---|---|---|
| Drug name and dose run together (especially problematic for drug names that end in "l" such as Inderal40 mg; Tegretol300 mg) | Inderal 40 mg Tegretol 300 mg | Mistaken as Inderal 140 mg Mistaken as Tegretol 1300 mg | Place adequate space between the drug name, dose, and unit of measure |
| Numerical dose and unit of measure run together (e.g., 10mg, 100mL) | 10 mg 100 mL | The "m" is sometimes mistaken as a zero or two zeros, risking a 10-to 100-fold overdose | Place adequate space between the dose and unit of measure |
| Large doses without properly placed commas (e.g., 100000 units; 1000000 units) | 100,000 units 1,000,000 units | 100000 has been mistaken as 10,000 or 1,000,000; 1000000 has been mistaken as 100,000 | Use commas for dosing units at or above 1,000, or use words such as 100 thousand" or 1 "million" to improve readability" |
| **DRUG NAME ABBREVIATIONS** | **INTENDED MEANING** | **MISINTERPRETATION** | **CORRECTION** |
| APAP | acetaminophen | Not recognized as acetaminophen | Use complete drug name |
| ARA A | vidarabine | Mistaken as cytarabine (ARA C) | Use complete drug name |
| AZT | zidovudine (Retrovir) | Mistaken as azathioprine or aztreonam | Use complete drug name |
| CPZ | Compazine (prochlorperazine) | Mistaken as chlorpromazine | Use complete drug name |
| DPT | Demerol-Phenergan-Thorazine | Mistaken as diphtheria-pertussis-tetanus (vaccine) | Use complete drug name |
| DTO | Diluted tincture of opium, or deodorized tincture of opium (Paregoric) | Mistaken as tincture of opium | Use complete drug name |
| HCl | hydrochloric acid or hydrochloride | Mistaken as potassium chloride (The "H" is misinterpreted as "K") | Use complete drug name unless expressed as a salt of a drug |
| HCT | hydrocortisone | Mistaken as hydrochlorothiazide | Use complete drug name |

| | | | |
|---|---|---|---|
| HCTZ | hydrochlorothiazide | Mistaken as hydrocortisone (seen as HCT250 mg) | Use complete drug name |
| MgSO4** | magnesium sulfate | Mistaken as morphine sulfate | Use complete drug name |
| MS, MSO4** | morphine sulfate | Mistaken as magnesium sulfate | Use complete drug name |
| MTX | methotrexate | Mistaken as mitoxantrone | Use complete drug name |
| NoAC | novel/new oral anticoagulant | No anticoagulant | Use complete drug name |
| PCA | procainamide | Mistaken as patient controlled analgesia | Use complete drug name |
| PTU | propylthiouracil | Mistaken as mercaptopurine | Use complete drug name |
| T3 | Tylenol with codeine No. 3 | Mistaken as liothyronine | Use complete drug name |
| TAC | triamcinolone | Mistaken as tetracaine, Adrenalin, cocaine | Use complete drug name |
| TNK | TNKase | Mistaken as "TPA" | Use complete drug name |
| TPA or tPA | tissue plasminogen activator, Activase (alteplase) | Mistaken as TNKase (tenecteplase), or less often as another tissue plasminogen activator, Retavase (retaplase) | Use complete drug names |
| ZnSO4 | zinc sulfate | Mistaken as morphine sulfate | Use complete drug name |
| **STEMMED DRUG NAMES** | **INTENDED MEANING** | **MISINTERPRETATION** | **CORRECTION** |
| "Nitro" drip | nitroglycerin infusion | Mistaken as sodium nitroprusside infusion | Use complete drug name |
| "Norflox" | norfloxacin | Mistaken as Norflex | Use complete drug name |
| "IV Vanc" | intravenous vancomycin | Mistaken as Invanz | Use complete drug name |
| **SYMBOLS** | **INTENDED MEANING** | **MISINTERPRETATION** | **CORRECTION** |
| ʒ | Dram | Symbol for dram mistaken as "3" | Use the metric system |
| ♍ | Minim | Symbol for minim mistaken as "mL" | |

| SYMBOLS | INTENDED MEANING | MISINTERPRETATION | CORRECTION |
|---|---|---|---|
| ×3d | For three days | Mistaken as "3 doses" | Use "for three days" |
| > and < | More than and less than | Mistaken as opposite of intended; mistakenly use incorrect symbol; "< 10" mistaken as "40" | Use "more than" or "less than" |
| / (slash mark) | Separates two doses or indicates "per" | Mistaken as the number 1 (e.g., "25 units/10 units" misread as "25 units and 110" units) | Use "per" rather than a slash mark to separate doses |
| @ | At | Mistaken as "2" | Use "at" |
| & | And | Mistaken as "2" | Use "and" |
| + | Plus or and | Mistaken as "4" | Use "and" |
| ° | Hour | Mistaken as a zero (e.g., q2? seen as q 20) | Use "hr," "h," or "hour" |
| ϕ or ∅ | zero, null sign | Mistaken as numerals 4, 6, 8, and 9 | Use 0 or zero, or describe intent using whole words |

**These abbreviations are included on The Joint Commission's "minimum list" of dangerous abbreviations, acronyms, and symbols that must be included on an organization's
"Do Not Use" list, effective January 1, 2004. Visit www.jointcommission.org for more information about this Joint Commission requirement.

 Report actual and potential medication errors to the ISMP National Medication Errors Reporting Program (ISMP MERP) via the
Web at www.ismp.org or by calling 1-800-FAIL-SAF(E).

APPENDIX E

# Top 100 Prescribed Medications

About the Top 100 Commonly Prescribed Medications. This list has been selected to be representative of the most commonly prescribed drugs for the year 2016 (see references). The list is arranged starting with the most prescribed prescription medication. It includes the brand name, generic name, and the drug's general class. Combination products have their individual ingredients listed.

| | BRAND NAME | GENERIC NAME | CLASS |
|---|---|---|---|
| 1 | Norco | hydrocodone and acetaminophen | opioid analgesic |
| 2 | Prinivil, Zestril | lisinopril | antihypertensive |
| 3 | Synthroid | levothyroxine | thyroid hormone |
| 4 | Norvasc | amlodipine | antihypertensive |
| 5 | Lipitor | atorvastatin | antihyperlipidemic |
| 6 | Prilosec | omeprazole | proton pump inhibitor |
| 7 | Zocor | simvastatin | antihyperlipidemic |
| 8 | Glucophage | metformin | antidiabetic |
| 9 | Amoxil | amoxicillin | antibiotic |
| 10 | Zithromax | azithromycin | antibiotic |
| 11 | Xanax | alprazolam | benzodiazepine |
| 12 | Microzide | hydrochlorothiazide | antihypertensive |
| 13 | Neurontin | gabapentin | anticonvulsant |
| 14 | Flonase | fluticasone propionate | nasal corticosteroid |
| 15 | Ultram | tramadol | opioid analgesic |
| 16 | Motrin | ibuprofen | nonsteroidal anti-inflammatory |
| 17 | Zoloft | sertraline | antidepressant |
| 18 | Deltasone | prednisone | steroid |
| 19 | Lopressor | metoprolol tartrate | antihypertensive |
| 20 | Toprol XL | metoprolol succinate | antihypertensive |
| 21 | Cozaar | losartan | antihypertensive |
| 22 | Lasix | furosemide | antihypertensive |
| 23 | Ambien | zolpidem | hypnotic |
| 24 | Celexa | citalopram | antidepressant |
| 25 | Percocet | oxycodone and acetaminophen | opioid analgesic |

| | BRAND NAME | GENERIC NAME | CLASS |
|---|---|---|---|
| 26 | Pravachol | pravastatin | antihyperlipidemic |
| 27 | Singulair | montelukast | leukotriene receptor antagonist |
| 28 | ProAir HFA, Ventolin HFA | albuterol | inhaled beta-2 agonist |
| 29 | Flexeril | cyclobenzaprine | skeletal muscle relaxant |
| 30 | Klonopin | clonazepam | benzodiazepine |
| 31 | Prozac | fluoxetine | antidepressant |
| 32 | Prinizide, Zestoretic | lisinopril and hydrochlorothiazide | antihypertensive |
| 33 | Tenormin | atenolol | antihypertensive |
| 34 | Protonix | pantoprazole | proton pump inhibitor |
| 35 | Mobic | meloxicam | nonsteroidal anti-inflammatory |
| 36 | Lexapro | escitalopram | antidepressant |
| 37 | Desyrel | trazodone | antidepressant |
| 38 | Augmentin | amoxicillin and clavulanate | antibiotic |
| 39 | Ativan | lorazepam | benzodiazepine |
| 40 | Cipro | ciprofloxacin | antibiotic |
| 41 | K-Dur, Klor-Con | potassium chloride | salt; treats hypokalemia |
| 42 | Coreg | carvedilol | antihypertensive |
| 43 | Keflex | cephalexin | antibiotic |
| 44 | Plavix | clopidogrel | anti-platelet |
| 45 | Bactrim | sulfamethoxazole and trimethoprim | antibiotic |
| 46 | Coumadin | warfarin | anticoagulant |
| 47 | Crestor | rosuvastatin | antihyperlipidemic |
| 48 | Flomax | tamsulosin | alpha-1 blocker |
| 49 | Zantac | ranitidine | $H_2$ antagonist |
| 50 | Naprosyn | naproxen | nonsteroidal anti-inflammatory |
| 51 | Diflucan | fluconazole | antifungal |
| 52 | Cymbalta | duloxetine | antidepressant |
| 53 | Roxicodone | oxycodone | opioid analgesic |
| 54 | Wellbutrin XL | bupropion XL | antidepressant |
| 55 | Effexor XR | venlafaxine ER | antidepressant |
| 56 | Zyloprim | allopurinol | antigout |
| 57 | Medrol | methylprednisolone | corticosteroid |
| 58 | Adderall | amphetamine salts IR | stimulant |
| 59 | Zofran | ondansetron | antiemetic |
| 60 | Kenalog | triamcinolone | topical corticosteroid |
| 61 | Nexium | esomeprazole | proton pump inhibitor |

| | BRAND NAME | GENERIC NAME | CLASS |
|---|---|---|---|
| 62 | Hyzaar | losartan and hydrochlorothiazide | antihypertensive |
| 63 | Valium | diazepam | benzodiazepine |
| 64 | Ergocalciferol | vitamin $D_2$ | vitamin |
| 65 | Elavil | amitriptyline | antidepressant |
| 66 | Paxil | paroxetine | antidepressant |
| 67 | Catapres | clonidine | antihypertensive |
| 68 | Tricor | fenofibrate | antihyperlipidemic |
| 69 | Glucophage XR | metformin XR | antidiabetic |
| 70 | Advair Diskus | fluticasone/salmeterol | inhaled beta-2 agonist/ corticosteroid |
| 71 | Fluvirin, Afluria, Fluzone | influenza vaccine | vaccine |
| 72 | Vibramycin | doxycycline | antibiotic |
| 73 | Amaryl | glimepiride | antidiabetic |
| 74 | Aldactone | spironolactone | antihypertensive |
| 75 | Maxzide, Dyazide | triamterene and hydrochlorothiazide | antihypertensive |
| 76 | Levaquin | levofloxacin | antibiotic |
| 77 | Valtrex | valacyclovir | antiviral |
| 78 | Tylenol #2, #3, #4 | acetaminophen and codeine | opioid analgesic |
| 79 | Lamictal | lamotrigine | anticonvulsant |
| 80 | Topamax | topiramate | anticonvulsant |
| 81 | Mevacor | lovastatin | antihyperlipidemic |
| 82 | Seroquel | quetiapine | antipsychotic |
| 83 | Flagyl | metronidazole | antibiotic |
| 84 | Vyvanse | lisdexamfetamine | stimulant |
| 85 | Phenergan | promethazine | antiemetic |
| 86 | none | folic acid | vitamin |
| 87 | Fosamax | alendronate | bisphosphonate |
| 88 | Glucotrol | glipizide | antidiabetic |
| 89 | Lantus Solostar | insulin glargine | long acting insulin |
| 90 | Cleocin | clindamycin | antibiotic |
| 91 | Xalatan | lantanoprost | ophthalmic antiglaucoma |
| 92 | Concerta | methylphenidate ER | stimulant |
| 93 | Vasotec | enalapril | antihypertensive |
| 94 | Lyrica | pregabalin | anticonvulsant |
| 95 | Tessalon Perles | benzonatate | antitussive |
| 96 | Inderal | propranolol | antihypertensive |
| 97 | Omnicef | cefdinir | antibiotic |

| | BRAND NAME | GENERIC NAME | CLASS |
|---|---|---|---|
| 98 | MS Contin | morphine | opioid analgesic |
| 99 | Adderall XR | amphetamine salts ER | stimulant |
| 100 | Imitrex | sumatriptan | antimigraine |

ER: extended release
IR: immediate release
XL: extended release
XR: extended release
References:
www.drugtopics.modernmedicine.com
www.online.lexi.com
Accessed in April 2017

# Index

Page numbers followed by *f* and *t* indicates figures and tables respectively

## E

## T